APPLICATIONS OF ELECTROENCEPHALOGRAPHY IN PSYCHIATRY

PARTICIPANTS

Ewald Busse, M.D.
Duke University, Durham, North Carolina

James Crawley, M.D.
Baylor University, Houston, Texas

Max Fink, M.D.
Missouri Institute of Psychiatry, St. Louis, Missouri

Robert L. Green, Jr., M.D.
Duke University, Durham, North Carolina

Charles E. Henry, Ph.D.
Cleveland Clinic, Cleveland, Ohio

Anton F. Heusler, M.D.
Missouri Institute of Psychiatry, St. Louis, Missouri

John R. Hughes, Ph.D.
Northwestern University, Chicago, Illinois

Peter Kellaway, Ph.D.
Baylor University, Houston, Texas

Margaret Kennard, M.D.
Manchester, New Hampshire

John Knott, Ph.D.
Iowa State University, Iowa City, Iowa

Robert Maulsby, M.D.
Baylor University, Houston, Texas

Walter Obrist, Ph.D.
Duke University, Durham, North Carolina

Charles Shagass, M.D.
Iowa State University, Iowa City, Iowa

Marvin J. Short, M.D.
Duke University, Durham, North Carolina

John A. Stern, Ph.D.
Washington University, St. Louis, Missouri

George A. Ulett, M.D.
Missouri Institute of Psychiatry, St. Louis, Missouri

William P. Wilson
Duke University, Durham, North Carolina

Thomas J. Word, A.B.
Missouri Institute of Psychiatry, St. Louis, Missouri

APPLICATIONS OF ELECTROENCEPHALOGRAPHY IN PSYCHIATRY

A Symposium

Edited by

William P. Wilson, M.D.

Duke University Press
Durham, North Carolina
1965

Library of Congress Catalogue
Card number 65–19449

Printed in the United States of
America by Kingsport Press, Inc.

PREFACE

The last decade has witnessed a revival of interest in the biological determinants of behavior. In spite of intensive efforts in the field of biochemistry, the major advances have occurred in neurophysiology where the relationship of the reticular system to consciousness and the limbic system to emotion have been of the greatest interest. Unfortunately, psychiatry is not blessed with an "experimental animal" for the anatomical complexity of the human brain, and the singular ability to communicate in a complex way make the meeting of the last of Koch's postulates impossible. In view of these limitations, it is necessary that we attempt to ascertain what differences may exist in the physiologic function of the brain in normal and diseased individuals. To date our most useful tool has been the electroencephalogram.

Since Berger's pioneering work in EEG, innumerable articles have been written about changes of cerebral electrical activity in mental disorders. Unfortunately a review of this literature has not been compiled since the publication of the *Bibliography of Electroencephalography* in 1948. Although there have been recent reviews of individual disease entities, it became apparent that a general review was indicated. In order to meet this need, a conference was organized under the joint sponsorship of the Research Committee of the APA and the Department of Psychiatry of the Duke University School of Medicine. The express purpose of this conference, held in Durham, North Carolina, November 18–19, 1962, was to attempt a compilation of the pertinent electroencephalographic investigations of mental disease and its treatment.

In planning this conference, it was recognized that a review of the literature relative to the effect of psychopharmacologic agents on the EEG was forthcoming as a supplement to the *EEG Journal*. Since it would be redundant to include this subject, original contributions were sought and are included.

As is so often the case, it is impossible to review the entire world literature. Several of the contributors to this symposium, therefore, reviewed only the English literature. However, the scope of the

v

papers is such that in all instances a comprehensive survey of the pertinent literature is available and will be most useful to both student and research worker.

In editing the manuscripts, an occasional duplication of references was found, a paper being cited as both an original publication and as an abstract in the "Society Proceedings" section of the *EEG Journal*. In such cases the abstract has been deleted from the list of references.

The editor is grateful to the participants of this symposium for their efforts which will meet a long recognized need, and to B. S. H. Harris III, who spent long hours checking the references included. In addition, the assistance of W. W. K. Zung, M.D., J. A. Hall, M.D., and Ethel Ashburn is acknowledged.

The good offices and financial support of The Schering Corporation, represented by Robert Burlew, M.D., and The Hoffman La Roche Company, represented by L. R. Hines, Ph.D., is acknowledged and appreciated.

Finally G. Ulett, M.D., and E. Busse, M.D., provided a conceptual framework for this symposium which fulfils a long recognized need.

CONTENTS

APPLICATIONS OF ELECTROENCEPHALOGRAPHY IN PSYCHIATRY

ELECTROENCEPHALOGRAPHIC CORRELATES WITH PERSONALITY

Charles E. Henry, Ph.D.

Papers on electroencephalography and personality have been appearing in the EEG literature from earliest years. Scattered through a wide variety of journals, the quantity has remained small, and the quality has often been less than outstanding.

The material in this report is reviewed under an imposed restriction needing explicit statement. The broad area of clinical psychopathology is largely excluded since it has been covered by other contributors to this volume. Thus some of the near-specific electrographic correlates of more spectacular disorder will follow this necessarily less exciting array. We will not dwell on the difficulty of obtaining a unanimous definition on the word *personality*, but if we interpret it freely to include behavior tendencies, temperament, and attributes, we can refer to a number of studies having at least indirect relevance to the topic.

In any attempt to set forth what is known about a particular aspect of the EEG it is well to consult Berger. Although he does not appear to have written about personality per se, he did anticipate subsequent work by noting the effects of fright, attention, anxiety, and sensory stimulation—all of which reduced the alpha rhythm. He clearly regarded the alpha rhythm as originating in the cortex but probably controlled from the hypothalamus. Further, he found that repeated records on the same individual were generally consistent (3).

This point is of some significance if one is interested in general correlations such as EEG and personality. It is necessary to remember the limitations, both philosophical and methodological, under which the first investigations were attempted. We were just getting accustomed to the idea that there was *any* detectable beat to the

3

cortex; the brain was just beginning to lose some of its "black box" inaccessibility. EEGs often were recorded with photographic rather than with inkwriting systems, were usually of very short duration, and utilized only single-channel "Lo-Fi" equipment.

The first firm hint of possible relationships between EEG and personality appeared in the *Cold Spring Harbor Symposium* for 1936, perhaps stimulated by Adrian's (1) comment of the year before: "It will be surprising if there are no differences in the mental and emotional constitution to correspond with such different behavior in the cortical machinery." [1] It was here that Hallowell Davis (13) mentioned the subsequently reported (52) broad interrelationship between the EEG and personality. The general theme is still as persuasive as any in the literature—and better than most. The original communication of Saul, Davis, and Davis (52) was read by title; it exists only in the *Transactions,* never too widely distributed, and probably rarely read in its brief entirety.

These workers determined the percent-time alpha (alpha index) from the occiput, recording through a broadly tuned 10-cycle filter, based on at least 30 seconds of record. Under standard conditions of response with the eyes closed they reported that "the alpha index and certain other features . . . are quite characteristic and constant for the majority of normal individuals." Thirty-one patients in psychoanalysis were retested after a 7-month interval; 25 had an alpha index within 10 points of the original value. All larger deviations (only 2 greater than 17 points) were toward a lower value of alpha and were not related to clinical changes occurring during therapy. The alpha distribution of 66 cases in analysis was similar to that of a control population of 200 normals—quite evenly distributed over the entire range.

The same investigators, searching for relationships between the alpha index and the emotional and instinctual trends of the individual as disclosed by psychoanalysis, noted two opposing trends. These related to an activity *vs.* passivity tendency in habitual actions and attitudes toward other persons, and toward food, work, sleep, and sex. Since both trends exist in the same individual, an assessment of relative strength was made (p. 168).

A high alpha index is characteristically associated with a passive, dependent, receptive attitude toward other persons, provided this attitude is freely accepted and not thwarted or inhibited internally. A person with

---

[1] We are indebted to Jasper's extraordinarily complete review in the *Psychological Bulletin* in 1936 (26) for the recall of this and much other early material.

a high alpha index may work to satisfy his desires but usually under protest, by force of circumstances, or by conscious effort. He usually desires and may actually require more than the average amount of sleep. Men who show a strong dependent attitude toward women, particularly to the mother, or a passive homosexual trend, typically show high alpha indices. Women with such strong, passive, dependent trends are also high. A sufficiently successful inhibition or "domestication" of fundamental instinctual activities suggests a high index. Such individuals are "solid citizens," patient workers and planners. In another type the strong fundamental receptivity is revealed by the results of thwarting—such as temper tantrums in some, and in others depression, even leading to attempts at suicide, although these symptoms are by no means pathognomonic. . . . Low alpha indices are usually associated with a consistent, well-directed, freely indulged drive to activity. This does not include the diffuse, hypomanic type of activity which is in the nature of a defense. A well-developed, active "reaction-formation" against an unacceptable underlying trend, such as passive desires, is strong indication of a low alpha index, even though the passive trends may be clearly apparent. An active "masculine" trend associated with a low index is active homosexuality in women. The homosexuality need not imply overt homosexual activities, but may be revealed in dreams and in life by identification and competition with men and envy of their masculinity, often reflected in masculine type of dreams and activity. A "primary" drive to activity which is not a reaction-formation also suggests a low alpha index.

Analysis of dream content was also helpful in revealing fundamental psychological trends. It was emphasized that these trends occurred in mixed amounts and that an understanding of opposing tendencies was necessary. "By careful study of case and dream material we have been able to predict the alpha indices of many subjects with an accuracy far exceeding chance."

Most experienced EEGers can recognize a certain validity to these statements; a number of patients "fit" nicely. The findings partially account for the paradox of individuals who seem overtly anxious, yet in the EEG laboratory display abundant rhythmic dominant alpha activity. (See also **4, 61**.)

The next presentation from these authors did not occur until 1949, when a longer paper was published in *Psychosomatic Medicine* (**53**) and a brief abstract appeared in the *EEG Journal* (**54**). The data basically reflect the material as of approximately 1942. They present a much more complete type of EEG classification and provide sufficient information to allow an understanding of their rating procedures. They add new cases for a total of 136, all with essentially normal EEGs. From information about the patient's life history and his character, they were able to predict successfully the type of EEG; they state that the more thoroughly such a patient was understood the more accurate was the EEG prediction. The reverse, viz., prediction of personality type from EEG, was not attempted. Again these workers found that very passive individuals had high alpha[2] EEGs; there were three times as many men as women in this group. Women with strong masculine trends generally had low-voltage fast or low alpha EEGs, and less consistently those women with active maternal drive had low alpha patterns; there were relatively few men with EEGs of this type. They added a third category consisting largely of frustrated, impatient, aggressive, demanding, and hostile women with mixed fast or mixed slow types of record; there were only two men with this constellation. The authors reiterated that a study of the dream life of the individual added significantly to the predictive accuracy. Of particular interest is the fact that, although some of these patients were studied over a five-year period, so long as the basic standard conditions of recording were used there was little change in the fundamental pattern. There was no pronounced shift from high alpha index to a low alpha index in any case despite on-going psychotherapy.

Because the findings in the above studies were quite explicitly and emphatically stated, it is not surprising that they have been quoted widely in the literature, generally meeting with rather greater acceptance by clinical psychiatrists than by electroencephalographers. This is illustrated by the critical reviews of Sisson and Ellingson (**60**), who discuss a wide range of material, covering the results of tests on penitentiary inmates, and reports on patients suffering from peptic ulcer and asthma, and the Rorschach responses of normal individuals (**16**). Rather surprisingly, neither of these comprehensive reviews mentions a study by Palmer and Rock (**46**), although it was first presented at a meeting of the Central EEG Society (**45**). Twenty-five men with a very high incidence of alpha activity were reported as having inadequate, schizoid, or immature personalities, being non-aggressive and conforming. They all had poor identification with fathers in early formative years; this lack of "crystallized experience" allegedly resulted in an idling brain that did not actively deal with life's problems in a masculine fashion. Another 15 men with

---

[2] This is the Type A EEG, not strictly synonymous with high alpha index. Careful attention to their original description of the EEG classification system would eliminate some misunderstanding.

passive personalities, but with adequate early father identification, did not show high alpha activity. The data do not permit a critical comparison with the more psychoanalytically oriented study and no additional material was found dealing with the notion of crystallized experience. It would be quite surprising if any such simple relationship existed.

One can agree with Sisson and Ellingson that subsequent workers have been too facile in their interpretation of the Saul, Davis, and Davis studies. The latter, however, should not be criticized for something that they never stated. The point is that EEG type was predicted with apparent accuracy from a knowledge of the personality. They noted that the converse, i.e., the prediction of personality type from EEG, had not been attempted although they had the impression that the relationship was reciprocal. Most specifically, since the point was emphasized by Sisson and Ellingson, Saul *et al.* made particular qualification that they were not sure that all individuals with high alpha EEGs were necessarily passive.

From another early paper of this era (1936) came findings phrased rather differently but also for a long time uncritically quoted. Lemere (**34**) had gained the impression, from repeated tracings on a group of 25 normal subjects, that good alpha waves appeared in the cyclothymic or manic-depressive type, whereas individuals of schizoid personality makeup showed poor alpha waves. The impression was further borne out by the records from 40 psychotic patients (no quantitative date given); mildly manic or depressed patients had good alpha rhythms, whereas schizophrenic patients "nearly always" showed poor alpha rhythm. The finding that 6 out of 13 patients with disseminated sclerosis complained of emotional instability, and that 5 of these 6 patients had a good alpha rhythm, furthered this conviction. Methodological and statistical details have never been available, and with the exception of a report by Yeager and Baldes (**75**), there has been little confirmation of Lemere's findings. Although we must avoid the more strictly psychiatric studies, it may be noted that Rubin (**50, 51**) found no percent-time alpha differences between normals and schizophrenics. More details of these early controversies are supplied in the very complete chapter by Lindsley (**37**) in the second volume of the Hunt *Personality and Behavior Disorders* handbooks.

From this early period, therefore, it was generally agreed that no obvious characteristic differences in the EEG differentiated the normal individual from his non-deteriorated brethren with psychiatric disorder, although as a group the latter showed a somewhat higher titre of deviant or abnormal record. It was hoped that a more searching and objective appraisal of personality might yield significant relationships, especially when combined with more quantitative indices of EEG.

In agreement with many other workers from Berger on, and reinforced by reports of similarity in identical twins (15, 39), Gottlober extended earlier observations (64) on the day-to-day consistency of EEGs by an inquiry into the relationship between alpha rhythms and personality (22). On the basis of subjective ratings and personality test scores, he selected a group of 67 normal subjects who were either extremely extroverted or extremely introverted. He concluded that "an organismic pattern in which a dominant-subdominant rhythm appears accompanied by an extroverted personality, as determined by our methods of rating, will be more common than one in which it appears accompanied by an introverted personality." Another and more quantitative but less quoted study of children, published in the same year by Lindsley (36), yielded no significant personality correlations. A critical analysis of the Gottlober data by Henry and Knott (24) pointed out that his sample was loaded with high alpha subjects and that *both* extroverted and introverted subjects tended to show a similar trend. They added a larger group of subjects, used the same rating scale, and found only a chance distribution of alpha-type *vs.* personality-type. A recombination of the data on all 147 cases yielded the following:

a. 58 per cent were high alphas; of these, 62 per cent were extroverted.

b. 42 per cent were low alphas; of these, 67 per cent were extroverted.

c. 64 per cent were extroverted; of these, 57 per cent were high alphas.

d. 36 per cent were introverted; of these, 62 per cent were high alphas.

They therefore concluded that there was an almost equal proportion of extroverts in both high and low alpha groups, as well as an almost equal proportion of high alpha subjects in both extroverted and introverted groups.

We come now to a miscellany of studies more or less directly relevant to this topic. There has been considerable interest in the EEGs of children with behavior disorder, a topic which we must neglect, but in passing we may wonder whether the failure to obtain sleep records in these personality-EEG studies might not have imposed a handicap comparable to that which occurred in studies of the behavior disorders. The analogy may be expanded to point up a methodological moral. Just as work on animals, first deeply anesthetized with barbiturates and later with other agents, then awake but restrained, and only recently unrestrained and unanesthetized, has led to a major expansion of our concepts, not only of sleep and wakefulness but also of the basic neurophysiology of the brain, so might similar inhibitory built-in experimental restrictions have limited our understanding of the EEG relationships in psychiatry. Unfortunately, evaluation of exciting clues derived from depth recording in man is still handicapped by the total absence of depth data from normal individuals.

Gallagher, Gibbs, and Gibbs (19) studied 200 normal fourteen- and fifteen-year-old boys at a private school. Personality was classified as poor, average, or good in the joint opinion of everyone from classmate to researcher; EEGs were classified on the Gibbs Spectrum Scale as of 1941. Most of these boys had dominant 10/sec alpha activity; divergence from this biological norm was associated with divergence from normal personality. Although there was no one-to-one relationship, and there were many exceptions, boys with unusually slow records were more likely to exhibit poor personalities, whereas those with dominant fast rhythms tended to have good personalities. Since athletic prowess was not mentioned, one can only speculate how these findings might be related to Kennard's finding (32) that normal subjects with deep reflexes of high threshold tended to have high-voltage slow dominant alpha rhythms and vice versa. This in turn is not obviously related to Thorner's findings (62) that flying ability among aviators decreased as the EEG deviated from the 10.5/sec alpha peak. We may note also the early admonitions and the included bibliography of Liberson with his justified emphasis on functional electroencephalography (35). For example, Cohn (7) found overbreathing and afferent stimulation useful in differentiating hyperemotional states by EEG.

To some extent these studies on normals, as well as on patients, may be considered as broadly involving the homeostasis of the whole body economy; our interest is on central factors, especially as repre-

sented by the EEG. The various central regulatory functions have
been considered in detail by Darrow and colleagues (**8, 9, 10,
11, 12**), who relate Bremer's "rhythm of repose" (**5**) to a combination of subcortical and vasoconstrictive regulatory effects. Also
germane in this context is Lindsley's activation theory of emotion
(**38**). There was a curious absence of speculation in a relevant
address by Davis (**14**) on the role of EEG activity. Denis Hill's
chapter on psychiatry in the Old Testament (**25**) contains a thought-
ful evaluation of EEG-personality relationships.

Some work has been done utilizing the variability and the responsiveness of alpha and other rhythmic features of the EEG. Usually
overlooked is the very early study of Travis (**63**), who attempted
to identify EEG changes associated with the temporal course of consciousness. Regular synchronized activity from the occiput was found
during mental blankness and during abstract thinking, whereas low-
voltage faster activity appeared with visual imagery and mental effort.
A classification of three types of alpha rhythm has long been used
in British laboratories (**21, 33, 70**). Individuals with P (persistent)
types are resistant to blocking by mental effort and tend to use
auditory, tactile, or kinesthetic rather than visual imagery. M (minus)
types show little alpha rhythms and use predominantly visual
imagery in solving problems. The R (responsive) types have the usual
reactive alpha rhythm. Subsequent studies (**59, 69, 70**) suggest a
generalized formulation that M-type subjects are predominantly visual
thinkers and P types are verbal thinkers, whereas R types used a
mixed imagery. The hypothetical example of the social and matri-
monial consequences of such differences, as presented in *The Living Brain* (**71**), is plausibly intriguing. These features are not apparent below the age of about 10; since there is a marked variation
in the EEG maturation rate, this offers a possibly rewarding area of
investigation in children.

There are other aspects of EEG which have been tentatively related to behavior, one of which was described by Walter under the
concept of versatility (**71**). Frequently analyzer spectra were reported
as showing greater variability among bright normals than among dull
patients, presumably indicating a more flexible and variable type of
scanning mechanism. A careful study by Ellingson *et al.* (**17**),
also using analyzer techniques, failed to substantiate this, although
it was noted that Wechsler-Bellevue scores may not constitute a good
index of "brilliance." Additional papers by Walter and J. Shipton

(58, 72) indicate optimism regarding the possibilities of the approach, but few firm findings. The various techniques of analysis yield data of a considerable order of complexity, difficult to condense to a readily understandable format. The many experimental papers in Supplement 6 of the *EEG Journal* (18) illustrate a variety of studies at least indirectly related to psychological phenomena.

Alpha persistence and other EEG features have been used in further exploratory studies of temperament and intelligence, especially by Mundy-Castle and colleagues. These efforts were critically reviewed with a pertinent bibliography in 1958 (42). They have only a peripheral bearing on our main theme and will, therefore, not be given in detail. One aspect is perhaps worth noting—the concept of primary-secondary temperament function. By primary is meant the immediate experience; secondary refers to the aftereffect which may be brought to bear on subsequent experiences. Mundy-Castle has argued that alpha frequency is related to the degree of secondary function, which in turn is related to the over-all excitability characteristic of the nervous system. He marshaled some support for low but consistent correlations between alpha frequency, alpha index, intelligence, mental-imagery type, alpha type, and a broad concept of temperament (40, 41, 43). There have been technical statistical criticisms (44, 55); a quantitative experimental study by R. Walter and Yeager (68) yielded only equivocal support for EEG changes in visual imagery. For tentative suggestions relating imagery type and alpha activity in a small sample of schizophrenic patients, see Rubin and Cohen (51).

Having surveyed much of the "old" literature of the first two decades, generally avoiding carping criticism, we may consider some of the more recent efforts. Earlier studies tend to be somewhat "clinical" in approach. There has been a gradual trend toward more experimental attack, using the EEG as one aspect of behavior, the latter being manipulated in something other than routine standard recording conditions. Ulett *et al.* (65) were interested in the use of EEG as an index of anxiety and its possible application to military selection. Previous studies had indicated that the main value of EEG was in detecting paroxysmal or other gross abnormalities. Through the use of analyzer data and photic stimulation, plus inquiry into the presence of subjective dysphoria, they were able to discriminate many of the anxiety-prone individuals. Some of their findings are "buried" in the School of Aviation Medicine *Reports*.

Their later publications (**27, 66, 67**) contain a sobering commentary on the surprising variability of reactions on repeated follow-up examinations—as many as 9 over a 3-year study of 182 normal young adults. Cases with deviant or disorganized spontaneous activity had no clinically apparent deficit, nor was there evidence of such even during EEG disruption induced by photic stimulation (**28**). This group of workers has also emphasized the hazards involved in obtaining representative control groups for such studies (**6**). We appear to be a long way from the confident use of the EEG in the prediction of relative performance within a group of individuals without pathology.

Another experimental approach involving the differential response to intravenous sodium amytal has been extensively exploited by Shagass. Although the technique was developed initially for use in psychiatry, subsequent papers have included references to anxiety and to personality characteristics. The procedure (**56**) involves injection of sodium amytal at a rate of 0.5 mg/kg every 40 seconds. The point of no appreciable further increment in frontal fast activity, which is usually related to the onset of slurred speech, is termed the "sedation threshold." This correlated highly with the clinical ratings of degree of tension in psychoneurotic but not in psychotic patients. A recent review and summary (**57**) of data dealing with sedation threshold reaffirmed a relationship to tension and manifest anxiety (high threshold) in both normal and psychoneurotic individuals. Personality characteristics were thought to involve hysterical-obsessive and extraversion-introversion axes. In support of this, Shagass found higher thresholds for the obsessive and introverted subjects. For the sake of completeness, and perhaps duplicating discussion in other chapters, we may note that sedation threshold reportedly had some predictive value in the selection of patients for electroshock therapy. Patients with neurotic depression (low threshold) had a better remission rate with EST. These studies illustrate how personality and functional EEG features may be involved in the understanding and therapy of psychiatric disorders. The basic concept underlying the work is that of central neuronal excitability.

There is a broad area of investigation which we have only mentioned, and one to which our European colleagues (somewhat neglected in this review) have contributed extensively. This involves the correlation of various EEG measures with a wide variety of psychological tests. The majority of these studies deal with psychiatric populations and emphasize diagnostic and prognostic features; relatively few are concerned with more normal personality. Virtually every issue of the *EEG Journal* contains references to electroencephalography and such testing, preponderantly in the "Society Proceedings" section, and only rarely appearing as complete papers. This suggests a certain negative or equivocal over-all trend of such research and indeed, such a conclusion is generally justified.

Thus, in an extensive thesis, Werre (**73**), who used the Bekkering Technique of EEG analysis, concluded that there were no unique relationships between EEG and psychological parameters. A more recent abstract (**74**) suggests that a certain grouping of psychological features may have meaning. Subjects with predominant alpha activity were characterized by extensivity (meaning durability, profoundness of feelings and strivings, etc.). Subjects with much beta activity were characterized by intensivity (vehemence, mobility of feelings and strivings).

There have been a large number of abstracts and some papers dealing with EEG and Rorschach scores. Various fragments of the total, complex, and elaborate Rorschach scoring system have been tentatively related to some aspect of EEG by one worker or another. Generally, these relationships were more likely to appear in clinical populations; e.g., the French monograph by Helman (**23**) dealt mostly with epilepsy. Sisson and Ellingson (**60**) selected 15 high and 15 low alpha cases, but found no significant differences between groups in Rorschach scoring categories. Kennard's review (**29**) in 1956 refers to an earlier thesis by Bennett (**2**) in which low alpha activity was related to total response and perhaps indirectly to anxiety. Kennard and colleagues have used Rorschach and other tests from a variety of normal, psychiatric, and prison groups (**31, 47**). They reported more theta *and alpha* activity in the prison group, which they then related to immature, passive, receptive personalities with acting-out tendencies. They have also used a unique display system wherein analyzer frequency data were plotted in superimposed form for all eight head regions (**30**). Psychiatric patients and anxious persons were reported to show less closely interrelated profiles for the various head regions.

All reviews touching on this area are variously incomplete. Existing studies are dispersed widely through the world literature, often in psychological journals, and often with no indication from the title that EEG data are included. No consistent and confirmed re-

lationships between EEG and Rorschach features were encountered
in the present survey.

The second portion of Supplement 6 of the *EEG Journal* contains a number of papers in French dealing with EEG and *com-
portement*. Among contributors not otherwise mentioned in this
review are Rémond and Lesèvre (**48**), who studied EEG and psychological reactions of air force recruits and truck drivers. EEG
features were classified in a system quite similar to Walter's visual
imagery scheme. The M-type subjects were hyperexcitable and emotionally unstable, the P types showed slow but stable psychomotor
performance, and the R types showed best performance and emotional stability. There was also a five-part multiple-authored report on groups of young soldiers, air force cadets, and neurotic
subjects. The cadets showed, as a group, less classically normal
EEGs with slightly slower alpha rhythm, more theta activity, and a
certain incidence of rolandic rhythms. The latter, beta and especially *arceau,* were often associated with aggressiveness and absence
of passivity. Alpha variants were regarded as "characteristic" of
psychopathic personality trends; theta and posterior slowing, and
slowing with hyperventilation, indicated immaturity and poor self-
control. Conclusions were couched in tentative terms, emphasizing
that relationships occurred between EEG and psychological complexes rather than between isolated or specific categories.

No review of this area of investigation would be complete if it
failed to comment on the massive interdisciplinary effort rather
briefly abstracted in the *EEG Journal* (**49**), and more fully in
Revue Neurologique (**20**). The title, "Report on the relations between the electroencephalographic variables and those expressing the
personality and the sensori-motor functions of 511 recruits, aged
20 years," indicates the scope of the nine abstracts. It seems probable that this is an extension, with a more sober evaluation of findings, of the material in Supplement 6. We shall note here only the
use of the Rosenzweig and MMPI scores, blended and filtered in
various combinations. The search for liaisons involved working from
contrasting EEG groups *vs.* psychological measures as well as the
converse procedure. Grey Walter has stated (**72**) that some seven
dimensions are necessary to express EEG variables. This joint effort
used 146 EEG categories, chi square, Pearsonian *r*, and even the
non-linear *eta* multivariate analysis. With so many manipulations
performed on so many data it was inevitable that some "significant"

relationships were found. Each contributor to this study displayed an admirable degree of restraint, somewhat unusual in work dealing with personality. The present effort could scarcely be more appropriately summarized and terminated than by quoting the conclusions as set forth by Gastaut (**49**, p. 227):

No relation exists between the EEG variables and those of the Rosenzweig tests and the intelligence tests. Some rare relations, slight and poorly organized, sometimes absurd, exist between the EEG variables and those of the MMPI.

These results, deceptive in spite of a comparatively advanced scrutiny, do not appear to depend on the selection of our EEG variables which consider all quantifiable aspects of electroencephalographic statics and dynamics in the present state of our knowledge. They seem, rather, to depend on the personality schemes provided by the psychometric tests used, schemes that are valid in themselves, but not adapted to a correlative study with electroencephalographic phenomena.

From this it appears that the primitive bioelectric function of the brain, simple and similar in the different stages of phylogenesis, can not be connected to immediate modes of apprehension of an entity as complex and phylogenetically recent as the human personality. This would explain the negativity of our results and of those of our forerunners, who, in 25 years of effort, have accumulated a multitude of positive factors, but so utterly contradictory that their algebraic sum is practically nil.

Far from abandoning the problem of correlations between the EEG and personality, our future task must therefore be the transformation of information obtained from each one of them, in order to render them comparable.

BIBLIOGRAPHY

1. Adrian, E. D. The electrical activity of the cortex. *Proc. Roy. Soc. Med.* **29**: 197–200, 1935.
2. Bennett, C. L. An experimental study of relationship between human electroencephalograms and certain Rorschach scoring categories. Dissertation, University of Southern California, 1951.
3. Berger, H. Über das elektrenkephalogram des Menschen. *J. Psychol. u. Neurol.* **40**: 160–179, 1930.
4. Brazier, M. A. B., Finesinger, J. E., and Cobb, S. A contrast between the electroencephalograms of 100 psychoneurotic patients and those of 500 normal adults. *Amer. J. Psychiat.* **101**: 443–448, 1945.
5. Bremer, F. Activité électrique du cortex cérébral dans les états de sommeil et de veille chez le chat. *C. R. Soc. Biol.* **122**: 464–467, 1936.
6. Brockway, A. L., Gleser, G., Winokur, G., and Ulett, G. A. The use of a control population in neuropsychiatric research (psychiatric, psychological, and EEG evaluation of a heterogeneous sample). *Amer. J. Psychiat.* **111**: 248–262, 1954.
7. Cohn, R. The influence of emotion on the human electroencephalogram. *J. nerv. ment. Dis.* **104**: 351–357, 1946.
8. Darrow, C. W. The electroencephalogram and psychophysiological regulation in the brain. *Amer. J. Psychiat.* **102**: 791–798, 1946.

9. Darrow, C. W. Psychological and psychophysiological significance of the electro-encephalogram. *Psychol. Rev.* **54:** 157–168, 1947.
10. Darrow, C. W. The relation of cerebral to autonomic activity in the conditioned emotional reactions of children. *Ann. N. Y. Acad. Sci.* **56:** 289–301, 1953.
11. Darrow, C. W., and Henry, C. E. Psychophysiology of stress. In: *A Survey Report on Human Factors in Undersea Warfare.* National Research Council, Washington, Chap. 20, pp. 417–439, 1949.
12. Darrow, C. W., Pathman, J., and Kronenberg, G. Level of autonomic activity and electroencephalogram. *J. exp. Psychol.* **36:** 355–365, 1946.
13. Davis, H. Some aspects of the electrical activity of the cerebral cortex. *Cold Spring Harbor Symp. Quant. Biol.* **4:** 285–291, 1936.
14. Davis, H. Homeostasis of cerebral excitability. *Electroenceph. clin. Neurophysiol.* **2:** 243–247, 1950.
15. Davis, H., and Davis, P. A. Action potentials of the brain in normal persons and in normal states of cerebral activity. *Arch. Neurol. Psychiat.* **36:** 1214–1224, 1936.
16. Ellingson, R. J. Brain waves and problems of psychology. *Psychol. Bull.* **53:** 1–34, 1956.
17. Ellingson, R. J., Wilcott, R. C., Sineps, J. G., and Dudek, F. J. EEG frequency-pattern variation and intelligence; a correlational study. *Electroenceph. clin. Neurophysiol.* **9:** 657–660, 1957.
18. Fischgold, H., and Gastaut, H. (Editors). Conditionnement et reactivité en électro-encephalographie. *Electroenceph. clin. Neurophysiol.,* Suppl. **6:** 1957.
19. Gallagher, J. R., Gibbs, E. L., and Gibbs, F. A. Relation between the electrical activity of the cortex and the personality in adolescent boys. *Psychosom. Med.* **4:** 134–139, 1942.
20. Gastaut, H., Bacher, F., Bert, J., Blanc-Garin, J., Fessard, A., Fraisee, P., Lee Van Goethem, M., and Roger, A. Relations entre les variables électroencephalographiques et celles experimant la personnalité et les fonctions sensori-motrices. Resultats d'une enquête effectuée sur une population homogène de jeunes adultes males ages de 20 ans. *Rev. neurol.* **101:** 320–390, 1959.
21. Golla, F., Hutton, E. L., and Walter, W. G. The objective study of mental imagery: I. Physiological concomitants. Appendix on new method of electroencephalographic analysis. *J. ment. Sci.* **89:** 216–223, 1943.
22. Gottlober, A. B. The relationship between brain potentials and personality. *J. exp. Psychol.* **22:** 67–74, 1938.
23. Helman, Z. *Rorschach et électroencephalogramme chez l'énfant épileptique.* Presses Universitaires de France, Paris, 1959.
24. Henry, C. E., and Knott, J. R. A note on the relationship between personality and the alpha rhythm of the electroencephalogram. *J. exp. Psychol.* **28:** 362–366, 1941.
25. Hill, D. Psychiatry. In: D. Hill and G. Parr (Editors), *Electroencephalography. A Symposium on Its Various Aspects.* Macdonald & Co., Ltd., London. Chap. 11, pp. 319–363, 1950.
26. Jasper, H. H. Electrical signs of cortical activity. *Psychol. Bull.* **34:** 411–481, 1937.
27. Johnson, L. C., and Ulett, G. A. Quantitative study of pattern and stability of resting electroencephalographic activity in a young adult group. *Electroenceph. clin. Neurophysiol.* **11:** 233–249, 1959.
28. Johnson, L. C., Ulett, G. A., Sines, J. O., and Stern, J. A. Cortical activity and cognitive functioning. *Electroenceph. clin. Neurophysiol.* **12:** 861–874, 1960.
29. Kennard, M. A. The electroencephalogram and disorders of behavior. A review. *J. nerv. ment. Dis.* **124:** 103–124, 1956.
30. Kennard, M. A., Rabinovitch, M. S., and Fister, W. P. The use of frequency analysis in the interpretation of the EEGs of patients with psychological disorders. *Electroenceph. clin. Neurophysiol.* **7:** 29–38, 1955.
31. Kennard, M. A., Rabinovitch, M. S., Schwartzman, A. E., and Fister, W. P. Factor of aggression as related to the electroencephalogram. *Dis. nerv. Syst.* **17:** 127–131, 1956.
32. Kennard, M. A., and Willner, M. D. Correlation between electroencephalograms and deep reflexes in normal adults. *Dis. nerv. Syst.* **6:** 337–342, 1945.
33. Kiloh, L. G., and Osselton, J. W. *Clinical Electroencephalography.* Butterworths, London, 1961.
34. Lemere, F. The significance of individual differences in the Berger rhythm. *Brain.* **59:** 366–375, 1936.
35. Liberson, W. T. Functional electroencephalography in mental disorders. *Dis. nerv. Syst.* **5:** 357–364, 1944.
36. Lindsley, D. B. Electrical potentials of the brain in children and adults. *J. gen. Psychol.* **19:** 285–306, 1938.
37. Lindsley, D. B. Electroencephalography. In: J. McV. Hunt (Editor), *Personality and the Behavior Disorders.* The Ronald Press Company, New York, Chap. 33, pp. 1033–1103, 1944.

38. Lindsley, D. B. Emotion. In: S. S. Stevens (Editor), *Handbook of Experimental Psychology.* John Wiley & Sons, Inc., New York, Chap. 14, pp. 473–516, 1951.
39. Loomis, A. L., Harvey, E. N., and Hobart, G. Electrical potentials of the human brain. *J. exp. Psychol.* **19**: 249–279, 1936.
40. Mundy-Castle, A. C. The relationship between primary-secondary function and the alpha rhythm of the electroencephalogram. *J. Nat. Inst. Personnel Res.* **6**: 95–102, 1955.
41. Mundy-Castle, A. C. The electroencephalogram and mental activity. *Electroenceph. clin. Neurophysiol.* **9**: 643–655, 1957.
42. Mundy-Castle, A. C. An appraisal of electroencephalography in relation to psychology. *J. Nat. Inst. Personnel Res.* Suppl. **2**: 1–43, 1958.
43. Mundy-Castle, A. C. Electrophysiological correlates of intelligence. *J. Personality.* **26**: 184–199, 1958.
44. Mundy-Castle, A. C. Comments on Saunders' "Further implications of Mundy-Castle's correlations between EEG and Wechsler-Bellevue variables." *J. Nat. Inst. Personnel Res.* **8**: 102–105, 1960.
45. Palmer, D. M., and Rock, H. A. High alpha incidence in the EEG and personality patterning. *Electroenceph. clin. Neurophysiol.* **3**: 374, 1951.
46. Palmer, D. M., and Rock, H. A. Brain wave patterns and "crystallized experiences." *Ohio med. J.* **49**: 804–806, 1953.
47. Rabinovitch, M. S., Kennard, M. A., and Fister, W. P. Personality correlates of electroencephalographic patterns: Rorschach findings. *Canad. J. Psychol.* **9**: 29–41, 1955.
48. Rémond, A., and Lesèvre, N. Remarques sur l'activité cérébrale des sujets normaux. La typologie électroencéphalographique dans ses rapports avec certains caractères psychologiques. *Electroenceph. clin. Neurophysiol.* Suppl. **6**: 235–255, 1957.
49. Report on the relations between the electroencephalographic variables and those expressing the personality and the sensori-motor functions of 511 recruits, aged 20 years. *Electroenceph. clin. Neurophysiol.* **12**: 224–236, 1960.
50. Rubin, M. A. A variability study of the normal and schizophrenic occipital alpha rhythm: I. *J. Psychol.* **6**: 325–334, 1938.
51. Rubin, M. A., and Cohen, L. H. A variability study of the normal and schizophrenic occipital alpha rhythm: II. The electroencephalogram and imagery type. *J. ment. Sci.* **85**: 779–783, 1939.
52. Saul, L. J., Davis, H., and Davis, P. A. Correlations between electroencephalograms and the psychological organization of the individual. *Trans. Amer. Neurol. Ass.* **63**: 167–169, 1937.
53. Saul, L. J., Davis, H., and Davis, P. A. Psychologic correlations with the electroencephalogram. *Psychosom. Med.* **11**: 361–376, 1949.
54. Saul, L. J., Davis, H., and Davis, P. A. Psychological correlations with the electroencephalogram. *Electroenceph. clin. Neurophysiol.* **1**: 515, 1949.
55. Saunders, D. R. Further implications of Mundy-Castle's correlations between EEG and Wechsler-Bellevue variables. *J. Nat. Inst. Personnel Res.* **8**: 91–101, 1960.
56. Shagass, C. The sedation threshold. A method for estimating tension in psychiatric patients. *Electroenceph. clin. Neurophysiol.* **6**: 221–233, 1954.
57. Shagass, C. Neurophysiological studies of anxiety and depression. *Psychiat. Res. Rep. Amer. Psychiat. Ass.* **8**: 100–117, 1958.
58. Shipton, J., and Walter, W. G. Les relations entre les activités alpha, les modes de pensée et les affinités sociales. *Electroenceph. clin. Neurophysiol.* Suppl. **6**: 185–202, 1957.
59. Short, P. L., and Walter, W. G. The relationship between physiological variables and stereognosis. *Electroenceph. clin. Neurophysiol.* **6**: 29–44, 1954.
60. Sisson, B. D., and Ellingson, R. J. On the relationship between "normal" EEG patterns and personality variables. *J. nerv. ment. Dis.* **121**: 353–358, 1955.
61. Strauss, H. Clinical and electroencephalographic studies: The electroencephalogram in psychoneurotics. *J. nerv. ment. Dis.* **101**: 19–27, 1945.
62. Thorner, M. W., Gibbs, F. A., and Gibbs, E. L. Relation between the electroencephalogram and flying ability. *War Med.* **2**: 255–262, 1942.
63. Travis, L. E. Brain potentials and the temporal course of consciousness. *J. exp. Psychol.* **21**: 302–309, 1937.
64. Travis, L. E., and Gottlober, A. How consistent are an individual's brain potentials from day to day? *Science.* **85**: 223–224, 1937.
65. Ulett, G. A., Gleser, G., Winokur, G., and Lawler, A. The EEG and reaction to photic stimulation as an index of anxiety-proneness. *Electroenceph. clin. Neurophysiol.* **5**: 23–32, 1953.

66. Ulett, G. A., Johnson, L. C., and Mills, W. B. Pattern, stability and relationship among "EEG" activation techniques. *Electroenceph. clin. Neurophysiol.* **10**: 768–769, 1958.
67. Ulett, G. A., Johnson, L. C., and Mills, W. B. Pattern, stability and relationship among electroencephalographic "activation" techniques. *Electroenceph. clin. Neurophysiol.* **11**: 251–266, 1959.
68. Walter, R. D., and Yeager, C. L. Visual imagery and electroencephalographic changes. *Electroenceph. clin. Neurophysiol.* **8**: 193–199, 1956.
69. Walter, V. J., and Walter, W. G. The central effects of rhythmic sensory stimulation. *Electroenceph. clin. Neurophysiol.* **1**: 57–86, 1949.
70. Walter, W. G. Normal rhythms—their development, distribution and significance. In: D. Hill and G. Parr (Editors), *Electroencephalography. A Symposium on Its Various Aspects.* Macdonald & Co., Ltd., London, Chap. 7, pp. 203–227, 1950.
71. Walter, W. G. *The Living Brain.* W. W. Norton and Co., New York, 1953.
72. Walter, W. G., and Shipton, J. La presentation et l'identification des composantes des rhythmes alpha. *Electroenceph. clin. Neurophysiol.* Suppl. **6**: 177–184, 1957.
73. Werre, P. F. The relationships between electroencephalographic and psychological data in normal adults. Thesis, Universitaire Pers., Leiden, 1957.
74. Werre, P. F., De Lange, J. W. N., and Storm Van Leeuwen, W. The relationships between electroencephalographic and psychological data in normal adults. *Electroenceph. clin. Neurophysiol.* **11**: 611, 1959.
75. Yeager, C. L., and Baldes, E. J. The electroencephalogram in organic and non-organic mental disorders. *Proc. Mayo Clin.* **12**: 705–712, 1937.

ELECTROENCEPHALOGRAMS IN PSYCHOPATHIC PERSONALITY AND IN MURDERERS

John R. Knott, Ph.D.

The earliest data relating EEG abnormalities to the category of psychopathic personality were contributed by Hill and Watterson in 1942 (18). Their total group data were based on 151 cases diagnosed as psychopathic personalities. The over-all extent of EEG abnormality which they reported was 55 per cent, while in a control group of 52 young adults only 15 per cent showed abnormalities by their criteria. It is interesting, however, to note that the criteria of abnormality used included the development of slow activity in response to overbreathing. At the present time (i.e., 1962), it is doubtful that most critical EEGers regard slow activity evoked by overbreathing (or prolonged or recurrent slow activity after overbreathing) as being truly abnormal, unless there is definite spike-wave, spike, or some other type of recognized seizure activity. The factors of low blood sugar and low CO_2 may well produce slow EEG phenomenon even in normal controls (4). The fact that Hill and Watterson did not obtain an equal proportion of such "activation" in their control group could possibly have been due to the time of day that the controls were examined, relative to their patient group, or to some other uncontrollable factors. However, if one deletes those EEGs ruled abnormal by this generous criterion, there still remains a difference between the controls and the psychopaths, with 51 of the 151 psychopaths presenting EEG abnormalities at rest while only 8 of the 52 controls showing abnormalities, a ratio of 33 per cent to 15 per cent.

Knott and Gottlieb (25) reported on the EEGS of 44 patients diagnosed as psychopathic personalities, using criteria of abnormality in reasonable accord with those of Hill and Watterson, although no weight was placed on slow activity associated with hyperventilation. The total incidence of EEG abnormality was 52 per cent. In a later study (**10**), the Gibbs Scale (**8**) was used to classify the EEGs of 100 psychopaths. Forty-two per cent of the cases yielded normal EEGs, 44 per cent showed "slightly abnormal" (S-1 or F-1), 10 per cent showed "very abnormal" (S-2 or F-2) EEGs, while 2 per cent exhibited frank paroxysmal seizure type episodes in their EEGs.

Inquiry into the distributions of normality-abnormality as they might be related to any particular type of psychopathy was made initially by Hill and Watterson (**18**). Sixty-six of their patients were classified as being "aggressive." Thirty-eight cases were classified as being "inadequate." Of the aggressive psychopaths, 44 per cent had abnormal EEGs at rest (i.e., without inclusion of the hyperventilation data in classification of abnormality). Only 23 per cent of the inadequate psychopaths presented with EEG abnormalities at rest. This finding led these authors to stress the relationship between aggressive features of the personality disorder and abnormalities in the EEG (see also **13**, **19**). The data of Knott and Gottlieb (**25**) did not appear to yield any apparent relationship of this type, and these latter authors cautioned against seeking EEG-personality relationships without large samples, even though their own findings seemed to suggest some relationships between sexual psychopathy and EEG anomaly. Simons and Diethelm (**42**), with a rather small total sample of 69, felt that some differences existed between types of psychopathy and distribution of EEG patterns. Patients with psychopathy "of a psychoneurotic" type ($N = 12$) and "of cyclothmic" type ($N = 7$) had normal EEGs. Those "with poor ethical standards" ($N = 11$), all of whom were aggressive, had moderately slow, abnormal EEGs. Those with "loose organization of personality and immaturity" ($N = 31$) had a mixture of EEG patterns although most were apparently normal. The inadequate group ($N = 8$) seemed loaded with records that were slower than normal.

Hill (**14**) has presented a more detailed description of EEG anomalies in psychopaths, with four types of activity which he considered "sensitive to the age factor" being found in normal children, and decreasing with age. These include: (1) central-temporal theta activity (excessive by adult standards), (2) focal posterior slow wave activity, (3) dominant theta activity in post-central areas, (4) "alpha variant" in occipital areas, with a subharmonic component, as first reported in detail by Goodwin (**9**). In addition, Hill considered another class of abnormality, composed of seizure-type paroxysmal electrical activity, insensitive to age: (1) fast spike and wave, and grouped spikes, (2) paroxysmal fast and slow rhythm, and (3) temporal spike foci.

Over the course of years there have been a few varying findings not in agreement with those of the workers mentioned above. Simon, O'Leary, and Ryan, (41) reporting on 96 cases in a military situation, were unable to discover any remarkably greater incidence of EEG abnormality in psychopaths than would be expected in a control group. Their records were classified on the Gibbs Scale, and they found that 72 per cent were within the normal range. This is only 12 per cent below the Gibbs et al. control "normal" EEG value (8). Simon et al. were unable to distinguish the EEGs of cases showing aggression and those who did not show outstanding symptoms of aggression. Nor was there demonstrable a relationship between the severity of the psychiatric disturbance and the degree of deviation of the EEG.

Collomb et al. (3) reported that a group of 43 psychopathic personalities were characterized, in EEG terms, by greater synchrony and higher amplitude of alpha activity, although alpha frequency of 8 per second was more often encountered than were faster alpha frequencies. Honke, Stromgren, and Zahle (20) did not find a remarkable incidence of anomaly in a group defined as "emotionally explosive." Kozaczewska and Kazanowska (28) found no evidence of pronounced EEG abnormality in a group of 71 cases diagnosed as psychopathic personalities, 55 of whom had normal records, and only 4 of whom were clearly abnormal. This latter group included 2 cases with "explosive" characteristics. These authors concluded that a strict selection of cases, rejecting all with any possible organic brain lesions, led to the amount of EEG abnormality being about that which occurred in control groups. It should be remarked, however, that in most of the earlier studies (including Hill and Watterson, Gottlieb and Knott, and Simons and Diethelm), all cases with clinically defined organic features were excluded. In the Knott and Gottlieb study, those with a presumably significant history of injury or illness were excluded.

In the original disclosures of Hill and Watterson, attempts were made to relate EEG abnormality in the patients to morbidity in the family constellation and to early head trauma in the patient. While there appeared to be certain clues in this study, perhaps the most important point brought out was that in the aggressive group of psychopaths there was a greater incidence of no positive history of head trauma than there was in the group of inadequate psychopaths. It is also interesting that there was no apparent relationship in the incidence of EEG abnormality in relation to positive head trauma in the aggressive and in the inadequate subjects. It merely seemed that the inadequates had a greater incidence of trauma.

Such problems were explored in detail by Gottlieb *et al.* (10) in a large group of children diagnosed as primary behavior disorder, and in an equally large group of young adults diagnosed as psychopathic personalities. Significant relationships between early injury and/or illness and the later demonstrated EEG abnormality were established. This finding led to the proposal that there were contributing factors, defined in terms of acquired characteristics (i.e., as sequelae of earlier traumatic events), which were brought about by apparently minor structural change. The obvious conclusion is that events in the past life of the patient which would normally be regarded as probably not out of the ordinary (measles, mumps, pertussis, presumably mild head trauma without unconsciousness or involving a relatively short lapse of consciousness, apparently minor birth trauma, etc.) do indeed relate to EEG abnormality. The obvious next question is, "Does this relate to the disorder of the personality?"

Gottlieb *et al.* (10) investigated factors in the constellation of the patients, as well as their immediate and remote families. If there was a positive family history of psychosis, maladjusted personality, chronic alcoholism, or epilepsy, there was a greater probability that the EEG of the patient would be abnormal. When a history of early illness or injury coincided with a positive family constellation, the probabilities of EEG abnormality were even greater.

Relationships which can be drawn back into the family suggest genetic factors. EEG investigations have been extended to include the parents of both children and adults, diagnosed either as primary behavior disorder or psychopathic personality (27). These investigations revealed some interesting relationships between EEGs of the parent and child. In the first place, the EEGs of the parents did not distribute as would be expected if they were drawn from a normal control population. Knott, Platt, Ashby, and Gottlieb reported an extensive study involving 86 children in which the EEGs of both true parents were classified as follows: (1) those cases where both parents showed normal EEGs, (2) those where one parent showed a normal EEG and the other one an abnormal EEG, and (3) those very few cases where both parents showed abnormal EEGs. As EEG abnormalities of the parents increased, there was a progressively increasing skewness away from the expected normal in the distribution of EEG types in the children. This rather clearly points to the probability that there must be factors of a genetic type. Kennard (23) has also brought forth data bearing on this point, although not statistically significant, including EEGs on the siblings of patients. In spite of the evidence suggesting genetic factors, however, Kennard argued strongly for environmental stress as a cause of similarity of EEG patterns in the patients and their families. This hypothesis has been evaluated in detail by Knott *et al.* (27), and rejected.

One should now turn back to the finding by Hill and Watterson (18) that the EEGs of the aggressive psychopaths did not appear to relate to early trauma, but instead tended to show certain features which could be regarded as "immature." These particularly include the presence of slow activity in the more posterior brain areas (occipital, posterior temporal, parietal). Over the course of time this has come to be called "the maturation defect." Hill (14) has stated the rationale of this term and set forth the criteria fairly clearly. Cohn and Nardini (2) have also commented upon this particular peculiarity of the EEGs of older children and young adults who show maladjustments in personality. Such an observation quite naturally leads one into an evaluation on the EEGs of children with disorders of adjustment, but it will not be our place to follow that line back to its direct origin. Aird and Gastaut (1) have made extensive observations on the posterior slow rhythms of children, adolescents, and adults. They reported "alpha variants" to have some relationship to emotional instability, with 50 per cent of alpha variant cases showing such characteristics. They regarded polyrhythmic, asymmetrical posterior 3-to-4-per-second activity as of no clinical importance, but believed it may indicate slow maturation. The immediate point of significance is that such slow posterior patterns tend to decrease and virtually disappear with age in normal children. The decrease with age in slow abnormalities in psychopaths has also been widely noted (14, 15). Nevertheless, the acceptance of *all* anomalies in the four classes of abnormality set forth by Hill (14) as "maturation defects" must bear closer scrutiny.

Over the course of time, changing interests in EEG, as well as changing examination procedures, have led to the discovery of the ubiquitous 14- and 6-per-second positive spike pattern (6). It has been shown by various investigators (26, 31, 32) that this EEG pattern is much more common in its pure form in psychiatric patients than in seizure patients, and that it is more common, proportionately, in a psychiatric than in any other referral group. There is a very large incidence of this particular EEG pattern in children and young adults diagnosed as "adjustment reactions," and this pattern correlates quite well with overt symptoms of aggressiveness. It is interesting to note that there are reports in the literature (21) relating posterior slow dysrhythmias in the awake subject with the incidence of the positive spike patterns in sleep. This finding has yet to be fully explored in psychopaths *per se*.

It is also interesting that the decline with age in the incidence of the positive spike pattern in psychiatric cases (26) more or less parallels the reducing incidence of slow rhythms in the EEGs of psychopaths which has been reported by Hill (15). One may indeed be able to accept the notion that there is a change in EEG patterns related to "maturation," but it is nevertheless important to consider, particularly in the case of the positive spike pattern, that these may be attributable in the first place to early, relatively mild types of cerebral insult. Apparent "improvement" in time could represent changes which are "maturational." Great complexity of analysis is introduced when one encounters less unique EEG patterns, such as theta rhythms, with some patterns in adults bearing a resemblance to those of younger groups. It is easy to assume that "slow" in the adult is a persistence of activity which is normal in younger "immature" ages. Perhaps some thought should be devoted to a consideration of relationships between acquired anomalies and the normalizing influence of time.

Turning now, relatively briefly, to the EEG characteristics of criminals, and particularly of murderers, one must mention the early studies done both in England and in America. One of the most complete early studies on criminal psychopaths was by Silverman (39), who reported a high incidence (53 per cent) of EEG abnormality in a prison group. A later study by Gibbs, Bloomberg, and Bagchi (7) was unable to show any particular deviation of the distribution of EEG types in a larger group of unselected prisoners. While it is always dubious to assume that if a man is in prison he is also a "psychopath," it does appear rather strange that this great disparity occurred, unless inadvertent sampling errors were involved. In this regard, refer also to the study by Simon, O'Leary, and Ryan (**41**). Kennard *et al.* (**24**) have also reported on the criminal psychopath, finding a greater incidence of EEG abnormality, seen as excessive theta activity, in a prison group particularly chosen to show psychopathy, than in a control group. Hill (**14**) has reported data indicating that of the four types of anomalies he regarded as showing "maturation defects," alpha variants and posterior temporal foci did not differ much from those of normal control subjects.

With relation to murder, one of the earliest and most fascinating reports, by Hill, Sargant, and Heppenstall (**17**), dealt with the case of a young man who had murdered his mother. There appeared to be some relationship in this young man's EEGs between the occurrence of slow activity and the level of the blood sugar. Whenever the blood sugar fell to a level below 100 mg/cc, EEG abnormalities appeared. Because the crime had been committed after the accused had been for some hours without food, and because he had also consumed a quantity of small beer, these investigators re-enacted the chemistry of the crime and were able to convince a jury that there may well have been an abnormal physiological condition of the brain, which in turn might have impaired the accused's judgment so as to "render him unable fully to appreciate the nature of the act." Some years later Hill and Pond (**16**) reviewed 105 cases of capital crimes in which EEG data were available. These authors stated that slightly more than one-half of the accused murderers showed abnormal EEGs, with a decrease in the proportion of abnormality up to the age of 40 (**30**). Hill (**14**), again using his four criteria of "maturation defect," demonstrated that a group of murderers ($N = 110$) showed excessive theta activity (22 per cent of cases) and a greater incidence of posterior temporal slow foci (8.2 per cent), than did control subjects ($N = 146$). In his series no outstanding incidence of paroxysmal patterns could be demonstrated, including temporal spikes.

These are findings of vital significance which should temper the over-ready generalizations which may be drawn from single case reports, from studies which are built upon apparently poor EEG technique, and from acceptance of inadequate criteria of abnormality.

Possibly because of the more routine acceptance of sleep EEG procedures in the United States, there were fairly early reports of

14-and-6 positive spike patterns in murderers. Gibbs and Gibbs (**6**) had four murderers in their initial series of 300 cases with 14-and-6. Other reports of this pattern in patients accused of crimes of violence and murder have appeared (**29, 37, 43, 44**). Knott and Niedermeyer (**26**) have demonstrated in a general psychiatric population, a relationship between aggression and the 14-and-6 pattern, but no relationship with psychiatric categories. Of the aggressives, three were murderers. Various authors (**6, 22, 34, 55**) have suggested that this EEG pattern has an organic etiology.

A most intriguing speculation on the significance of the 14- and 6-per-second positive spike pattern in murderers has been recently offered by Woods (**48**). He assumes a causal relationship between the phenomenon of positive spiking in sleep and "the assault on the organic matrix of ego-functioning." His hypothesis is that "the dysrhythmia itself does not induce violence, but rather that it serves as a biologically determined stress on an already impoverished ego. . . . (T)here is the emergence of primitive non-neutralized aggression, with the violent acting-out of conflict previously held in check by the defensive system of the ego. This is contrasted to epilepsy, where the presence of a seizure discharge provides a short-circuiting mechanism with considerable relief of tension."

To one who operates inside the fields of neurophysiology and neuroanatomy, this speculation has neuromythological over- and undertones. It is difficult to conceive of a "dysrhythmia" seen almost only in the special physiological conditions of drowsiness and sleep as producing "stress" on the "ego," unless one postulates that the specific dysrhythmic activity does occur during the aggressive act, and postulates pathways, over which are conducted anomalous patterns of electrical impulses, terminating in the nuclear masses of the brain that are the anatomical and neurophysiological equivalents of the "ego."

A more parsimonious hypothesis would propose that there is some particular brain area which, when damaged, is capable of producing positive spikes during the neurophysiological states associated with drowsiness and/or sleep. Gibbs and Gibbs suggest the thalamus or hypothalamus, Refsum *et al.* (**35**) the rhinencephalon, and Grossman (**11, 12**) possibly the cortex. This same brain area also may be involved in the anatomical-physiological circuits determining emotional reactivity and when damaged or otherwise rendered incapable of normal function may yield emotional hyper-reactivity as a symptom incorporated into the organism's behavioral repertoire. These two symptoms, the one electrical and the other behavioral, are unrelated in time but are related in terms of their being indices of malfunction of brain circuitry related to emotional reactivity.

In conclusion, the rather scattered threads of evidence derived from electroencephalographic evaluations of psychopaths and murderers indicate that there is an aggregate of patterns suggesting maturational, and/or acquired, and/or inherited deviation of cerebral neurophysiological activity. The challenge to the clinician, however, is not in the demonstration of a statistical trend for a group, but lies in the evaluation of each individual patient.

As electroencephalographic evidence may be applied to any individual case, abnormal findings may provide a lead toward previously suspected organic factors which may be documented by more incisive inquiry or by re-evaluation of historical information. Nevertheless, the modification by maturation of trauma-induced EEG anomaly must still be taken into account, although present knowledge about such modification is so slim that further investigation, rather than further speculation, is necessary. Conversely, one must ponder the problem of trauma-induced modulation of already existing EEG abnormalities, whether maturational or genetic in origin. These genetic factors are themselves poorly understood, and their mechanisms totally unknown, although their presence has been amply demonstrated.

Consequently, the application of EEG techniques to individual cases is still fraught with speculation. Nevertheless, healthy and intelligently directed speculation on the interacting roles of genetic, maturational, and acquired determinants of cerebral physiology can set the stage for a broad, rewarding field of clinical investigation. It is to be hoped that a re-review of the present status of the problem may encourage new interests and new efforts which will fill the gaps in our knowledge and provide the psychiatrically oriented electroencephalographer (and the electroencephalographically oriented psychiatrist) with a firm and meaningful basis for understanding individual patients.

BIBLIOGRAPHY

1. Aird, R. B., and Gastaut, Y. Occipital and posterior electroencephalographic rhythms. *Electroenceph. clin. Neurophysiol.* **11**: 637–656, 1959.
2. Cohn, R., and Nardini, J. E. The correlation of bilateral occipital slow activity in the human EEG with certain disorders of behavior. *Amer. J. Psychiat.* **115**: 44–54, 1958.

3. Collomb, H., Bert, J., Plas, R., and Guilloux, G. Comparative study of electro-encephalographic findings collected from 274 male patients with ages ranging from 19 to 25. *Electroenceph. clin. Neurophysiol.* **12**: 229–230, 1960.
4. Davis, H., and Wallace, W. M. Factors affecting changes produced in electroencephalogram by standardized hyperventilation. *Arch. Neurol. Psychiat.* **47**: 606–625, 1942.
5. Gibbens, T. C. N., Pond, D. A., and Stafford-Clark, D. A follow-up study of criminal psychopaths. *J. ment. Sci.* **105**: 108–115, 1959.
6. Gibbs, E. L., and Gibbs, F. A. Electroencephalographic evidence of thalamic and hypothalamic epilepsy. *Neurology.* **1**: 136–144, 1951.
7. Gibbs, F. A., Bloomberg, W., and Bagchi, B. K. Electroencephalographic study of criminals. *Amer. J. Psychiat.* **102**: 294–298, 1945.
8. Gibbs, F. A., Gibbs, E. L., and Lennox, W. G. Electroencephalographic classification of epileptic patients and control subjects. *Arch. Neurol. Psychiat.* **50**: 111–128, 1943.
9. Goodwin, J. E. The significance of alpha variants in the EEG and their relationship to an epileptiform syndrome. *Amer. J. Psychiat.* **104**: 369–379, 1947.
10. Gottlieb, J. S., Ashby, M. C., and Knott, J. R. Primary behavior disorders and psychopathic personality: 1. Correlations of the electro-encephalogram with family history and antecedent illness or injury. *Arch. Neurol. Psychiat.* **56**: 381–400, 1946.
11. Grossman, C. The role of "cortical laminar blocking" in the origin of evoked and spontaneous "positive bursts." *Electroenceph. clin. Neurophysiol.* Suppl. **3**: 61, 1953.
12. Grossman, C. Laminar cortical blocking and its relation to episodic aggressive outbursts. *Arch. Neurol. Psychiat.* **71**: 576–587, 1954.
13. Hill, D. Cerebral dysrhythmia: Its significance in aggressive behavior. *Proc. Roy. Soc. Med.* **37**: 317–330, 1944.
14. Hill, D. EEG in episodic psychotic and psychopathic behavior. A classification of data. *Electroenceph. clin. Neurophysiol.* **4**: 419–442, 1952.
15. Hill, D. Psychiatry. In: D. Hill and G. Parr (Editors), *Electroencephalography. A symposium on its various aspects.* MacDonald and Co. Ltd., London, Chap. 11, pp. 319–363, 1950.
16. Hill, D., and Pond, D. A. Reflections on one hundred capital cases submitted to electroencephalography. *J. ment. Sci.* **98**: 23–43, 1952.
17. Hill, D., Sargant, W., and Heppenstall, M. E. A case of matricide. *Lancet.* **1**: 526–527, 1943.
18. Hill, D., and Watterson, D. Electroencephalographic studies of psychopathic personalities. *J. Neurol. Psychiat.* **5**: 47–65, 1942.
19. Hodge, R. S. Impulsive psychopath: A clinical and electro-physiological study. *J. ment. Sci.* **91**: 472–476, 1945.
20. Honcke, P., Stromgren, E., and Zahle, V. Elektrencephalographische Untersuchungen an Psychopathen. *Arch. Psychiat. Nervenk.* **183**: 55–63, 1949.
21. Hughes, J. R., Gianturco, D., and Stein, W. Electro-clinical correlations in the positive spike phenomenon. *Electroenceph. clin. Neurophysiol.* **13**: 599–605, 1961.
22. Kellaway, P., Crawley, J. W., and Kagawa, N. A specific electroencephalographic correlate of convulsive equivalent disorders in children. *J. Pediat.* **55**: 582–592, 1959.
23. Kennard, M. A. Inheritance of electroencephalogram patterns in children with behavior disorders. *Psychosom. Med.* **11**: 151–157, 1949.
24. Kennard, M. A., Rabinovitch, M. S., and Fister, W. P. The use of frequency analysis in the interpretation of the EEGs of patients with psychological disorders. *Electroenceph. clin. Neurophysiol.* **7**: 29–38, 1955.
25. Knott, J. R., and Gottlieb, J. S. The electroencephalogram in psychopathic personality. *Psychosom. Med.* **5**: 139–142, 1943.
26. Knott, J. R., and Niedermeyer, E. The "fourteen and six" pattern. Some comments on its clinical correlates. *Proc. Amer. EEG Soc. Electroenceph. clin. Neurophysiol.* **15**: 161, 1963.
27. Knott, J. R., Platt, E. B., Ashby, M. C., and Gottlieb, J. S. A familial evaluation of the electroencephalogram of patients with primary behavior disorder and psychopathic personality. *Electroenceph. clin. Neurophysiol.* **5**: 363–370, 1953.
28. Kozaczewska, W., and Kazanowska, J. Clinical symptomatology and EEG correlations in a selected group of psychopaths. *Electroenceph. clin. Neurophysiol.* **14**: 582, 1962.
29. Mills, W. B. Paroxysmal 14 and 6/sec. spike discharges and clinical cases, including a teenage murderer. *Electroenceph. clin. Neurophysiol.* **8**: 344, 1956.
30. Mundy-Castle, A. C. The EEG in 22 cases of murder or attempted murder, together with a discussion of the possible significance of alphoid rhythms. *Electroenceph. clin. Neurophysiol.* **8**: 162, 1956.

31. Nicholson, J. M., and Knott, J. R. Sleep EEGs in psychiatric patients. *Electroenceph. clin. Neurophysiol.* **9:** 174–175, 1957.
32. Niedermeyer, E., and Knott, J. R. Psychiatric implications of the 14 and 6 positive spike pattern of the EEG. *Proc. III World Congr. Psychiat.* **1:** 439, 1961.
33. Pond, D. A. EEG in behavior problem children. *Electroenceph. clin. Neurophysiol.* **10:** 198, 1958.
34. Poser, C. M., and Ziegler, D. K. Clinical significance of 14 and 6 per second positive spike complexes. *Neurology.* **8:** 903–912, 1958.
35. Refsum, S., Presthus, J., Skultad, A., and Östensjö, S. Clinical correlates of the 14 and 6 per second positive spikes. *Acta psychiat. scand.* **35:** 330–334, 1960.
36. Roth, G. Das persistierende juvenile EEG. *Psychiatria.* **136:** 195–203, 1958.
37. Schwade, E. D., and Geiger, S. G. Matricide with electroencephalographic evidence of thalamic or hypothalamic disorder. *Dis. nerv. Syst.* **14:** 18–20, 1953.
38. Schwade, E. D., and Otto, O. Homicide as a manifestation of thalamic or hypothalamic disorder with abnormal electroencephalographic finding. *Wisconsin med. J.* **52:** 171–174, 1953.
39. Silverman, D. Clinical and electroencephalographic studies on criminal psychopaths. *Arch. Neurol. Psychiat.* **50:** 18–33, 1943.
40. Silverman, D. The electroencephalogram of criminals. *Arch. Neurol. Psychiat.* **52:** 38–42, 1944.
41. Simon, B., O'Leary, J. L., and Ryan, J. J. Cerebral dysrhythmia and psychopathic personalities. *Arch. Neurol. Psychiat.* **56:** 677–685, 1946.
42. Simons, D. J., and Diethelm, O. Electroencephalographic studies of psychopathic personalities. *Arch. Neurol. Psychiat.* **55:** 619–626, 1946.
43. Stehle, H. C. Thalamic dysfunction involved in destructive-aggressive behavior directed against persons and property. *Electroenceph. clin. Neurophysiol.* **12:** 264–265, 1960.
44. Winfield, D. L., and Ozturk, O. Electroencephalographic findings in matricide (A case report). *Dis. nerv. Syst.* **20:** 176–178, 1959.
45. Winkler, G. E., and Kove, S. S. The implications of electroencephalographic abnormalities in homicide cases. *J. Neuropsychiat.* **3:** 322–330, 1962.
46. Wissfeld, E. EEG changes in epileptoid psychopaths. *Electroenceph. clin. Neurophysiol.* **5:** 121, 1953.
47. Wissfeld, E., and Kaindl, E. Über die Deutung und den Wert abnormer EEG-Befunde bei psychopathischen Persönlichkeiten. *Nervenarzt.* **32:** 57–66, 1961.
48. Woods, S. M. Adolescent violence and homicide: Ego disruption and the 6 and 14 dysrhythmia. *Arch. gen. Psychiat.* **5:** 528–534, 1961.

THE ELECTROENCEPHALOGRAM
IN PSYCHIATRIC DISORDERS
IN CHILDHOOD

Peter Kellaway, A.M., Ph.D., James Crawley, M.D.,
and Robert Maulsby, M.S., M.D.

The electroencephalogram in the early days of its development proved to be a great disappointment to those psychiatrists and other investigators who rushed to the study of the brain waves as a possible fountainhead of diagnostic, nosologic, and prognostic information in the study of psychiatric disorders. This disappointment was largely a consequence of the real limitation of the technique as it was practiced at that time and as it still is being used today (8). Perhaps the disappointment need not have been so overwhelming had the expectations been less and the approach to research more critical. However, even in the face of these disappointments, the heuristic value of electroencephalographic studies in psychiatry has been significant. Particularly in children, many "bits" of information obtainable from the electroencephalogram could be diagnostically useful or could lead to a new understanding of some of the common disturbances of autonomic function, behavior, mentation, and performance.

This paper is not the end product of a critical investigation of any specific aspect of the subject with which it deals, but is rather an attempt to define the usefulness of EEG in child psychiatry and to elaborate upon certain poorly understood aspects of electroencephalographic abnormalities encountered in children. It is based upon a broad experience in clinical pediatric electroencephalography, specific research in this field, and the authors' experience in dealing with these problems in a clinic in which many patients with such disorders are evaluated and treated.

More than 36,000 children have been studied electrographically in our laboratories in the past 15 years. Many of these children have had multiple studies. Approximately 60 per cent of the patients were referred for study because of problems which may be said to have psychiatric significance. These include, for example, disorders of behavior, learning, communication difficulties, personality problems, episodic attacks of pain or other purely subjective symptoms, and real or apparent mental incapacity.

On the basis of our own studies and work reported by others, we believe that there are four major areas in which electroencephalographic studies may provide the clinical psychiatrist with either specific diagnostic data or an indication that the symptom complex under consideration has an organic basis. These are: (1) episodic pain and autonomic dysfunction without evidence of organic disease; (2) ictal-psychic, perceptual, and experiential symptoms; (3) behavioral aberrations due primarily to organic cerebral dysfunction; and (4) "pseudo-mental retardation" and disorders of communication or perceptual integration of similar cause. The electroencephalogram can also be of more value than almost any other laboratory test in confirming or suggesting a diagnosis of intoxication, particularly intoxication with ataractic agents, which currently are being used extensively.

APPARENT PSYCHOPHYSIOLOGIC REACTIONS OF ORGANIC ORIGIN

It is not uncommon for children to complain of abdominal pain to avoid an unwanted event such as going to school, being required to eat a particular food, or being asked to go to bed. Abdominal pain is also a complaint which is commonly used by children to get attention or sympathy. The so-called separation syndrome seen in the young child parted from the family for the first time, perhaps when he reaches the age at which he is sent to school, often involves a complaint of pain, usually abdominal, which seems designed to keep the child at home. Such complaints are usually recognized for what they are by the parents or the physician.

However, in our studies of a particular electrographic abnormality known as the 14- and 6-per-second positive spike pattern (12, 13) we found that many children have genuine attacks of abdominal pain or headache (or both of these symptoms) as the chief manifestation of a disorder of cerebral origin. These attacks are presumably due to paroxysms of abnormal neuronal discharge and are, therefore, often referred to as "convulsive equivalent" phenomena. The pain is frequently accompanied by evidence of hyperactivity or irritability of the autonomic nervous system. The severity of the symptoms varies considerably among these patients. Many of the less severe cases are mistaken for a feigned or functional disorder. Since emotional tension or stress is likely to trigger these attacks of pain, the organic nature of the child's complaint is often not discovered unless electroencephalographic studies are carried out. In some cases, however, the pain is obviously disabling, or the associated autonomic disturbances, such as pallor, sweating, body temperature elevation, nausea and vomiting, etc., are so obvious that the attacks become a matter of concern and the child is taken to a physician.

The syndrome of paroxysmal pain and autonomic dysfunction was initially recognized as a clinical entity by British physicians and was called the "periodic" syndrome (24). There was no objective evidence of the cerebral origin of the symptoms, however, until investigation of the EEG abnormality known as the 14- and 6-per-second positive spike pattern. This syndrome characteristically occurs in a patient who is between 5 and 16 years of age. In about one-third of the patients a head injury or febrile illness may have preceded the onset of the symptoms by a variable period of time. The patient is otherwise normal and has normal intelligence. Without immediate precipitating cause, he begins to have attacks of abdominal pain and headache. These attacks are usually brief, lasting several minutes or less, but occasionally they persist for several hours. There is sometimes a prodrome of irritability or mild confusion, and the attacks themselves are variously accompanied by anorexia, nausea, vomiting, pallor, and dizziness. Less frequently, the patients may exhibit alteration in body temperature (particularly mild fever), lethargy, and partial or complete loss of consciousness. The symptoms and signs of autonomic dysfunction usually follow the headache and abdominal pain, but in some cases pallor, sweating, nausea, or vomiting initiates the attack. Although many symptoms are found in patients with this disorder, the clinical pattern in an individual patient tends to be stereotyped and does not vary significantly from one attack to another. This stereotyped pattern and the characteristic electroencephalographic abnormality are of primary importance in establishing the diagnosis.

Specific etiologic factors have not been established for this syndrome, and pathologic studies are lacking because of its benign clinical course. In the group of patients we have studied, no significant etiologic data could be discovered in the majority (63 per cent). However, 20 per cent of these patients had suffered mild or moderate head injuries and 17 per cent had been clinically diagnosed as having viral encephalitis. We have carried out serial EEG studies on many of these patients, the initial examinations being done during the acute phase of encephalitis or within several days following head injury. Several weeks or months after the acute EEG abnormality subsides, the 14- and 6-per-second positive spike pattern appears, followed by the specific symptom complex described above. Our initial report of this syndrome in 1959 summarized our data in a series of 450 cases (12). Since that time we have accumulated over 2500 cases.

It is important to recognize that the severity and character of the symptoms are quite variable among the patients included in this group. In individual patients, however, the attacks are likely to be quite similar, although some variation in duration or severity does occur, even as with frankly epileptiform attacks. In many cases the usual attacks are so mild that investigation is not carried out until a prolonged or severe episode occurs. Not infrequently, however, the pain is so incapacitating or the associated autonomic disturbance so disabling that the parents seek medical attention early in the course of the illness. Some patients are subject to what may be called the "full-blown" or complete syndrome, having episodes of abdominal pain accompanied by headache, various autonomic disturbances, alterations in consciousness, deterioration in learning capacity, and a change in behavior. More commonly, these children have attacks which are "fractions" of the total syndrome. These may consist of episodes of abdominal pain, episodes of purely autonomic disturbance, or any combination of these.

In our community, EEG studies are now an almost routine part of the clinical evaluation of a child with symptoms of this type. Presumably as a result of this, the number of children having had exploratory abdominal surgery or extensive radiologic examinations has diminished during the past several years.

The following case history is an example of the total syndrome:

Case 1. A 9-year-1-month-old Negro boy was the product of a normal pregnancy delivered at full term. Labor and delivery were normal and he developed normally. He had no injuries and no illnesses except mumps and rubeola. He was referred to the clinic approximately one year after the onset of attacks which began with a cramping mid-epigastric pain followed promptly by nausea and vomiting. Approximately ten minutes later, he developed bifrontal headache and dizziness. He then felt warm and his face became flushed. Oral temperature had been recorded on several occasions during these attacks and varied between 100.2 and 101.8 degrees. The entire episode usually lasted from 30 to 45 minutes, the symptoms then disappearing spontaneously. The patient was usually lethargic for several hours after cessation of the attack, and he often fell asleep. Attacks of this type occurred about every other week, but he also had more frequent episodes consisting only of abdominal pain and dizziness, lasting several minutes and occurring several times each week. Prior to the onset of these attacks, the child had been well-behaved and had done well in school. His parents noted that at the time these symptoms made their appearance, his behavior also changed. He developed an aggressive, hostile attitude toward his younger siblings, particularly a brother who was 1½ years younger than the patient. Although his brother had not yet been injured, the patient had physically attacked him on numerous occasions and had threatened to kill him. These attacks of aggressive, hostile behavior were unprovoked and, following each outburst, the patient was

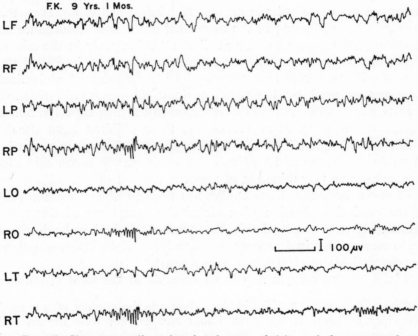

Case 1. Sleep recording showing bursts of 14- and 6-per-second positive spikes.

remorseful and unable to explain it. Although he had previously done well in school, he had failed the semester prior to his being seen in the clinic.

Physical and neurological examination and X ray of the chest and skull were within normal limits. The sleep electroencephalogram revealed frequent episodes of the 14- and 6-per-second positive spike abnormality; the waking record showing frequent irregular high-voltage fused slow waves and transients in the occipital leads.

DISORDERS OF COMMUNICATION OR PERCEPTUAL INTEGRATION AND "PSEUDO-MENTAL RETARDATION"

During the past three years we have studied more than 1,000 children who were failing in school. Approximately 40 per cent of these patients had significant EEG abnormalities. These abnormalities were varied and will be described in more detail below. Clinical evaluation of these children who are performing poorly in school and who also have various EEG abnormalities reveals the following consistent characteristics: the poor school performance is out of proportion to the measured intelligence of the child, the performance level is "patchy" and may vary even at different times of the same day, the attention span is short, and there is marked distractibility. In addition, these children exhibit a subtle disturbance in communication, involving reading, writing, and number identification, which can be considered to be a general disorder of sensorimotor integration.

Poor school performance is a difficult problem, particularly when the measured intelligence is adequate and when the difficulty appears to involve a specific disability, such as failure to learn to read or the more general and less specific factors known as disorders of visual-motor integration. We believe that combined clinical, electrographic, and psychological evaluation of these patients may, in the future, be very revealing and may provide clues to rational therapy. In this paper the discussion will be limited to the EEG findings. The absolute necessity of obtaining sleep records must be stressed, as many of the electrographic abnormalities seen in these patients (as well as in other clinical entities) appear only in sleep or are greatly accentuated during sleep. This observation has been stressed by us previously, and the procedures for obtaining proper sleep recordings in infants and children have been described (3).

Because the electrographic abnormalities seen in this group of patients are quite varied, and because it is possible that various types of cerebral dysfunction can give rise to the syndrome of poor school performance, a program of detailed clinical, electrographic, and psychologic study of these patients should be undertaken. The most frequent EEG abnormalities seen in these patients are: (1) occipital or occipito-temporal slow fused and sharp random waves (occipital slow dysrhythmias); (2) the 14- and 6-per-second positive spike abnormality, alone or associated with occipital slow dysrhythmias; and (3) foci of random spike discharge, particularly in the temporal and occipital regions.

It is important to recognize that these abnormalities may occur as the only objective evidence of cerebral dysfunction. These patients have no history of seizures, no abnormality in the neurologic examination, and often have no history to suggest that the child has suffered a cerebral insult at any time. As we have pointed out elsewhere (23), more than 40 per cent of children with occipital foci do not have seizures. In nearly 50 per cent of these cases the etiology of the focus cannot be determined. The absence of a history of brain injury or of neurological abnormality cannot be considered conclusive evidence that organic brain dysfunction does not exist. On the other hand, the possibility of electrographic abnormality is greatly increased (6) if there is even minimal evidence of neurologic abnormality or if there is history of brain injury, infection, or other insult.

The following case summaries are presented to illustrate the character and variety of electrographic abnormalities which are seen in children who are having communication and learning problems:

Case 2. A white girl who was 14 years and 3 months of age was referred because of failure in school. The child had a normal birth and developmental history. There was no history of serious illness. At the age of 17 months, she fell out of the door of a parked automobile and struck her head on the concrete driveway. There was a scalp laceration but no skull fracture. The injury was followed by unconsciousness for three to five minutes and lethargy for several hours. The patient vomited twice immediately following the injury. She was hospitalized for two days, but there was no apparent residual. She had never had seizures or other evidence of neurologic abnormality. The child had done well until she entered school, the difficulty becoming evident only when she reached the second grade. This problem consisted of an apparent inability to transfer information, from either the spoken word or from reading, to paper. Early in her school career the patient had

had neurological, ophthalmological, and audiological studies. Her I. Q. was measured at 108. She was normal physically. The electroencephalo-gram revealed a focal spike discharge in the left parietal region and episodes of 14- and 6-per-second positive spikes. Both of these abnor-malities appeared only in sleep, the waking record being within normal range for her age.

Case 3. An eight-year-old white boy was the product of a normal pregnancy. Delivery was by breech presentation, but there were no neonatal difficulties. His growth and development had been normal. Ap-proximately one year before the patient was referred for poor school work, he had suffered a mild blow to the occipital region which made him "dazed" but not unconscious. One month later he had one noc-turnal seizure. The onset of this attack was not witnessed, but when his mother reached him, he was having a generalized convulsion which was more marked on the left side. He was hospitalized following this seizure, but no physical abnormalities were discovered. He had appar-ently recovered completely one day following the attack. This attack occurred just after the child had entered the third grade in public school. He had done well before, but after this seizure his school work de-

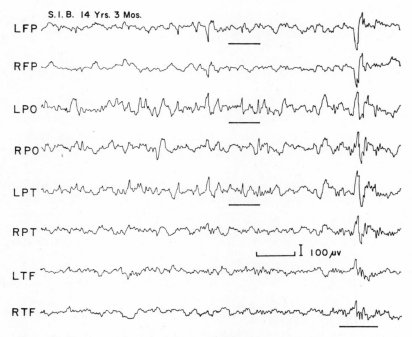

S. I. B. 14 Yrs. 3 Mos.

LFP

RFP

LPO

RPO

LPT

RPT

I 100 μv

LTF

RTF

Case 2. Sleep tracing showing a left parietal spike focus and 14- and 6-per-second positive spikes.

teriorated progressively. The child was distractible, hyperactive, and seemed unable to apply himself to a learning situation for any period of time. While he was not specifically a behavior problem, his restlessness and hyperactivity interfered with normal classroom routine, and the teacher found it necessary to discipline him frequently. An electroencephalogram was performed after he had failed the first semester of his third year in school. This showed an almost continuous abnormality of the slow spike and slow wave type, probably originating in the right frontal lobe but showing wide areal reference. Following the electroencephalographic study, the child was treated with Dilantin. He has been on this drug for eight months and, during this time, has completed the third grade successfully.

Case 4. This case demonstrates a similar clinical picture but with different electrographic findings. This patient is a seven-year-two-month-old white male who had a normal birth but whose developmental milestones were slightly retarded. At the age of nine months, the child fell out of bed, striking his head, but was apparently not injured. He was also struck on the head at the age of three years, but again was

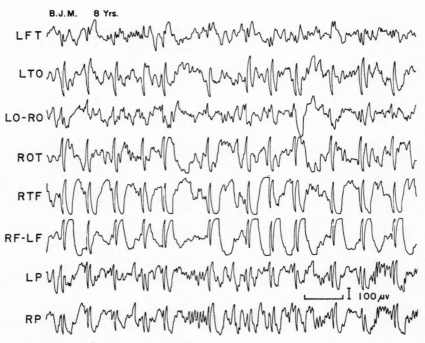

Case 3. Slow spike-and-wave abnormality with localization to the right frontal area.

apparently uninjured. The child was referred for evaluation because of very poor performance in school. He was in the first grade and was failing all subjects. He was considered to have normal intelligence, but at school he refused to talk to the teacher or to the other children. At home he talked normally with his parents and other siblings, but when he was upset or angry, he would go to his bedroom and remain he was reading, however, and did not retain the material adequately. had no seizures. The clinical impression was of early juvenile schizophrenia. The electroencephalogram showed a paroxysmal spike-and-wave dysrhythmia of the type generally associated with absence seizures.

Case 5. This boy was referred because of inadequate school work resulting from a spotty and poorly sustained level of performance. He is a white male of 11 years of age who was adopted shortly after birth. No details of the prenatal or natal history were known. The child was an avid reader and could read big words and pronounce them correctly. He did not have good comprehension of what he was reading, however, and did not retain the material adequately. On some days he was unable to perform a simple arithmetic problem correctly, but on other days he could perform 20 to 30 problems without error. At such times he seemed to do better if the problem

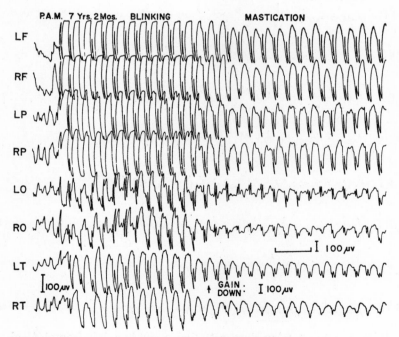

Case 4. Three-per-second spike-and-wave pattern.

were read to him than if he had to read it himself. On occasion
he confused addition and subtraction. His motor and visual-motor
coordination were also variable. At times he was able to copy words
accurately and to spell them correctly, but at other times he was
unable to copy or to spell even simple words. He was well behaved
when he was alone or with adults, but with children he became
overactive. He participated in group play, but if he did not under-
stand the game or if he was not winning, he became angry and
started to fight. He slept poorly and had frequent bad dreams
and nightmares. He awakened several times each week, frightened and
crying. After being awake for two or three minutes, he became
quiet and went back to sleep. He had had no seizures and no serious illnesses. His I.Q. was rated at 95, but the testing psychologist
was dubious about the accuracy of this evaluation because of marked
variability of the patient's responses. The school problem was complicated by numerous emotional disturbances in the family. The father
had had three surgical operations during the year before the child was
seen. During this year the maternal grandmother died and the family's
home was almost destroyed by a storm. Neurological examination was
normal with the exception of poor coordination and poor performance

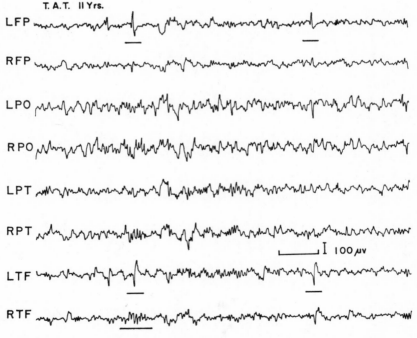

Case 5. Sleep tracing demonstrating a random left frontal focal
spike discharge and 14- and 6-per-second positive spikes.

of rapidly alternating movements. He used a pencil very awkwardly and attempts to copy figures demonstrated poor visual-motor coordination and defective visual perception. The electroencephalogram was abnormally slow, showed an active focus of spike discharge in the left frontal region, and revealed numerous episodes of the 14- and 6-per-second positive spike abnormality in sleep.

Case 6. This case is clinically similar to the preceeding one, but with different electroencephalographic findings. This eight-year-five-month-old white boy's electroencephalogram showed independent focal spike discharges in the right and left occipital regions in sleep. The waking record was also abnormal because of frequent high-voltage slow and sharp fused wave forms in the occipital leads on both sides. This child was sent for evaluation because of unsatisfactory school work. His birth and early developmental histories were normal. Except for small stature, he was not considered abnormal until his second year in school, when it was found that he was completely unable to handle numbers and had constantly failed arithmetic. His handwriting was poor and he often transposed let-

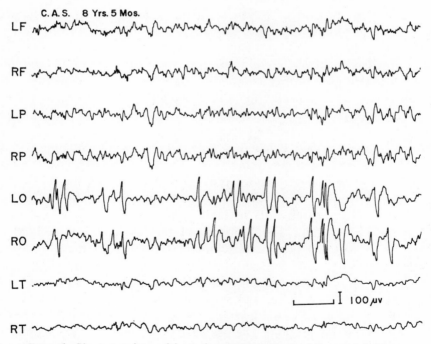

Case 6. Sleep tracing with active independent right and left occipital spike discharges.

ters. A repeat electroencephalographic examination was carried out four months after the initial study, during which time the child had been treated with Dilantin. The record showed some improvement in that the slow fused and sharp activity in the occipital regions was less marked, but the focal spike discharges in the left and right occipital regions were essentially unchanged. During this time there had been improvement in the child's school performance, but he had been receiving special tutoring in addition to medical therapy.

The electrographic abnormalities are the manifestations of various types of known cerebral pathology, but in some instances, no specific pathology has been established. The importance of these abnormalities in understanding a complex problem, such as poor school performance, lies in their ability to provide a guide in the diagnostic consideration of such patients. The presence of electroencephalographic abnormality of any type in a child who is performing poorly in school should affect our consideration of the possible primary role of emotional disturbance, lack of motivation, or merely poor inherited intellectual capacity. Recognition of subtle disturbances of cerebral function revealed by electroencephalography is important because the attitude of physician, parent, and teacher is changed by the realization that the child has an organic cerebral disorder. Thus the usual techniques of punishment or reward for performance are ineffective in such children, and pressure exerted by parents and teachers may further compound the problem by producing tension and emotional upset in both the child and other members of the family. This is apt to result in still poorer school performance because these children often show a tendency to react to such pressures by exaggerated behavioral responses. The school failure may then be complicated by a behavior disorder of psychogenic type.

Because electroencephalographic abnormalities of the kind described above are associated in some patients with frank seizure disorders, we have empirically treated a number of these patients with anticonvulsant drugs. The rationale of this therapy is based upon our belief that the poor intellectual performance of these children may be the result of one or both of two possible conditions. The first condition is the presence of a brain lesion resulting in destruction of neural tissue and functional deficit in a neural system specifically involved in the learning process, in communication, or in sensori-motor integration. The second condition is the consequence of an irritative discharge arising from a cerebral lesion. This discharge interferes with the function of subjacent or even distant neural elements, thus disturbing or preventing their normal participation in integrated motor or sensory functions.

It is fashionable, especially among classically trained neurologists, to speak disparagingly of what they call "treating the EEG." Despite the absence of overt seizures, our experience suggests that patients who have difficulty in learning and who have epileptiform abnormalities in their electroencephalograms should be given a therapeutic trial on anticonvulsant medication. This is not "treating the EEG" but is an attempt to determine whether drugs which are known to suppress or limit the spread of abnormal brain discharges will result in improvement of function. The results of such therapeutic trials in these patients is variable, as might be expected. In some patients a satisfactory response occurs promptly, while there is no improvement or the change is doubtful in others. This variability may well reflect the presumed dual cause for poor school performance in these patients. Those whose failure is based primarily upon subclinical epileptiform discharges respond satisfactorily and those whose disturbed function is the manifestation of a destructive lesion show no response or a poor response.

In the group of children with EEG abnormalities whose chief difficulties are related to learning and communication, the spectrum of poor performance ranges from relatively minor problems of visual-motor integration to what might be called a state of "pseudo mental retardation." This term is used to characterize a disorder in which constant subclinical epileptiform discharges so impair mental performance that the patient is considered to be mentally retarded. Frank epileptic seizures may or may not occur in these patients.

Case 7. An eight-year-two-month-old white girl was referred for evaluation because of presumed mental retardation. The patient was the product of a normal first pregnancy. Labor was prolonged but delivery was normal and the patient's condition in the neonatal period was satisfactory. The parents first became concerned about the child's condition when she was five or six months old and appeared to be unable to sleep for more than two hours at a time, waking eight to ten times during every night. Development was slow—the child did not walk alone until she was 16 months of age and did not say understandable words until she was approximately two years of age. She was hyperactive and distractible and was "unable to be quiet long enough to learn." At the time she was initially seen, she was unable to read and could not write her name. She could print the alphabet with prompting. The parents described her as affectionate and sweet; but, if she was reprimanded, she would go to her room and talk to herself in the mirror, complaining about what her parents had done. Neurological examination was within normal range.

The electroencephalogram revealed paroxysmal bursts of generalized irregular spike-and-wave activity which lasted 3 to 4 seconds and which occurred every 20 to 50 seconds. Each burst was followed by a long episode of occipital slow activity of irregular and sharp configuration. After this electroencephalogram was performed, the child was placed on anticonvulsant medication and a repeat study demonstrated great reduction in the paroxysmal spike and slow wave bursts and marked reduction in the interburst dysrhythmia, normal occipital alpha activity appearing intermittently. Concomitant with the improvement in the electrographic findings, there was improvement in mental performance. The child remained in special education classes but was making progress and had learned elementary reading and writing. The apparently autistic behavior that was present prior to therapy had completely disappeared.

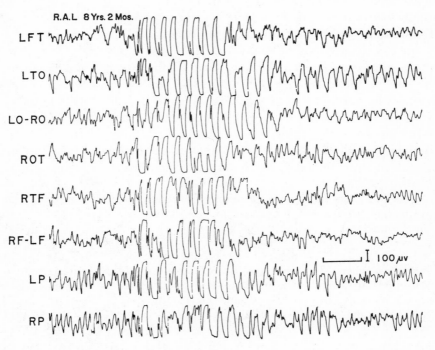

Case 7. Irregular spike-and-wave activity with a slow background.

BEHAVIOR DISORDERS

As has been illustrated in the case histories presented above, behavior disorders often complicate primary learning and communication problems in children. Early workers in clinical electroencephalography found electrographic abnormalities, particularly occipital slow dysrhythmias, in a significant number of children with behavior disorders (**9, 17, 16, 15**). Electroencephalographic abnormality was very early reported in patients with what Kahn (**10**) has called "organic drivenness," a hyperkinetic, impulsive, and compulsive behavior pattern sometimes associated with outbursts of sudden, unprovoked, aggressive, and destructive acts. Other workers subsequently added additional descriptive features to this profile: distractibility, short attention span, excessive curiosity, and overfriendliness.

This descriptive profile characterizing the child with organic behavior disorder has stood the test of time, and children showing all or many of these behavioral patterns show a high incidence of electroencephalographic abnormality. Detailed study of the electroencephalograms in these patients has shown that generalized or occipital slow dysrhythmias are not a constant or even the most common electrographic abnormality (**14**). When sleep studies are done, almost any type of electrographic abnormality may appear. In most of these patients it is impossible to predict what the EEG will show. The organic behavior syndrome is specific only in that it points to behavioral disturbances based upon organic cerebral dysfunction. It is not specific in terms of the nature, extent, or location of the underlying cerebral pathology, although all such cases may have in common a lesion, as yet undiscovered, of a particular neural system.

The pathophysiologic background of organic behavior disorder is probably similar to that which underlies abnormal learning capacity. Thus, the abnormal behavior may arise from a chronic destructive lesion and be the result of damage or continuing dysfunction of neural systems which are specifically involved in the elaboration of emotional responses and behavioral expression. The behavioral abnormality may also arise as the expression of an irritative neuronal discharge in parts of the brain which are particularly involved in behavior, such as the hypothalamus and the entorhinal portions of the temporal complex. The latter patients are subject to paroxysms of rage or furors of aggressive and destructive activity. Children with this type of behavioral attack commonly show, in their electro-encephalograms, either the 14- and 6-per-second positive spike abnormality (7) or temporal spike foci (22, 5). Other transient modifications of behavior and affect have been shown by chronic depth electrode studies to occur in association with prolonged sub-clinical epileptiform activity confined to the hippocampus and possibly the insular cortex in patients who have psychomotor seizures (2, 11, 20). Although never proved to occur, it seems quite possible that ictal discharge manifested only in terms of behavior and affect could exist in a patient who was never known to have had an overt epileptic seizure.

It is apparent that both chronic non-ictal organic behavior and behavioral outbursts related to paroxysmal neuronal discharges may coexist in a single patient. It is a well-documented fact that patients with lesions of the temporal lobe often exhibit chronic behavioral and personality disturbances as well as episodic seizures that have primary psychic and behavioral manifestations (18, 19).

It is generally stated that children rarely have psychomotor seizures or by inference, temporal foci. Recent studies indicate that these findings are not rare, although the clinical patterns of the attacks are not always similar to those seen in adults (1). Epilepsy of focal origin accounts for more than one-third of all epilepsy in children and temporal foci constitute about 42 per cent of all foci seen.

Case 8. A typical example of a child with a temporal spike focus illustrates both paroxysmal and chronic behavioral abnormality of bizarre character. This patient was a white boy, aged eight years seven months. He was referred for evaluation because of staring episodes with laughing and head shaking, and prolonged periods of sulky, taciturn, mute behavior followed by less withdrawn periods in which he was slow to respond and showed much perseveration of thought and speech. The child had been normal until he was approximately seven years of age, when he had a prolonged bout of unexplained high fever, headache, and brief episodes of confusion. The behavioral change followed the febrile illness by about two months. The patient was initially seen by a psychiatrist, who diagnosed childhood schizophrenia. Neurological consultation was obtained and physical examination was normal. The electroencephalogram revealed an active left temporal spike focus which was present in both the waking and sleep records but was much more active in sleep.

Following electroencephalographic study, the child was treated with Mysoline and the episodes of staring, unusual laughter, and head shaking stopped. His behavior also improved, but the child con-

tinued to be a moderately withdrawn boy who was often uncooperative, anxious, and ill at ease, particularly with strangers.

Stereotyped automatisms, such as picking at the clothes, are often
fairly obvious clues to a diagnosis of temporal-lobe epilepsy, but
sometimes the behavioral manifestations of epileptiform discharges
are not so easy to recognize in children. The child may, for example, begin to have episodes in which he grimaces briefly or rolls
his eyes up in a peculiar way, as in a habit or tic, or as if he were
"just acting silly." He may have forced laughter which is inappro-
priate to the situation or other mannerisms which are difficult to
evaluate, such as coughing, clearing his throat, gagging, chewing,
or puckering movements of the mouth. Sometimes the child may
be subject to episodes of altered consciousness with a staring facial
expression. These are often interpreted by parents as daydreaming.
If such episodes occur frequently throughout the day or seem prolonged, the child may be thought to be autistic and a diagnosis of
schizophrenia may be considered, as in the case described above.

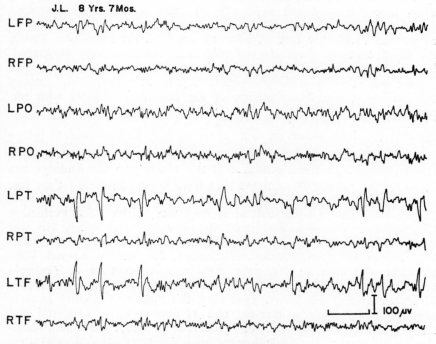

Case 8. Active left temporal spike focus in sleep.

While temporal-lobe abnormalities in the EEG are the most common findings in children having symptoms of this type, temporal foci are not the only electrographic abnormalities that are seen in such cases. Similar bizarre behavioral symptoms may occur in children who show generalized spike-and-wave patterns or, less commonly, the 14- and 6-per-second positive spike abnormality.

Case 9. This case illustrates a clinical history which could well be accounted for by a temporal-lobe abnormality but which showed bursts of 3-per-second spike-and-wave activity which occurred frequently during repeated recordings. This child was an 11-year-6-month-old white boy who was referred because of prolonged episodes of staring, unresponsiveness, pursing of the mouth, and blowing of his breath through his pursed lips. These episodes had begun when the child was 7½ years old but occurred only infrequently until about six months prior to his evaluation in the clinic. At the time of the increased frequency and duration of these episodes, his school work declined appreciably, but he had not yet failed. He also began to exhibit secretiveness of behavior, was unpredictable, and seemed dull and uninterested in his environment. During these episodes, described by his parents as "trancelike," the patient would sometimes respond to verbal requests, but the response would be poorly carried out and, when motor activity was involved, the child would frequently drop objects, spill liquids, etc. The physical examination and past history, as well as the family history, were all negative. As mentioned above, the electroencephalogram showed frequent, sometimes very prolonged, bursts of 3-per-second spike, polyspike, and slow wave activity. The patient was treated with phenobarbital and Zarontin. This therapy brought about complete cessation of the abnormal episodes with improvement in school work.

Behavior disturbances in older children may be the residual symptom of brain damage which was manifested by "organic drivenness" in earlier life. In these adolescents the electrographic findings are often not as "specific" as those that have been considered thus far.

Case 10. This 12-year-old white boy was referred for evaluation because of a sexual assault upon his seven-year-old sister. He was the product of the second normal pregnancy of a mother who had had four subsequent normal pregnancies. He was a normal baby and was well until he was four years of age, when he had rubeola accompanied by fever, stiff neck, mental confusion, and an episode of stupor lasting 12 hours. Following this illness, the child became unmanageable, easily distracted, and extremely active. He did not sleep well and often laughed or "jabbered" in sleep. He would sometimes sit up suddenly while asleep, as if he were startled, and then would lie down and go back to sleep. He has always done poorly in school, the mother saying that she has to go to the school two to three times a week to talk to the teacher. In addition to this sexual assault on his sister, he had set numerous fires in the house in closets, garbage cans, trash barrels, etc. The mother stated that no matter what reprimands or punishment the child was subjected to, he continued to be stubborn, unmanageable, and overbearing. He preferred to play with younger children, particularly girls.

About a year and one-half before his being seen in the clinic, he had an episode of unconsciousness preceded by extreme anger. He fell to the floor, his eyes fell back, and saliva drooled from his mouth. He was unconscious for two to three minutes and was slightly cyanotic, then aroused spontaneously and seemed normal.

Neurological examination was normal except for poor coordination. The electroencephalogram revealed abnormal fast activity and spindling, which was present both awake and during sleep. Overventilation produced a marked increase in this spindling activity.

INTOXICATION STATES

The extensive use of a group of drugs that are generally referred

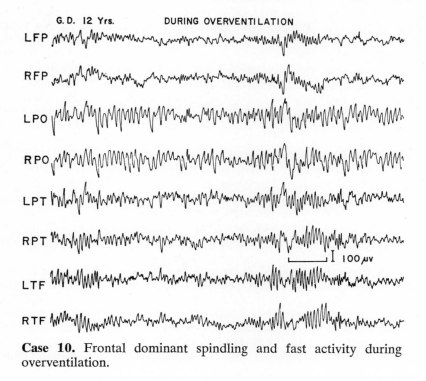

Case 10. Frontal dominant spindling and fast activity during overventilation.

to as ataractics or psychotropic agents has given rise to a problem in differential diagnosis in some of the patients who received them. These drugs are commonly used in the treatment of a wide variety of symptoms and at times it is difficult to determine whether symptoms the patient may develop while on medication are due to a psychological disturbance or an organic brain disease, or are the result of idiosyncratic response or overdose of the drug being used in therapy. Much too frequently, these drugs are prescribed indiscriminately. The dose the patient is given, or takes himself, may be excessive, at least for that particular patient. The pharmacology and mode of action of many of these agents are poorly understood, and toxic symptoms are quite variable and often bizarre.

The electroencephalogram can provide insight into the nature of the problem in an individual patient, and not infrequently will point toward drug intoxication even when it is not suspected (**21**).

Case 11. A case in which the diagnosis of drug intoxication was initially unsuspected is presented here. This child was a 10-year-7-month-old white child who was brought to the clinic by her mother because of episodes of confusion and lethargy alternating with episodes of hyperactivity. The mother gave a history of a normal pregnancy but of a prolonged labor. She stated that there had been difficulty in getting the child to breathe and that the baby was kept in the hospital for two weeks after delivery. Developmental milestones had been delayed and the child had always done poorly in school, although she had passed each year until the year she was seen in the clinic. There was also a history of hyperactivity, and the child had been seen in another clinic because of this when she was six years of age.

Examination revealed a dull, heavy-lidded 10-year-old. She responded to, but seemed uninterested in, her surroundings. Tests of coordination and rapidly alternating movements were poorly performed. The gait was wide-based, but the patient did not stagger. The initial impression was of brain damage from the anoxic episode at birth.

Routine laboratory studies, X rays, and EEG were obtained. All were normal except for the EEG, which revealed a high-voltage mixed slow and fast dysrhythmia.

After these studies had been obtained, the patient's mother was questioned specifically about drug ingestion and she then revealed that she had been giving the child three to four 400 mgm meprobamate tablets daily for 3 months. The mother had been given a prescription for this drug for herself because of nervousness and she felt that it would calm the hyperactivity of the patient.

The drug was withdrawn and the episodic confusion, lethargy, and incoordination disappeared. The patient continued to be somewhat slow mentally.

Children who are not psychotic but who are subject to transient emotional stress may react in a fashion similar to that of an immature adult. If this involves ingestion of sedative-type drugs, a prompt diagnosis may determine the difference between recovery or death.

Case 12. A boy of 11 years 6 months was discovered unconscious in his bed one morning by his mother and brought to the hospital emergency room immediately. Except for profound coma, the physical examination was normal. There was no evidence of trauma. Blood, urine, and cerebrospinal fluid examinations were all normal. The electroencephalogram showed continuous high-voltage 18-to-22-per-second activity in all leads, a finding seen in intoxication with various sedative drugs.

After this test had been carried out, the mother discovered that approximately 15 capsules of methyprylon (Noludar) which she used as a sedative were missing. The presumed cause for this suicide attempt was a disagreement between the parents, overheard by the child, during which they discussed separation and divorce.

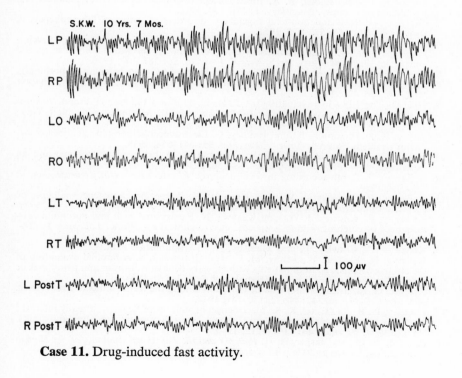

Case 11. Drug-induced fast activity.

SUMMARY

This paper has attempted to outline the usefulness of the electro-encephalogram in the understanding of various complicated symptoms or symptom complexes in which psychiatric evaluation of the patient is likely to be required. The information that the EEG may provide the physician, as well as its limitations, has been described. Further avenues for investigation, combining clinical psychiatry, electroencephalography, and psychological testing, have been suggested.

The value of providing unsuspected information is less important than the avenues of research which are indicated.

BIBLIOGRAPHY

1. Bloomquist, C., and Kellaway, P. The natural history of temporal foci in children. *Electroenceph. clin. Neurophysiol.* **15:** 151, 1963.
2. Brazier, M. A. B. Depth recordings from the amygdaloid region in patients with temporal lobe epilepsy. *Electroenceph. clin. Neurophysiol.* **8:** 532–533, 1956.
3. Crawley, J., and Kellaway, P. The electroencephalogram in pediatrics. *Pediat. Clin. N. Amer.* **10:** No. 1, 17–51, Feb., 1963.
4. Gibbs, E. L., and Gibbs, F. A. Electroencephalographic evidence of thalamic and hypothalamic epilepsy. *Neurology.* **1:** 136–144, 1951.
5. Gibbs, F. A. Ictal and non-ictal psychiatric disorders in temporal lobe epilepsy. *J. nerv. ment. Dis.* **113:** 522–528, 1951.
6. Gottleib, J. S., Ashby, M. C., and Knott, J. R. Primary behavior disorders and psychopathic personality. 1. Correlations of electroencephalogram with family history and antecedent illness or injury. *Arch. Neurol. Psychiat.* **56:** 381–400, 1946.
7. Henry, Charles E. Positive spike discharges in the EEG and behavior abnormality. In: G. H. Glaser (Editor), *EEG and Behavior.* Basic Books, Inc., New York, Chapter XIII, pp. 315–344, 1963.
8. Hill, D. The EEG in psychiatry. In: J. D. N. Hill and G. Parr (Editors), *Electroencephalography: A Symposium on Its Various Aspects.* Macmillan Co., New York, 1963.
9. Jasper, H. H., Solomon, P., and Bradley, C. Electroencephalographic analyses of behavior problem children. *Amer. J. Psychiat.* **95:** 641–658, 1938.
10. Kahn, E., and Cohen, L. H. Organic drivenness: A brain-stem syndrome and an experience. *New. Engl. J. Med.* **210:** 748–756, 1934.
11. Kellaway, P. Depth recording in focal epilepsy. *Electroenceph. clin. Neurophysiol.* **8:** 527–528, 1956.
12. Kellaway, P., Crawley, J. W., and Kagawa, N. A specific electroencephalographic correlate of convulsive equivalent disorders in children. *J. Pediat.* **55:** 582–592, 1959.
13. Kellaway, P., Crawley, J. W., and Kagawa, N. Paroxysmal pain and autonomic disturbances of cerebral origin: A specific electro-clinical syndrome. *Epilepsia.* **1:** 466–483, 1960.
14. Kellaway, P., Crawley, J., and Maulsby, R. L. Unpublished data.
15. Knott, J. R., Platt, E. B., Ashby, M. C., and Gottleib, J. S. A familial evaluation of the electroencephalogram of patients with primary behavior disorder and psychopathic personality. *Electroenceph. clin. Neurophysiol.* **5:** 363–370, 1953.
16. Kreezer, G. Electrical phenomena of the brain among the feeble minded. *Proc. Amer. Ass. Ment. Deficiency.* **42:** No. 2, 130–141, 1937.
17. Lindsley, D. B., and Cutts, K. K. Electroencephalograms of "constitutionally inferior" and behavior problem children: Comparison with those of normal children and adults. *Arch. Neurol. Psychiat.* **44:** 1199–1212, 1940.
18. Penfield, W. G., and Jasper, H. H. *Epilepsy and the Functional Anatomy of the Human Brain.* Little, Brown and Co., Boston, 1954.

19. Penfield, W. G., and Kristiansen, K. *Epileptic Seizure Patterns.* C. C. Thomas, Springfield, 1951.
20. Petersen, M. C., Bickford, R. G., Sem-Jacobsen, C. W., and Dodge, H. W. The depth electrogram in schizophrenic patients. *Proc. Mayo Clin.* **28:** 170–175, 1953.
21. Schneider, J., Perrin, J., and Sifferman, A. EEG changes in psychiatric patients under the continued action of psychotropic drugs. *Electroenceph. clin. Neurophysiol.* **15:** 135, 1963.
22. Scott, J. S., and Masland, R. L. Occurrence of "continuous symptoms" in epilepsy patients. *Neurology.* **3:** 297–301, 1953.
23. Smith, Jean M. B., and Kellaway, P. Occipital foci in children: An analysis of 452 cases. *Electroenceph. clin. Neurophysiol.* **15:** 1047, Dec., 1963. (Abstract)
24. Wylie, W. G., and Schlesinger, B. The periodic group of disorders in childhood. *Brit. J. Child. Dis.* **30:** 1–21, 1933.

A REVIEW OF THE POSITIVE SPIKE PHENOMENON

John R. Hughes, M.A. (Oxon.), Ph.D.

In 1951 Gibbs and Gibbs (16) described an electroencephalographic pattern called 14- and 6-per-second positive spikes, presumably arising from the thalamic-hypothalamic region and found mainly in adolescents and young adults with a history of attacks of pain, rage, and various vegetative disorders. Since that time, this EEG pattern has become extremely controversial and has received extensive criticism. Many factors have contributed to the controversial nature of the positive spike phenomenon. First of all, almost all epileptiform spikes seen on the EEG are known to be negative in polarity, and the positivity of the spikes under discussion suggested to some electroencephalographers that this pattern was actually artifactual. Secondly, the frequencies of 14/sec and 6/sec that were named to describe the pattern were viewed suspiciously by the more neurophysiologically oriented electroencephalographers who looked for the expected harmonic relationship between these two frequencies. In addition, the symptoms associated with this electrographic pattern were varied and featured largely subjective (7, 42) complaints which are commonly considered psychiatric or functional. Finally, relatively few electroencephalographers have carefully examined this pattern and only those few have been in a position to make positive statements regarding the phenomenon. Investigators from the many EEG laboratories that not only fail to use electrodes on the posterior temporal areas but also fail to utilize a monopolar type of recording during light-sleep states will neither see positive spikes nor be likely to recognize them if they do appear.

The plan of this review is to present a summary of the data on positive spikes that are available in the literature and to evaluate these data with special reference to the factors that have contributed to the controversial nature of the positive spike phenomenon.

54

GENERAL DESCRIPTION OF POSITIVE SPIKES

Positive spikes usually appear maximal on the posterior temporal areas during a drowsy or light-sleep state. Figure 1 shows an example of these spikes as they appear in a prominent downward deflection, indicating a positive polarity when the posterior temporal electrode is referred to a relatively inactive area, the ear. The spikes appear in bursts at a frequency of approximately 14–16/sec and also at approximately 6–8/sec.

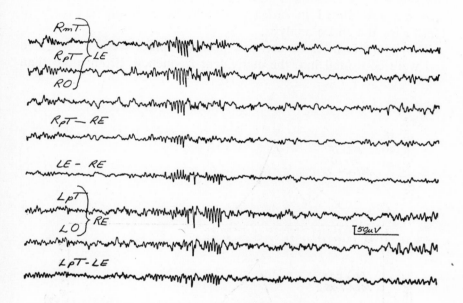

Figure 1. EEG showing the positive spike phenomenon. The first three channels show a recording from the midtemporal, posterior temporal, and occipital areas on the right, referred to the contralateral ear. The fourth channel shows a recording from the right posterior temporal area, referred to the ipsilateral ear. Channel 5 shows the activity recorded between the left and right ears. Channels 6 and 7 show a recording from the posterior temporal and occipital areas on the left, referred to the contralateral ear, and the last channel from the left posterior temporal area, referred to the ipsilateral ear. Note the downward-directed positive spikes, maximal on the posterior temporal areas, first on the right then on the left, and appearing at both the slow (6–8/sec) and fast (14–16/sec) forms.

1. Data from Tape Recorder

In order to investigate some of the details of the electro-
physiological characteristics of positive spikes, our laboratory tape-
recorded many of these spikes simultaneously from both posterior
temporal areas from five different patients with the use of a Ber-
lant 2-channel or a Mnemotron 4-channel FM tape recorder (35).
The recorder was played back into a Tektronix cathode-ray oscil-
loscope and the scope traces were photographed with a Grass
kymographic camera. Calibrated sine waves, from a signal generator,
checked with a General Radio audio frequency meter, were also
recorded and filmed in order to check the resulting accuracy of
1-msec for the entire analysis.

The intervals in msec between positive spikes were investigated
and were converted into the equivalent frequency. From more than

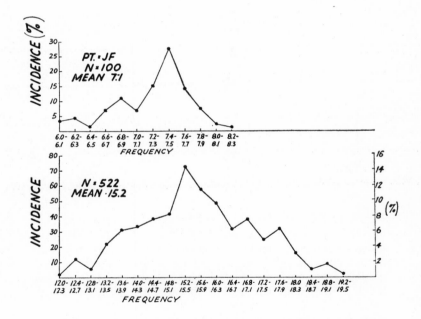

Figure 2. Incidence of various frequencies of the slow and
fast forms of the positive spike phenomenon (pt. J.F.).
Note that the slow form shows a frequency-range of 6.0
to 8.3/sec with the mean of 7.1/sec and the fast form
shows a range of 12.0 to 19.5/sec with the mean of 15.2/
sec.

2,000 intervals measured, two major frequency ranges appear: the slow form, ranging from 6.0 to 8.3/sec, and the fast form, ranging from 12.0 to 19.5/sec. Figure 2 shows the distribution of equivalent frequencies from one given patient. The mean frequency of the slow form was 7.1/sec and the mean frequency of the fast form was 15.2/sec.

Table I records the mean frequencies of both forms from the five different patients. The five means of the slow form vary from

Table I. Means of Slow and Fast Forms of Positive Spikes

Pt.	Slow		Fast	
	Mean	No.	Mean	No.
F. W.	7.3	12	15.8	200
J. F.	7.1	100	15.2	522
J. W.	7.2	6	14.7	28
E. R.	6.9	252	14.9	585
J. M.	6.7	35	14.3	371
Grand mean & total no.	7.0	405	15.3	1706

6.7/sec to 7.3/sec with the grand mean of 7.0/sec; the five means of the fast form vary from 14.3/sec to 15.8/sec with the grand mean of 15.3/sec. From these data it appears that the frequencies of positive spikes may vary considerably, but the slow form tends to appear at approximately 7/sec. This accurate analysis essentially confirms the results of the frequency counts derived from a more gross analysis on EEG paper (**34**). The relatively common frequency of 7/sec supplies evidence that the slow and fast forms are harmonically related. However, the present analysis shows that the fast form appears more frequently at 15/sec than 14/sec. The apparent discrepancy regarding the possible harmonic relationship between two wave forms with mean frequencies of 7/sec and 15/sec is resolved by the examination of the changes that occur within a given burst of positive spikes. When the frequencies of the first 6 spikes in a burst of the fast form were determined, the average frequency was found to be 15.5/sec (pt. E.R.). Since the average frequency for the entire burst was 14.9/sec in this case, the frequency, therefore, decreased at the end of the burst at the time when the fast form tends to convert to the slow form. The slow form appears, on the average, after 69 per cent of the burst has occurred. At that time the burst has slowed down nearer to 14/sec when the subharmonic 7/sec tends to appear. Although the frequency of the fast form tends to change during the burst, there is a tendency for the average frequency to be maintained. For example, if a given interval between two spikes in the early part of a burst shows a frequency less than 14/sec, the next interval will show, on the average, a frequency of 16.4/sec and therefore will maintain the mean frequency near 15/sec.

Although the spikes seen on the two posterior temporal areas are often completely independent (**15**, **16**, **22**, **26**), at times they appear to be transmitted from one side to the other. Figure 3 shows an example of transmission between the two sides. In this figure spikes appear independently on the right side, transmit to the left after a latency of approximately 14 msec, occur independently on the left, and then appear synchronously on the two sides. Also, in this figure, examples are seen of a harmonic of the fast form, 28–34/sec, which also at times shows transmission to the opposite side.

Figure 4 shows the incidence of various times for the transmission of positive spikes from one side to the other. Synchrony is fairly common, as are transmission times of 7, 14, and 21 msec,

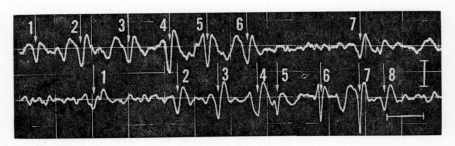

Figure 3. Data from tape recording of positive spikes from both posterior temporal areas. The right posterior temporal area is shown on the upper channel and the left posterior temporal area on the lower channel, each referred to the contralateral ear. Independent spikes of the fast form appear on the right with evidence of transmission to the left. Right-sided spikes #2, 4, 5, and 6 show transmission to the left as spikes #1, 2, 3, and 4, after transmission times of 15, 13, 14, and 14 msec, respectively. After spike #4 on the left, note that independent spikes appear on the left and that a harmonic of the fast form appears between #4 and 5 and also between #7 and 8 (29.4/sec). Synchronous spikes are seen at #7 from both sides. Time calibration is 50 msec and voltage calibration is 50 μV.

especially 14 msec. The absolute values here are only coincidentally the same as the frequencies usually noted in positive spikes, but these values do help to emphasize again that the complex neural system responsible for these spikes operates with harmonic and subharmonic principles, including harmonics of transmission time. Wherever positive spikes actually originate, one may assume that the time for transmission from the locus on one side to the corresponding locus on the opposite side is commonly 14 msec. It may be only coincidental that Williams (**88**) found that the transmission time for the spike in 3/sec spike and wave complexes from thalamus to cortex (and vice versa) was usually 14 msec.

The probable mechanism of transmission has been investigated. Whether a spike appears on the contralateral side appears unrelated to the amplitude of the ipsilateral spike, since the average peak-to-peak amplitude of transmitting spikes was 52.8 μV, while the average amplitude of non-transmitting spikes was a similar value of 54.8 μV. Transmission appears to occur after a number of spikes appear on one side, as seen in Figure 5, suggesting a temporal summation as the mechanism of transmission.

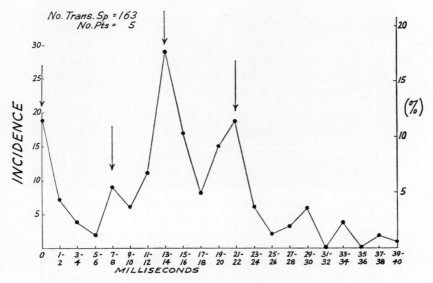

Figure 4. Incidence of transmission times of positive spikes from one side to the other. Note that bilateral spikes tend to be synchronous or tend to show transmission times of 7, 14, or 21 msec.

Other evidence suggests that spikes seen on both sides may be related to each other or perhaps a third locus. Figure 6 illustrates an example of bilateral positive spikes as they gradually move nearer toward synchrony. The last spike from both sides appears at intervals shorter than the average, and these latter spikes approach bilateral synchrony. Only rarely is the opposite tendency noted, when the spikes on the two sides become progressively more asynchronous toward the end of a bilateral burst.

In conclusion, this investigation of the neurophysiological characteristics of the positive spike phenomenon was undertaken in the hopes that these data might aid in the actual localization of the discharges within the brain. The present analyses does not allow

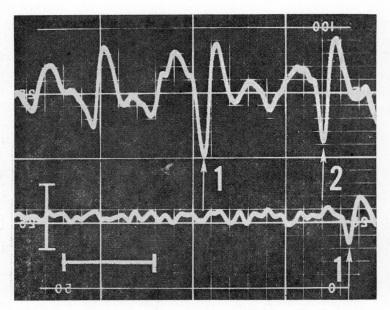

Figure 5. Transmission of positive spikes from one side to the other. Note that a number of spikes appear on the right side (top) and finally show evidence of transmission after 14 msec from #2 (top) to #1 (bottom). Note from the top channel that #2, which shows transmission, is slightly lower in amplitude than #1, which shows no transmission. Amplitude is likely not a significant factor in the transmission of positive spikes from one side to the other. Time calibration is 50 msec and voltage calibration is 50 μV.

for a definite designation of a brain area as the actual locus of positive spikes, but does provide a suggestion that the actual locus of these spikes on one side is an area which commonly shows transmission after 14 msec to the corresponding locus on the opposite side. The discussion regarding the actual frequencies of the positive spikes has no bearing on the important electro-clinical relationships that will be mentioned later, nor do these data invalidate many of the characteristics of these spikes that have been previously described in the literature. The discussion regarding the frequencies seems justified, however, for the sake of accuracy and in order to avoid misleading misconceptions and gain neurophysiological evidence that might aid in the eventual localization of the spikes within the brain. It may also aid in the day-to-day recognition of the wave form in routine clinical EEG. In addition, this analysis

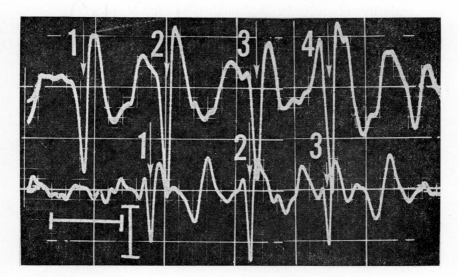

Figure 6. Positive spikes from the two sides tending toward synchrony. The time separation between right-sided spikes (top) #1 and 2, 2 and 3, and between 3 and 4 is 62, 65, and 55 msec, respectively. The time separation between left-sided spikes (bottom) #1 and 2, and between 2 and 3 is 71 and 56 msec, respectively. The transmission time between #2 (top) and #1 (bottom) is 12 msec, between #3 (top) and #2 (bottom) is 4 msec, and between #4 (top) and #3 (bottom) is 2 msec. Note also the evidence for harmonics of the fast form (28–34/sec). Time calibration is 50 msec and voltage calibration is 50 μV.

shows that many of the characteristics of positive spikes fit commonly accepted neurophysiological principles.

2. Data from Routine EEG Recording

Data acquired from routine EEG recording have suggested that the slow and fast forms of the positive spike phenomenon are harmonically related (34). Positive spikes at 6/sec did certainly appear in this study, but spikes at 7/sec were more commonly seen. Another group of investigators (81), using data from routine EEG recordings, failed to confirm this finding, but found, incidentally, that the 7/sec form and never the 6/sec form appeared in cases with sleep disorders. Grossman (31) had previously suspected the harmonic relationship of the two frequencies and had referred to the slow form as the 6–7/sec positive spikes.

Positive spikes appear on both sides at one time or another in the majority of records. Although Refsum *et al.* (73) found only 41.7 per cent of records bilateral, Koizumi *et al.* (49) found 59 per cent, Albernaz (1) 60 per cent, Gibbs and Gibbs (16) 84 per cent, and later (26) 91 per cent, and Millen and White (62) found 90.9 per cent bilateral. It seems possible that the longer time that the record is run, the more likely this figure approaches 100 per cent. Although these bursts usually appear on both sides, a clear predominance exists for the appearance of right-sided positive spikes. Hughes *et al.* (37) found 73 per cent of records with more spikes on the right, 18.3 per cent with more on the left, and 8.7 per cent equal on the two sides. Previously, other data (1, 16, 62) had suggested a right-sided preference, reconfirmed recently by Niedermeyer and Knott (68) and Metcalf (58).

Positive spikes appear mainly in the drowsy and light-sleep states, but according to Shimoda *et al.* (81) may be activated at times by hyperventilation or diphenhydramine. Rarely these spikes may appear during the resting, waking state. Gibbs and Gibbs (16) claimed that 3 per cent of cases with positive spikes show these bursts during the waking record, and later (26) these authors raised this value to 8 per cent after analyzing more cases. Recently, Gibbs (25) claimed that in young children positive spikes are primarily a deep-sleep pattern, but shift to a light-sleep pattern in older children and finally appear commonly in the waking state of adults. Among adults over 40 years of age with positive spikes, 46 per cent showed these bursts during the waking state. Poser and Ziegler

(72) found only 1.4 per cent of cases with positive bursts in waking records, Koizumi *et al.* (49) found 2 per cent, and Albernaz (1) reported a 1.2 per cent incidence. These values are, however, sufficiently low that laboratories specializing only in waking records will likely miss positive spikes completely.

The incidence of the slow form (6–8/sec), the fast form (14–16/sec), and both forms of positive spikes in the same record has received only moderate attention. Although one group of investigators (73) reported that a slight majority of cases (51.4 per cent) showed only the slow form, most authors (1, 16, 62, 68, 75) have found that the majority of cases (55–80 per cent) showed both forms in the same record. As in the case of the incidence of bilateral bursts, it seems likely that the longer that the record is run, the more likely that both forms will appear. Gibbs (25) has reported that the slow form is more common during the first year of life; thereafter, the fast form is more common, except after the age of 40, when the slow form again predominates. Earlier Gibbs and Gibbs (16) had indicated that the slow form appeared more frequently in the deeper states of sleep, while the fast form was more common during the lighter states of sleep.

3. Other Abnormalities in Records with Positive Spikes

Among abnormalities seen in records with positive spikes the most common appears to be slow activity in the posterior regions. Without specifying the locus of the slow activity, Poser and Ziegler (72) found it in 30 per cent, Refsum *et al.* (73) in 36.1 per cent, and Shimoda *et al.* (81) in 36.3 per cent of their positive spike cases. The posterior locus for the slowing, especially the occipital areas, was designated by Kellaway *et al.* (43) in more than 50 per cent of cases and by Hughes *et al.* (37) in 39 per cent of cases. In the latter study a right-sided predominance of posterior slow waves was also noted, especially in cases showing predominantly right-sided positive spikes. Left-sided slowing was seen especially in cases showing positive spikes mainly on the left. The conclusion of Kellaway *et al.* (43) that posterior slowing, commonly noted in cases with positive bursts, is a co-related abnormality seems justified. Consistent with this conclusion is the finding by these authors that the general clinical correlations were essentially unchanged in positive spike cases with or without posterior slow waves. Although unlikely, the latter findings may also indicate that posterior slow waves are of no significance in the positive spike phenomenon. The same authors (43) concluded that another co-related abnormality is the excessive response to hyperventilation, also noted by others (37, 72, 91). Hyperventilation is also said to activate positive spikes in 15.5 per cent of cases showing these bursts, according to Shimoda *et al.* (81). Other related abnormalities may be sharp sleep transients and independent intertemporal sleep spindles, which Little (50) claimed are frequently found in records with positive spikes.

Finally, the incidence of clear epileptiform discharges, other than positive spikes, becomes significant, especially in view of the possible epileptiform nature of the positive spike phenomenon itself. The incidence of clear discharges in cases with positive bursts includes the values of 3 per cent (16), 7 per cent (75), 10 per cent (81), 14 per cent (37), and 27 per cent (62, 72). Poser and Ziegler (72) have concluded that no significant differences can be found clinically between positive spike cases with and without epileptiform activity.

4. General Symptomatology

The general symptomatology in cases with positive spikes has been a subject of common agreement by all investigators who have systematically studied this phenomenon (6, 9, 16, 20, 26, 37, 43, 45, 49, 58, 68, 72, 73, 79, 80, 89). Three types of symptoms are generally found in cases with positive spikes: (1) autonomic dysfunction, (2) behavior disorder and (3) convulsive phenomena.

5. Autonomic Dysfunction

The prominence of autonomic symptomatology in cases with positive spikes provides one of the reasons for the presumption that the locus of these spikes is within the thalamic-hypothalamic region. Autonomic is used as a descriptive, not an explanatory, term. In patients with these spikes the incidence of autonomic symptoms was 53.7 per cent in the report of Kellaway *et al.* (43), 64.7 per cent in Shimoda's study (80), and 66.1 per cent in the report of Hughes *et al.* (37). The values of 19.8 per cent of Poser and Ziegler (72) or 34.8 per cent of Shimoda *et al.* (81) would seem to be too low, but their method of categorizing symptoms allowed patients to be placed in only one of the various symptom-categories. As another indication that autonomic symptoms are associated with the positive spike phenomenon, a significant incidence of these bursts has been reported in cases with various autonomic disorders. Among patients with peptic ulcers 6 per cent showed positive spikes, and among patients with periodic functional disorders of the gastrointestinal tract 20 per cent showed these spikes (47). With patients whose chief complaint was abdominal pain 36 per cent (61) to 42 per cent (78) showed this electrographic entity. In pediatric patients with episodic abdominal pain and headaches, Kellaway et al. (44) found 86 per cent with positive spikes.

One study disclaimed any significant association of these autonomic symptoms with the positive spike phenomenon (86). This study involved four different groups: one showing positive spikes as the only abnormality, one with these spikes and other abnormalities, another with abnormalities other than positive spikes, and a normal group. Each patient was placed in one of two categories, according to whether he gave a history of 0–1 or 2–3 symptoms of headaches, abdominal pain, and vertigo. With a 2×2 table, no statistically significant differences were found. However, the number of patients in each of the four groups was so small that to achieve a p value less than 0.05, at least 77 per cent of the positive spike group and no more than 27 per cent of the normal group would have to fall in the category showing 2–3 of these autonomic symptoms. In addition, these authors stressed the relationship between the occurrence of autonomic symptoms in both the mother and the patient. Since a significant relationship was found between the occurrence of symptoms in the mother and patient in the normal group, but not in the group with positive spikes and other abnormalities, this relationship was said to be most likely due to an environmental "rubbing off" of psychogenic symptoms rather than to a constitutional factor or "epileptic equivalent." However, the data on which the authors based their conclusions referred to the presence of headache alone and not to autonomic symptoms in general, as was implied. The emphasis by Walter and his colleagues on the necessity of controlled groups in studies of this sort constitutes an important contribution in this paper.

Table II shows the incidence of various autonomic symptoms in patients with positive spikes. Some of the variability of the values seen in this table is likely explained by the differences among investigators in the definition of various terms, in the population of their sample, etc. This table shows that the most common autonomic symptom found in patients with these bursts is headache. The next most common symptoms are abdominal pain, vertigo, and syncope. Various investigators (**9, 26, 78**) have pointed out that more than one of these autonomic symptoms may occur at the same time. Sheeby *et al.* (**78**) indicated that headaches and syncopal attacks often accompany abdominal symptoms, while Gibbs and Gibbs (**26**) pointed out that vertigo unrelated to posture is often followed by headaches in patients with positive spikes. Gibbs and Gibbs (**26**) have also pointed out that these same autonomic symptoms at times constitute auras to frank convulsive activity, and that many of the patients with "autonomic epilepsy" actually show positive spikes in their

Table II. Autonomic Symptoms in Patients with Positive Spikes

Head-ache	Abd. pain	Vertigo	Syncope	Vomit.	Nausea	GI	Others	Pts.	Reference
6%	6%	6%	4%					156	Metcalf (**57**)
13.4	2.6							343	Niedermeyer & Knott (**68**)
21.1		8.7	9.2				25.7	814	Shimoda (**80**)
26	16		11	5	11			19	Millen & White (**62**)
31.3	24.3	23.5	17.4	9.6	8.7		22.6	115	Hughes *et al.* (**37**)
38.8		30.6	12.5			22.2	19.4	72	Refsum *et al.* (**73**)
		11.5	30.0	8.2	3.5		19.2*	427	Gibbs & Gibbs (**26**)
45.3		13.0	12.2	2.9	9.3			139	Glenn & Knuth (**28**)
1st†	4th†	2nd†	3rd†					115	Brown (**6**)
								2200	

* Pain.   † In incidence.

EEG. Sheeby *et al.* (**78**) have indicated that disorders of consciousness are frequently seen before and after the autonomic attacks, while Kellaway *et al.* (**44**) have also emphasized that lethargy and sleep, likely postictal phenomena, frequently follow these autonomic attacks. The latter authors inferred that their "paroxysmal pain syndrome" is epileptiform in character. The periodicity and the stereotyped character of the attacks of abdominal pain, at times occurring while the patient was engaged in pleasurable activity, constitute reasonable evidence for this conclusion. The duration of these autonomic attacks usually ranged from 1 to 45 minutes, but 10 per cent of these patients gave histories of attacks lasting for more than two hours.

6. Behavior Disorder

The association of behavior disorders with the positive spike phenomenon has been evident from most studies. Table IIIA summarizes the degree of association, according to whether the behavior disorder is listed as the major complaint or whether it is simply included in the clinical history. The table shows that nearly 20 per cent of patients with positive spikes will show a behavior disorder as the major complaint. Some form of disturbed behavior, however, is included in the history in over 60 per cent of cases showing these

Table IIIA. Incidence of Behavior Disorder in Cases with Positive Spikes

	%	Cases with positive spikes	Reference
	12	156	Metcalf (57)
	15	427	Gibbs & Gibbs (26)
	15.3	72	Refsum *et al.* (73)
1. Behavior disorder	17	136	Poser & Ziegler (72)
as major complaint	18.7	343	Niedermeyer & Knott (68)
	22	98	Koizumi *et al.* (49)
	25.2	814	Shimoda (80)
	26	19	Millen & White (62)
Total	19.8	2065	
2. Behavior disorder	61.7	115	Hughes *et al.* (37)
included in history	63	19	Millen & White (62)
Total	61.9	134	

bursts. Table IIIB also shows that among a population of behavior disorders the incidence of positive spikes is approximately 30 per cent, confirmed in our own laboratories. Of course, the values in this table are very much dependent on the population sample, definition of terminology, etc. It would seem that a simple operational definition of behavior disorder would be adequate, i.e., behavior that is sufficiently disturbed to be listed among the chief complaints of a patient brought to the hospital or to a physician's office. Since the range of values seen in Table IIIB does not appear to be

Table IIIB. Incidence of Positive Spikes in Cases with Behavior Disorder

%	Cases with behavior disorder	Reference
23	48	Garneski (13, 14)
29	100	Low and Dawson (52)
31.2	298 (psychiat. ref.)	Niedermeyer & Knott (69)
31.4	146	Poser & Ziegler (72)
30.2	592	

extreme, the problem of variability in the population sample and in the definition of terms would not seem to be very significant.

One team of investigators (86) concluded that they were unable to find any outstanding area of significant difference between the children with positive spikes and other groups studied (see autonomic dysfunction above). In the attempt to determine whether there was something unique about the personality of the child with positive spikes, 263 items were checked from the histories of both the patient and the parents. All of these items were then grouped into five different categories representing a type of item cluster or symptom pattern, although, in a number of instances, a given item was found in more than one category. The five categories were aggressive behavior, organic symptomatology, emotional symptomatology, disturbed mother syndrome, and disturbed family syndrome. For each patient the applicable items in each category were simply enumerated and a mean value was determined for each category for the four different groups of patients. Statistical studies revealed that in the category of emotional symptomatology the group with positive spikes as the only abnormality showed a significantly lower mean score than the normal group or the abnormal group. In addition, in the category of aggressive behavior the mean score of the group with positive bursts and other abnormalities was significantly higher than for the normal group or for the abnormal group. These results are entirely consistent with the conclusions of other investigators who have pointed out that patients with positive spikes frequently show a blunted affect and also aggressive behavior. However, Walter *et al.* (86) reported, somewhat paradoxically, that they were unable to find any outstanding area of significant difference between the children with these spikes and the other groups studied. In another report from the same laboratory, Koegler *et al.* (48) claimed that they found no difference in the aggressive and impulsive behavior shown by children with positive spikes compared to the control groups. Again, the reviewer is unable to reconcile this statement with the results published from the same laboratory in the paper by Walter *et al.* (86). However, Koegler and his colleagues discussed the great difficulty in the evaluation and measurement of behavior and emphasized the need for improvement of methods for quantification of behavior and psychopathology. These latter points constitute an important contribution by these authors.

Various characteristics have been emphasized in the behavior disorders seen in patients with positive spikes.

a. **Conditions before the act.** Although some patients with behavior disorders who show positive spikes have unremarkable psychological pasts, many of the patients with severe behavior disorders have suffered significant psychiatric trauma. Schwade and Geiger (**75**) have emphasized that the emotionally traumatized past or present, sparked by some related or seemingly unrelated act, sets up conditions for the impulsive action often seen in these patients. Winfield (**89**) has also pointed out that insignificant stimuli, at times, seem to precede these acts of aggression. Schwade and Geiger (**75, 76**) further analyzed that these patients show a deep threat to the safety of their egos and a threat to their environmental status, usually associated with an early disturbance of parent-child relationship. Metcalf (**57**) has expressed a similar idea by the suggestion that these patients with positive spikes who show behavior disorders frequently demonstrate a combination of continual anger directed toward the people who have deprived them and a counterattack against a world that they think threatens to destroy them. From a number of other reports the two terms that seem to characterize so many of these patients are impulsivity and compulsivity. Schwade and Geiger (**74**) have emphasized that an extreme kind of compulsion is shown by these patients likely on the basis of some undeniable need. Woods (**93**) has pointed out that these patients show an obsessive preoccupation with impulses and frequently show a feeling of an overwhelming and uncontrollable urge whose tension cannot be relieved until the act associated with the urge is completed. The latter author presented a case of a patient who, for a few years, had overpowering impulses to destroy and kill and finally did murder his cousin. The author suggested that in this type of case there was an impoverished ego with a translation into action of impulses previously held in check by some defensive system.

b. **The act itself.** In the descriptions of the behavior itself there is an impressive consistency among the various investigators who have studied this aspect of the positive spike phenomenon. Short descriptions of the various types of behavior include hyperactivity, nightmares, temper tantrums (**92**), nocturnal agitation (**9**), destructive behavior (**89**), rage and destructive anti-social actions

(57), and assaultiveness, which is skilfully directed and executed (16). The description of Woods (93) featured episodes of bizarre, impulsive, destructive, and aggressive behavior which was out of proportion to the precipitating factor; and, once started, the patient showed an inability to stop or deflect the direction of this impulse. Stehle (82) has studied patients who have committed murders of family members, caused serious physical injury, been responsible for extreme property damage by setting fires and other means, and who have made serious homicidal or suicidal attempts as an expression of impulsive, uncontrolled, but apparently well-directed behavior. Henry (32) had previously emphasized that positive spikes correlate well with a history of behavior disorder, especially with those aspects of behavior having to do with self-control, response to authority, and emotional stability. Niedermeyer and Knott (69) have stated that the presence of impulsivity appears to be the best correlate of the positive spike phenomenon.

Longer and more complete descriptions of the behavior of patients showing positive spikes with a history of impulsive acts have been given by Schwade and Geiger (74). These authors have emphasized the outbursts of impulsive and unrestrained, violent behavior which may vary from sudden outbursts of rage with destruction of objects in the environment to the extreme of mutilation, attempted murder, or murder. Clinically, the onset of the disturbed behavior appears to be abrupt and lasts only a brief time with rapid dissipation of the act. In 1956 Schwade and Geiger (75) presented additional information regarding the type of behavior seen in these patients. Again, these authors emphasized that the behavior was characterized by impulsivity, inability to establish controls, violent action of varying degrees, and inability to change the direction of the act until it was completed. Among the many different forms in which this behavior may manifest itself, the following acts were commonly seen: uncontrollable cruelty to children and animals without remorse for the act, near panic reactions with extreme destructiveness, impulsive running away from home or school, larceny, fire-setting, attempted suicide or aggressive behavior without adequate motivation, and sexual misbehavior with excitement rising to explosiveness or violence, including murder. In touching upon a most delicate legal point Schwade and Geiger suggest that these behavior disorders, when severe, are comparable to a grand mal seizure, in that the patient has no more control over his behavior than an epileptic has over a grand mal attack. Later (**76**) these authors asked the difficult questions, "If there is no recall can a patient be responsible for the act?" and "Can an individual 'acting out' an organic disorder be held legally responsible?" However, they (**75**) had previously emphasized that the attacks seen in patients with positive spikes are not to be confused with psychomotor seizures in which attacks are usually autistic, confused, and without coordination. Cases with positive spikes show impulsive acting out in which attacks are performed with a considerable degree of skill and precision. This interesting contrast with psychomotor seizures had been previously emphasized by Gibbs and Gibbs (**26**).

The probability that any given electrographic abnormality would commonly appear among patients who have committed murder is, of course, extremely remote. Yet, from many different papers in the literature, there is an impressive compilation of data on patients who have committed murder who also show the positive spike phenomenon. Gibbs and Gibbs (**26**) pointed out that in their series four murderers had an epileptiform type of record and all of these showed positive spikes. In addition, in their series of 1,612 epileptics only four had abnormal sexual behavior and all of these patients had positive spikes. Schwade and Otto (**77**) presented a case of a boy who killed a playmate, later likely drowned his younger brother, and still later probably drowned a young girl, and finally brutally cut another boy with glass. Walker (**84**) presented a case of a boy who drowned a small child who was a complete stranger to him. Other cases of murderers who showed positive spikes include a 13-year-old boy who shot his mother (**92**), a 15-year-old boy who murdered his sister (**93**), a teenage murderer (**65**), and two murderers of family members (**82**), in addition to four other murderers (**75, 76**). The conclusion that all cases with positive spikes have strong tendencies toward murder or that all murderers are likely to have positive spikes is, of course, absurd. However, this list of patients who have exhibited the most violent of disturbed human behavior emphasizes the point that close attention must be paid to some of these patients and that, in some instances, the symptomatology associated with the positive spike phenomenon cannot be considered relatively benign.

c. Conditions after the act. Descriptions of the events that follow the impulsive act are varied, but considerable agreement can be found in the reports from various investigators. Schwade and Geiger (75) pointed out that, although some patients remembered and were aware of their acts, other patients had no memory of the events. They further emphasized that most of the patients were without any demonstrable feeling tone. The same lack of guilt or anxiety in patients with positive spikes and a history of behavior disorder has been noted by Winfield and Ozturk (92), who stated later that these patients were often unable to give reasonable motivation for their act (89). Woods (93) pointed out that the patients with positive spikes may have some difficulty in remembering their behavior, but usually show no real amnesia and, if pressed, frequently remember the details. This latter investigator also emphasized the striking flattening of affect shown by the patient while he is discussing his own behavior. The absence of remorse or regret was characteristic of these patients, who often differentiated right from wrong except in the area of their own aggressive behavior, which was often shallowly rationalized. Stehle (82) has labeled this type of response commonly seen in cases with positive spikes "thalamic affect," referring to a marked degree of coldness, blunting, psychic indifference or lack of feeling tone, in addition to the lack of appropriate concern, remorse, guilt, or self-criticism. One patient described by Schwade and Otto (77) admitted to no lapse or gap in his memory and showed concern about his murdered victim only because the crime had hurt his reputation. In the case presented by Walker (84) the patient told his story after the murder without any sign of remorse or emotion.

Since patients with positive spikes and behavior disorders frequently have histories of psychological trauma, it is important to determine whether or not their disordered behavior can be completely explained on the basis of the psychological trauma alone. Schwade and Geiger (75) felt that the impulsivity, the immediate lack of traceable motivation, and no more than a transient response to individual therapy (9) with simultaneous therapy of the parents exclude this type of behavior from the field of pure psychodynamics. Their conclusion that the data indicate organic pathology as contributive, if not causative, is worthy of consideration. Most of the data, however, seems to indicate that both organic and psychiatric factors play significant roles in patients with positive spikes who show extreme behavior disorders. Although many investigators have seen cases of behavior disorder with positive spikes without any history of significant psychiatric trauma (**80**), the majority of these patients with behavior disorders have clear psychiatric histories. Other investigators (**33, 68, 93**) have pointed out that usually both psychological and organic factors appear to be necessary for the emergence of this extreme disordered behavior. Woods (**93**) added that it is not, therefore, surprising to find "normal" behavior in some cases with positive spikes. He feels, probably correctly, that the abnormality associated with positive spikes usually does not, by itself, induce violence, but rather serves as a crucial, biologically determined stress in an already impoverished ego, allowing for the breaking through of impulses previously held in check by some defensive system. In the discussion of patients with behavior disorders who show positive spikes, the "law of parsimony" must be used with great caution. Since these cases of severe behavior disorder usually appear to represent an example of the complicated interplay between organic and psychiatric factors, psychologically oriented investigators will likely have great difficulty in explaining this disordered behavior solely on psychiatric grounds, while neurologically oriented investigators will usually have similar difficulty explaining the behavior solely on organic grounds.

The previous discussion has emphasized that patients with positive spikes tend to exhibit symptoms of behavior disorder and/or various forms of autonomic dysfunction. An experiment conducted in our laboratories with Drs. I. Jacobs, L. Baumel, D. Carboy, and L. Sobocinski was designed to investigate the type of autonomic changes seen during experimentally induced anxiety in patients with behavior disorders and positive spike phenomenon (Hughes *et al.*, **39**). It was hoped that this experiment would provide evidence regarding the essential character of the complaints frequently noted in patients with positive spikes.

Three groups of patients were included in the study: (1) 25 behavior disorders with positive spikes in their EEGs, (2) 25 behavior disorders without positive EEG spikes (henceforth referred to as the non-positive spike group), and (3) 25 normals without neurological or psychiatric complaints.

The conditions during the experiment could be divided into three categories: (1) basal state, (2) experimentally induced anxiety state, and (3) recovery state. After earphones and various electrodes were attached to the patient the basal state began; it consisted of a five-minute period when the patient was told to sit quietly and relax. The anxiety state lasted approximately five minutes and could be divided into five subdivisions: (1) an instructional period when the patients were told that they were going to be given material for reading aloud, that they would be asked questions regarding the content, and that they should do their very best in this task; (2) a period of normal reading of grammar-school material about spiders and their webs; (3) a period of delayed feedback when the patients heard what they read 1/4 second after they read it; (4) a period of questions by the experimenters regarding the content of the material that was read and regarding the reasons for an alleged poor performance by the patients; and (5) reading of nonsense material without delayed feedback. The delayed feedback in period three was accomplished with an Ampex tape recorder, which recorded the reading, delayed it by 1/4 second, and then played it back into the earphones worn by the patients. The recovery state began with an explanation to the patients that the test was designed to make them anxious and that they had, in fact, performed excellently on this difficult task, that the test was finished, and also that they should relax for five minutes.

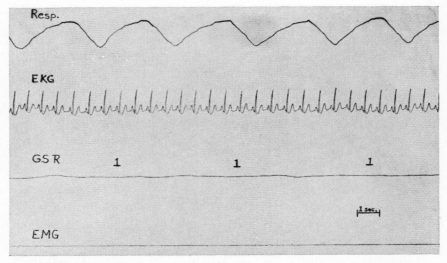

Figure 7. Example of the record taken on patients subjected to experimentally induced anxiety. The first channel records respiration, the second EKG, the third GSR with values noted from readings taken directly from the Psychogalvanoscope. The last channel records the EMG from the forehead.

Four different measures were recorded on a 4-channel Medcraft modified EEG machine. The EKG and respiration rate were recorded in a conventional manner. The EMG from the forehead was of little value and now should be disregarded. The galvanic skin response, GSR, was recorded directly on a DC channel of the modified EEG machine, but for greater accuracy, values from the constant current psychogalvanoscope of Stoelting Co. were read and noted on the EEG paper at least every five seconds, or whenever a noticeable change occurred. Figure 7 is an example of the type of record that was obtained.

Figure 8 illustrates the changes in respiration rate. On the left of the figure, the means of the absolute values are noted for the basal, anxiety, and recovery periods with respiration rate per minute represented on the vertical axis. For each of the three groups (the positive spike group, the non-positive spike group, and the normal group) the respiration rate increased during the anxiety period, represented here as a mean for the entire period, and returned near the basal level during the recovery period. On the right another way of representing the data is noted, in the form of the means of

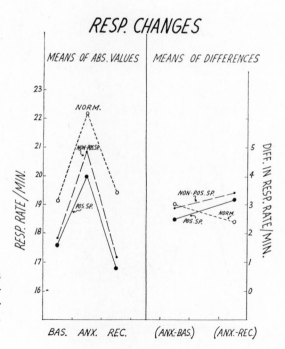

Figure 8. Respiration changes recorded from patients subjected to experimentally induced anxiety. See text for details.

the differences between the values during anxiety and the other two conditions, with the use of the highest value during anxiety. On the horizontal axis are represented the difference between anxiety and basal values, and also the difference between anxiety and re- the figure, the means of the absolute values are noted for the basal, covery values. The nearly horizontal lines here indicate that the values during recovery closely approached the basal level.

Figure 9 shows the changes in the EKG rate. On the left of anxiety, and recovery periods with EKG rate per minute repre- sented on the vertical axis. For all three groups of patients the EKG rate increased during the anxiety period, with the use again of the mean for the entire period, and returned to near-basal levels during recovery. On the right the differences between the anxiety and basal and also between anxiety and recovery states are noted with the use of the highest value during anxiety. The nearly horizon- tal lines indicate that values during recovery closely approached the basal values for all three groups of patients.

Figure 10 graphically illustrates the values for the GSR. On the left of the figure, the means of the absolute values are noted for the basal, anxiety, and recovery periods for the three different groups

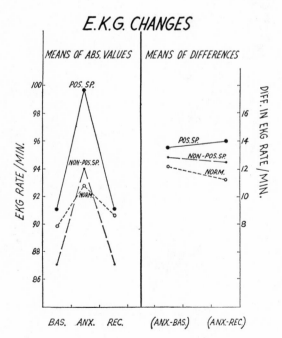

Figure 9. EKG changes re-corded from patients sub-jected to experimentally in-duced anxiety. See text for details.

of patients. The vertical axis shows the mean relative GSR values. During the basal period the values for the positive spike group were significantly higher than for the two other groups ($p = .043$ and $.007$ from the Mann-Whitney U Test). During the anxiety period with the use of the mean for the entire period, the value for the positive spike group was significantly higher than for the non-positive spike group ($p = .047$) and during recovery the value for the positive spike group was significantly higher than for the two other groups ($p = .017$ and $.004$).

Figure 10 has shown that the positive spike group had higher values during the anxiety period, but also that higher values appeared during the basal period. We were concerned whether or not the positive spike group would show any differences from the two other groups during anxiety, except of course, the differences in the absolute values noted during the basal period. In other words, did the high value for the positive spike group during anxiety reflect only the high value during the basal period or were there

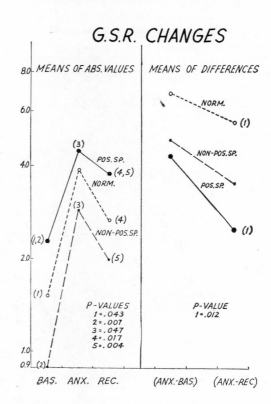

Figure 10. GSR changes recorded from patients subjected to experimentally induced anxiety. See text for details.

real differences between the groups in response to the anxiety? For this question we used a non-parametric statistic, the inversion-non-inversion test, which disregarded the *absolute* values of the basal period and concerned itself as to whether values steadily and progressively increased above the basal level during each of the five subdivisions of the anxiety period. Note that the values for the positive spike group showed a statistically significant difference above chance level at a p value less than the .01 level, indicating that GSR values during the five subdivisions of the anxiety period were not just random fluctuations. The non-positive spike group showed a p value at less than the .05 level and the normal group more than the .05 level. This test indicates that regardless of the absolute basal values the positive spike group tended to show steadily increasing GSR values to a greater degree than the two other groups during the anxiety period, this difference being statistically significant at a p value less than .01.

Table IV. Inversion-Non-Inversion Test for Anxiety

Groups of pts.	Invers.	Non-invers.	p
Pos. Sp.	140	235	< 0.01
Non-Pos. Sp.	156	219	< 0.05
Norm.	162	212	> 0.05

Possibly the most significant point on the left part of Figure 10 is the differences in the slope of the lines from the anxiety values to the recovery values. The slope of these lines indicates the relatively slow return of the positive spike group toward the basal level. On the right of Figure 10 this point is demonstrated by the means of the differences between the highest anxiety value noted and the basal and recovery values. On the horizontal axis are represented the difference between anxiety and basal values and also the difference between anxiety and recovery values. For the positive spike group, contrasted with the other two groups, there is a much larger difference between anxiety and basal values than between anxiety and recovery values. This large difference is another indication of the slow return toward basal levels during the recovery period. A statistically significant difference ($p = .012$) is seen between the positive spike and normal control groups for the differences between anxiety and recovery values. Table V demonstrates this important point in another way. This table shows for the three different groups the average percentage of recovery of the GSR values after the anxiety period, calculated for each patient and then averaged. During the recovery period the positive spike group returned only 59 per cent of the way back toward the basal level, the non-positive spike group back to 78 per cent, and the normal group returned 96 per cent, almost the entire way back to the basal level. Although a statistically significant difference was not achieved between the values of the positive spike and non-positive spike groups, the difference between the values of the positive spike and normal groups is statistically significant with a p value of .002.

Table V. Recovery of GSR to Basal State after Anxiety State

Means of $\dfrac{(\text{Anx-Rec.})}{(\text{Anx-Bas.})} \times 100$

Groups of pts.	%	p
(1) Pos. Sp.	59.9	
(2) Non-Pos. Sp.	78.2	$(1, 2) = 0.16$
(3) Norm.	96.2	$(1, 3) = 0.002$

In summary, we believe that the most interesting feature in this experiment is the relatively slow recovery toward basal values after anxiety for the patients with positive spikes. These patients prominently react to anxiety-producing stimuli but do not easily recover from their exaggerated response. This perseveration of the response, or failure to recover from the effects of anxiety, may possibly represent the nature of the behavior disorder seen in the positive spike phenomenon. This possibility is presently under further investigation.

7. Convulsive Phenomena

Most investigators dealing with positive spikes have emphasized that patients showing this electrographic entity not infrequently show convulsive attacks. In this case the reference is to the type of attack that is universally considered epileptic in character. Table VI shows the results from many different laboratories regarding the number of patients with positive spikes who have shown frank convulsions. With a sample of over 1,900 patients with positive spikes the average incidence of these patients with convulsions is over 41 per cent, although the result from the study of Gibbs and Gibbs (26) tends to weight this percentage toward the higher values. However, Gibbs (23) later published graphs which show this value to be lower. The most common type of attack would seem to be the grand mal seizure, but psychomotor attacks, petit mal, and Jacksonian seizures are also seen at times. Regardless of the actual incidence of patients with positive spikes who show frank convulsive phenomena, seizures are sufficiently common in these patients to suggest that the positive spike phenomenon at least may be related to an epileptiform disorder. In their original, classical paper Gibbs and Gibbs (16)

Table VI. Positive Spike Patients with Convulsive Phenomena

% with convuls.	Grand mal	Psycho-motor	Petit mal	Jack-sonian	Focal	Other	No. with pos. sp.	Reference
20.7							29	Walter et al. (86)
25.7							156	Metcalf (57)
26.3							19	Millen & White (62)
	10.1		4.3				139	Glenn & Knuth (28)
26.5	17.3		5.0		4.0		98	Koizumi et al. (49)
27.0	11.3	1.7	7.0	5.2		3.5 (febrile)	115	Hughes et al. (37)
30.7	11.6					19.1 (attacks of uncon.)	241	Kellaway et al. (43)
32.9	23.0		6.9		3.0		135	Shimoda et al. (81)
37.9	15.2	4.1	0.9		3.5	14.2	343	Niedermeyer & Knott (68)
41.7	27.8	15.3				9.7 (unreal feelings)	72	Refsum et al. (73)
42.6							136	Poser & Ziegler (72)
67	55.5	4.0	1.4	2.3	3.0	0.9	427	Gibbs & Gibbs (26)
41.5 (weighted mean)							1910	

stated that it was no more surprising that convulsions appear as an accompaniment of thalamic and hypothalamic disorders than that convulsions appear as an accompaniment of sensory Jacksonian seizures. Although some investigators, especially Niedermeyer and Knott (68), have claimed that patients with positive spikes who also have convulsions usually have a second EEG abnormality, Poser and Ziegler (72) have shown that 40 per cent of patients with positive spikes alone showed convulsions, while similarly 44.7 per cent of cases with these bursts and other abnormalities had convulsions.

An important related question is whether or not the symptoms of behavior disorder and autonomic dysfunction, commonly seen in patients with positive spikes, are epileptiform in character. This difficult question has been cautiously avoided by many investigators, but must be dealt with on both practical and theoretical grounds. Gibbs and Gibbs (16) claimed that 87 per cent of their patients with positive spikes had an ictal type of symptom, and they preferred to call these symptoms "epileptoid." Continuing with the discussion of the same general point, these authors argued that since the manifestation of the disorder takes the form of spike activity, the disorder should be considered epileptic in type. They also pointed out, however, as Niedermeyer and Knott (**68**) later emphasized, that positive spikes are not strictly a seizure discharge because they rarely are associated with an immediate clinical seizure. Gibbs and Gibbs (**16**) do mention one case in which these spikes occurred in the waking state each time a patient gagged or coughed. Finally, these investigators claimed that positive spikes correlate with an epileptic type of clinical disorder and concluded that these spikes could be properly considered as evidence of a deep-lying epileptic focus. Later, Gibbs *et al.* (**18**) reported that positive spikes were found twice as often in cases with mental retardation without convulsive phenomena as in cases with mental retardation and convulsive phenomena. Although the authors admitted that these data suggested that the positive spike pattern was non-epileptic, they stated that they believed this abnormality could be classified as epileptic or, at least, epileptiform.

Kellaway *et al.* (**43**) have made important contributions to the discussion on the possible epileptiform character of the positive spike phenomenon. In agreement with Gibbs and Gibbs (**16**), they pointed out that positive spikes are only a sign of a disorder, unlike the 3/sec spike and wave of petit mal epilepsy, which is a seizure discharge in and of itself since it actually accompanies a clear clinical seizure. In the opinion of the reviewer, however, since most positive spikes occur only during the light-sleep state and rarely during the waking state, no proper evaluation can be given to the possible subjective changes that might accompany positive spikes. Even if these spikes prove to be unassociated temporarily with any clinical changes, this conclusion would not militate against their possible epileptiform nature. Of course, the interictal, single, isolated temporal-lobe discharge is also only a sign of a disorder and does not

usually accompany a clinical temporal-lobe seizure. Kellaway *et al.*
(43) also pointed out that patients with positive spikes in their
sleep records show hypersynchronous slow activity during their clinical attacks. These same hypersynchronous slow waves are frequently
seen, of course, during the clinical attacks of temporal-lobe epileptics. The authors conclude that the underlying lesion, of which the
electrical abnormality is a manifestation, apparently is generally epi-
leptogenic in that it is usually associated with clinical and electrical
abnormalities of paroxysmal character. During the next year Kellaway *et al.* (44) summarized their excellent arguments regarding
the nature of positive spikes. They argued that some of the characteristics of the paroxysmal pain syndrome with autonomic symptomatology are very suggestive of an epileptiform disturbance—in this
case, a spontaneous, paroxysmal, neuronal discharge involving cerebral elements of specific sensory or autonomic function. The authors
pointed out that the attacks of headaches, abdominal pain, and
various other types of autonomic disturbances appear sudden in
onset and are brief in duration, affecting an otherwise normal child.
The interictal period was again said to be associated with an EEG
pattern which is epileptiform in type and which changes during the
attack to an EEG pattern that is classically epileptiform with paroxysmal slow bursts of activity. In addition, the authors pointed out that
these autonomic disturbances are occasionally accompanied by alteration in consciousness or even by loss of consciousness. Following
the report of Kellaway (40), Druckman (11) studied patients with
attacks called convulsive equivalents, with or without loss of consciousness, or associated with convulsions or psychomotor attacks.
Positive spikes proved to be the most significant EEG finding in
these cases which also showed paroxysmal slow waves and excessive hyperventilation responses.

Hughes *et al.* (37) have briefly dealt with this question regarding the possible epileptiform character of the positive spike
phenomenon. They pointed out that from the electrographic point
of view the positive spikes are as sharp and paroxysmal as sharp
waves associated with the more classical forms of epilepsy. Their
conclusion was that the determination of whether these patients with
positive spikes should be considered epileptic or not awaits a careful definition of clinical epilepsy. The reviewer agrees with Gibbs
(25), who stated that what we now call the borderland of epilepsy
will ultimately be recognized as "true" epilepsy and a considerable

area which lies beyond the present boundaries of the borderland
will be later considered part of the main territory.

POSITIVE SPIKES IN VARIOUS
NON-EPILEPTIFORM DISORDERS

Positive spikes have been occasionally found in patients with
various non-epileptiform disorders. Winfield *et al.* (**91**) claimed

Table VII. Patients with Positive Spikes with Various Non-epileptic
Disorders

% with pos. sp.	Disease	Reference
75	12 pseudohypertrophic musc. dys.	Winfield *et al.* (**91**)
26	242 cerebral palsy without convul.	Gibbs *et al.* (**19**)
16	50 asthmatic children	Blatman & Metcalf (**4**)
6	50 peptic ulcer	Kirschbaum & Stehle (**47**)
Single cases	Cardiovascular	
	cardiac sinus arrhythmia	Metcalf (**57**)
	pulseless disease	Poser & Ziegler (**72**)
	cardiac anomalies	Poser & Ziegler (**72**)
	Endocrinological	
	diabetes insipidus	Refsum *et al.* (**73**)
	diabetes mellitus	Poser & Ziegler (**72**)
	hyperthyroidism	Poser & Ziegler (**72**)
	hyperthyroidism	Condon *et al.* (**10**)
	hyperthyroidism (2)	Shimoda *et al.* (**81**)
	Systemic & diffuse CNS disease	
	Friedreich's ataxia	Millen & White (**62**)
	multiple sclerosis	Stephenson (**83**)
	Huntington's chorea	Poser & Ziegler (**72**)
	progressive cerebellar degen.	Stephenson (**83**)
	phenylketonuria	Low *et al.* (**53**)
	phenylketonuria	Poser & Ziegler (**72**)
	Hodgkin's dis.	Glenn & Knuth (**28**)
	chorea	Glenn & Knuth (**28**)
	phenylpyruvic oligophrenia	Fois *et al.* (**12**)
	chronic polyneuritis	Stephenson (**83**)
	polyneuropathy	Poser & Ziegler (**72**)
	Miscellaneous	
	breath-holder	Low *et al.* (**54**)
	congenital deafness	Millen & White (**62**)
	retinal degeneration	Poser & Ziegler (**72**)
	hepatic coma	Poser & Ziegler (**72**)

that 9 of 12 children with pseudohypertrophic muscular dystrophy
showed these spikes, in addition to 3 of 7 mothers of those same
children. Although some of the illustrations published in this paper
were not entirely convincing, it is interesting to consider Winfield's

suggestion that hypothalamic-endocrine dysfunction may be related to both positive spikes and muscular dystrophy. Table VII lists other studies that have dealt with positive bursts in various diseases. Gibbs *et al.* (**19**) showed that 26 per cent of cases with cerebral palsy without clear clinical convulsions had positive spikes. The authors pointed out that many of these patients had ictal type of complaints, but no clear-cut epilepsy. In a very interesting study Blatman and Metcalf (**4**) showed that 16 per cent of 50 asthmatic children showed positive spikes in their EEG. They pointed out that the asthmatics with this EEG abnormality showed a unique behavioral and clinical picture contrasted to the patients who did not show this pattern. The onset of the asthmatic attacks of patients with positive spikes was often strikingly related to their own emotional needs. These patients were also aggressive, destructive, disobedient, uncooperative and showed little remorse for this behavior and, therefore, were considered severe management problems. It is interesting that these patients were improved with phenobarbital and Dilantin, showing an appreciable improvement in their behavior as well as a decrease in the frequency and severity of their wheezing. Shimoda (**80**) has also pointed out that positive spikes are occasionally seen in cases of asthma, in addition to various dermatological disorders. Table VII also lists 24 patients with these spikes and various cardiovascular, endocrinological, systemic, and diffuse central nervous system diseases. In most of these cases the central nervous system was likely diffusely involved.

INCIDENCE OF POSITIVE SPIKES

Table VIII records the incidence of the positive spike phenomenon in various types of population samples. The variability, even within each type of population sample, likely represents to a great extent the lack of common or standard conditions between different laboratories. Some reports, for example, did not make clear whether only sleep records or all records were considered. Other reports failed to mention the age range of the population sample. In Table VIII it may be observed that the closer the population sample approaches the type of patient that most commonly shows positive spikes, the higher the incidence appears. Since positive spikes appear mainly in adolescents, the population sample of adult referrals alone showed a very low incidence. A slightly higher percentage was found with a sample of all referrals that included the pediatric population, but the values differed according to whether all records or only sleep records were considered. With only pediatric referrals

Table VIII. Incidence of Positive Spike Phenomenon

Population sample	No. of pts.	% with pos. sp.	Reference
1. Adult referrals	14,000	0.54	Kellaway et al. (**43**)
	2,500	1.3	Stephenson (**83**)
2. All referrals	10,000	1.4	Shimoda et al. (**81**)
	1,600	2	Garneski & Green (**15**)
	2,346	3	Refsum et al. (**73**)
		3	Brown (**6**)
	6,677	5.1	Niedermeyer & Knott (**68**)
	2,209	6.4	Poser & Ziegler (**72**)
(all records)	2,198	11.4	Hughes (**36**)
(sleep records)	1,500	12.0	Albernaz (**1**)
(sleep records)	38,084	13.6	Gibbs (**25**)
(sleep records)	1,000	13.9	Glenn & Knuth (**28**)
(sleep records)	1,398	17.9	Hughes (**36**)
3. Pediatric referrals	547	4	Millen (**60**)
		10.2	Kellaway et al. (**44**)
(aged 10-20 yrs.)		10-12	Brown (**6**)
(non-psychi.)	1,300	12	Metcalf (**57**)
(neurol.)		15.8	Low & Dawson (**53**)
	1,476	19.8	Niedermeyer & Knott (**69**)
4. Pts. with abnormal EEGs	720	4.4	Garneski & Green (**15**)
	1,357	10.5	Poser & Ziegler (**72**)
(all records)	1,385	18.5	Hughes (**36**)
(sleep records)	880	28.4	Hughes (**36**)
5. Pts. with abn. EEGs under 20 yrs.	614	18.0	Poser & Ziegler (**72**)
6. Pts. with abn. EEGs aged 11-20 yrs.	259	25.2	Poser & Ziegler (**72**)
7. Psychiatric referrals (adult)	168	20	Nicholson & Knott (**67**)
(pediatric)	135	20	Metcalf (**57**)
(pediatric)	100	29	Low & Dawson (**53**)
(pediatric)	108	31.4	Poser & Ziegler (**72**)
	298	31.2	Niedermeyer & Knott (**69**)
8. Pts. with "epileptiform" EEG		35.6	Hughes et al. (**37**)
9. Problem children in school	181	58.6	Weir & Anderson (**87**)
10. "Atypical seizures"	682	68.4	Gibbs (**25**)
11. Impulsive children (organic)		72	Schwade & Geiger (**75**)

as the sample, the incidence of cases with positive spikes usually was between 10 and 20 per cent. In the case of patients with abnormal EEGs, this value was usually higher than 10 per cent, but it was again significant whether the sample included all abnormal records or only abnormal sleep records. Poser and Ziegler (72) found that 18 per cent of patients with abnormal EEGs under 20 years of age showed positive spikes, but in the restricted age range of 11 to 20 years this value increased to 25 per cent. If only psychiatric referrals constituted the population sample, the incidence was usually near 30 per cent. If only epileptiform records were considered, the incidence was as high as 35 per cent. Finally, Weir and Anderson (87) found that 58.6 per cent of problem children in school had positive spikes and Schwade and Geiger (75) reported that in the sample of impulsive children, in whom organicity was suspected, 72 per cent showed these spikes.

CONTROL STUDIES

The question of the incidence of the positive spike phenomenon among "normal" individuals is extremely important. Some data have been published on this question, but further investigation is desperately needed. The opinion of the reviewer is that all studies on "normal controls" will remain essentially incomplete until a battery of psychological tests, a psychiatric interview, and a careful history are included, together with both a waking and sleeping EEG. Unfortunately, individuals have been included in the category of "normal" simply by whether they have managed to stay out of an institution or out of a hospital.

Some data are available on the incidence of positive spikes in "normal" individuals. In their original 1951 paper Gibbs and Gibbs (16) stated that 2.7 per cent of 300 normal individuals showed these spikes. This figure was very close to the 2.3 per cent of Kellaway et al. (43), based on 1,000 normal children. Schwade and Geiger (76) reported that 1.5 per cent of 300 controls showed positive spikes, and later rechecking revealed that most of these positive cases had histories of "temper tantrums." Niedermeyer and Knott (68) emphasized a similar point by indicating that "normals" with positive spikes are potential candidates for showing the symptoms usually associated with these spikes. Kellaway et al. (43) emphasized the same point that some children who show positive spikes without any symptomatology often develop clear clinical symptoms later. In a population sample of normal public school children Metcalf (58) reported that 9.7 per cent of 31 cases had positive spikes in their EEG and in the same report this author claimed that

21 per cent of 70 children in a longitudinal study showed these spikes. However, the children in the latter study were not chosen by any criteria of normalcy, but because they were born within a certain period of time. Recently Gibbs (25) has stated that 21 per cent of "unselected controls" of 5-14 years of age showed positive spikes, but he has emphasized that the children with these spikes should not be considered "normal." As Gibbs has indicated, positive spikes in certain age groups may be as common as certain childhood diseases, but the fact that they are common does not mean that they may not constitute a significant abnormality.

Cases with positive spikes have also been compared to cases without this pattern but with some suspected cerebral abnormality. Refsum *et al.* (73) found that patients with positive spikes had headaches and dizziness twice as often and had gastrointestinal complaints, syncope, pallor, and behavior disorder three times as often as patients without positive spikes but with a probable cerebral lesion.

Hughes *et al.* (37) compared two groups of behavior disorders, one with and one without positive spikes. Generally, patients with these spikes had a more disordered EEG, especially with lower frequencies of the background rhythm, higher incidence of the classical types of epileptiform discharges, and also a higher incidence of diffuse slow activity during hyperventilation. In addition, a significantly higher percentage of cases with positive spikes had a history of head injury and complained of autonomic dysfunction in addition to their behavior disorder.

SEX RATIO

Table IX records the sex ratio of patients with positive spikes. The table shows that all of the studies except one indicate a higher

Table IX. Sex Ratio in Positive Spike Patients

% Males	No. with pos. sp.	Reference
45.8	136	Poser & Ziegler (72)
50.4	814	Shimoda (80)
54	300	Gibbs & Gibbs (16)
55.6	72	Refsum *et al.* (73)
57.8	135	Shimoda *et al.* (81)
59.5	180	Albernaz (1)
60.8	343	Niedermeyer & Knott (68)
70.4	115	Hughes *et al.* (37)
75	135	Metcalf (57)
89.5	19	Millen & White (62)

incidence in males. As the authors of one study (37) have pointed out, approximately twice as many males as females are found in consecutive admissions to a hospital (59). Other factors would seem to account for the predominance of positive spikes in males. Since behavior disorders are seen so prominently in cases with the positive spike phenomenon, males might be expected to have more opportunity to exhibit drastic action because of their relatively greater freedom of behavior. Thus, their disordered behavior usually comes more often to the attention of the authorities of law and order, like those in children's court, who may refer these patients for an EEG. In addition, significant head injuries, which are found as the most common presumed etiology, may be expected to appear more prominently in males, again because of the relatively greater freedom of behavior and vigor of play.

AGE

Table X summarizes the published data on the age distribution of the patients with positive spikes. The table shows that the youngest patient is usually only a few years of age and the incidence of patients with positive spikes under the age of five is about 3 to 4 per cent. The mean peak age of the positive spike phenomenon varies according to the population sample. With a pediatric population the mean peak age is about 9 to 10 years, but in a sample from the general population the peak age seems to be about 14 to 15 years. Some studies show the incidence over the age of 25 to be from 5 to 8 per cent, but other studies record higher values for the incidence over 30 years of age. The general conclusion from this table is that the positive spike phenomenon is primarily a teenage disorder.

MENTAL STATUS

Little information is available regarding mental status of patients with positive spikes. Hughes et al. (37) found that 20 per cent of the patients with these spikes had IQ's below 80 on a composite of performance and verbal psychological tests. Millen and White (62) considered 26.3 per cent of their patients with positive bursts mentally retarded, and Refsum et al. (73) reported that 34.8 per cent of their patients had IQ's below the average. Niedermeyer and Knott

(68) categorized 13.7 per cent of their patients as cases with dementia. These studies are no more than suggestive and further work is necessary along these lines before any definite conclusions can be stated. Further studies that are related to this question, at least indirectly, included the report of Gibbs *et al.* (18), who found twice as many cases with positive spikes among 1,118 cases who were mentally retarded without epilepsy as were found in a comparable mentally retarded group with epilepsy. Brant (5) found only one

Table X. Age Distribution in Positive Spike Patients

1. Youngest	
1½ yrs.	Poser & Ziegler (72)
1½	Kellaway *et al.* (43)
1½	Schwade & Geiger (75)
1⅔	Niedermeyer & Knott (68)
2	Metcalf (58)
3	Hughes *et al.* (37)
4	Millen & White (62)
2. Under 5 years	
Rare	Winfield (89)
2.6%	Hughes *et al.* (37)
2.8	Glenn & Knuth (28)
3	Metcalf (57)
3.5	Gibbs & Gibbs (26)
4.4	Niedermeyer & Knott (68)
5.1	Poser & Ziegler (72)
6	Kellaway *et al.* (43)
3. Peak age	
a. Pediatric population	
5-10 yrs.	Millen & White (62)
9-10	Winfield (89)
9-10	Kellaway *et al.* (43)
10½-12	Kellaway *et al.* (44)
b. General population	
11-20 yrs.	Poser & Ziegler (72)
14	Metcalf (58)
15.5	Hughes *et al.* (37)
15-20	Gibbs & Gibbs (26)
61% > 15	Refsum *et al.* (73)
4. Over 25 years	
5%	Metcalf (57)
7	Niedermeyer & Knott (68)
7.8	Hughes *et al.* (37)
5. Over 30 years	
9.2%	Poser & Ziegler (72)
11	Albernaz (1)
19.3	Glenn & Knuth (28)
22	Gibbs & Gibbs (16)
30	Shimoda *et al.* (81)
30	Koizumi *et al.* (49)

case with positive spikes among 23 cases of mental retardation without epilepsy and without cerebral palsy.

PRESUMED ETIOLOGY

Table XI summarizes the data available in the literature regarding the presumed etiology for the positive spike phenomenon. Clearly, the most common etiology is head injury and values range from 15 per cent to 55 per cent with an over-all average of approximately 27 per cent. However, Kellaway (41) pointed out that the development of the positive spike phenomenon is not closely correlated with the severity of the injury. One of the inherent difficulties in the subject of presumed etiology is the variation in the definition of terms. In one study (37) head injury was strictly defined to include only patients who had previously suffered either a skull fracture or a concussion, which was defined as a head injury producing unconsciousness. In that study the incidence of patients with positive spikes who had suffered a head injury was as high as 40 per cent, compared to the lower value of 30 per cent found in patients with temporal-lobe epilepsy (39). The next most common presumed etiological factor seems to be encephalitis. Again, the different definition of terms likely accounts for part of the range of values seen in the table, and whether or not the diagnosis of encephalitis requires laboratory confirmation would seem to be an important factor here. Recently Gibbs (25) has emphasized that some of the common childhood diseases may be followed by the appearance of positive spikes. Nine per cent of 112 children who did not show these bursts before measles developed them after the disease. In addition, 18 per cent of asymptomatic post-poliomyelitis cases showed these spikes, contrasted to 49 per cent of the symptomatic cases.

Other possible etiological factors have been noted. Metcalf (57, 58) stated that the incidence of positive spike phenomenon is significantly higher among prematures than full-term infants. Specifically, Lubchenco and Metcalf (55) reported that 35 per cent of prematures with sleep records showed positive spikes. Tumors have occasionally been reported as the presumed etiology of this abnormality. The earliest report was by Stephenson (83), who presented the details of two subcortical tumors in patients with positive spikes. Later Refsum et al. (73) mentioned two cases with subcortical tumors, Glenn and Knuth (28) referred to one case with a craniopharyngioma, and Bevilacqua and Little (2) reported on two cases of hypothalamic tumors. Inherited factors would not seem to play a more important role in the case of positive spikes than in the case of focal epilepsy. This was the conclusion of Gibbs and Gibbs (26), who reported that 7 per cent of near relatives of patients with positive spikes also had this same abnormality. Kellaway et al. (43) reported that no more than 2 per cent of cases with positive bursts had a family history of any kind of disorder referrable to the nervous system. Also, Millen and Winters (63) presented a case of identical twins who showed positive spikes and also stated that they found five families in their population of 275 cases with this same abnormality in two or more members of the family. Reference to other presumed etiological factors is found in one case by Metcalf (57) and one case by Naoi et al. (66), who recorded these spikes after electroconvulsive treatment, but not before this procedure. Walter (85) mentioned a case, involved with an anesthetic accident, who was comatose for 24 hours and later was found to have positive spikes. Gibbs and Gibbs (16) mentioned three cases with vascular accidents and two cases with carbon monoxide poisoning who later developed these spikes.

Table XI. Presumed Etiology of Positive Spikes

Head injury	Enceph. or menin.	Birth inj. or premat.	Others	No. of Cases	Reference
14.6%			19.8% (organic CNS disease)	136	Poser & Ziegler (72)
20.8	9.4%	5.4%	7 (family hist. of epilepsy)	427	Gibbs & Gibbs (26)
20.9	17.7		2 (family hist. of nerv. sys. dis.)	550	Kellaway et al. (43)
26.3		10.5		19	Millen & White (62)
37	3	4	2 (tumors)	72	Refsum et al. (73)
40	3.5	5.2		115	Hughes et al. (37)
55.4	5.0	5.8	1 (tumor)	139	Glenn & Knuth (28)
27%				1458	

ACTUAL LOCUS OF POSITIVE SPIKES

In their original report Gibbs and Gibbs (16) concluded that the locus of the positive spikes was likely within the thalamic and hypothalamic region. One of the reasons for this conclusion revolved around the supposition that the 14/sec positive spikes most likely represented the rectification (without the negative phase) of normal 14/sec sleep spindles, which appear to be controlled from the thalamic-hypothalamic region. In addition, the diffuse distribution of these spikes throughout the scalp leads suggested that the spikes were mediated by the non-specific thalamic efferent system. The positive polarity of the bursts also suggested a subcortical origin. However, Bishop (3) claimed that the positivity, indicating that the critical electrode is at a distance from the active region, is correct only under certain circumstances, and that negativity, in some circumstances, can indicate activity at a distance, dependent upon the position of the electrode relative to the path of current flow. Finally, the clinical symptoms seen in patients with the positive spike phenomenon suggested the thalamic-hypothalamic locus. Kirschbaum and Stehle (46, 47) specifically pointed out that the gastrointestinal symptoms that are sometimes seen in patients with positive spikes, especially peptic ulcers, suggest the possible cor-

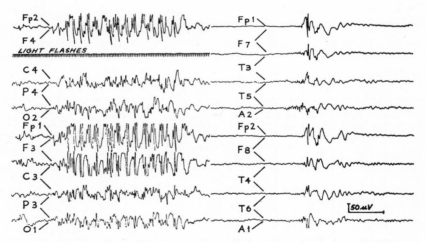

Figure 11. EEG from patients showing both 3/sec spike-and-wave complexes and the positive spike phenomenon. The first half of the figure shows irregular 3/sec spike-and-wave complexes (with some multiple spikes) induced by light flashes, which are monitored on Channel 2. The second half of the figure shows a drowsy record with positive spikes seen from the left posterior temporal area (Channel 4) immediately followed by abortive bilateral spike-and-wave complexes.

relation between the gastric disorders and thalamic-hypothalamic disorders.

The occasional close relationship between the positive spike phenomenon and the bilaterally synchronous spike-and-wave complexes of centrencephalic epilepsy may supply suggestive evidence for the locus of positive spikes. Although Gibbs (25) has pointed out that the two wave forms rarely appear in the same patient, positive spikes and spike-and-wave complexes appear at times to be related when seen in the same patient. Figure 11 is a sample of the EEG from one of our patients who showed symptomatology referrable to both centrencephalic epilepsy and the positive spike phenomenon. This figure shows that positive spikes may immediately proceed the occurrence of bilaterally synchronous spike-and-wave complexes, which are commonly assumed to arise from diencephalic structures (70). Some of the figures published by Chieffi and Fois (9) show these same two wave forms in a given EEG. Although many different neural systems may activate paroxysms arising from diencephalic areas, the occasional close relationship between these two wave forms suggests that both may arise from closely related structures, possibly diencephalic.

The localization of tumors in cases with positive spikes has provided suggestive evidence that the actual locus of these bursts is within the diencephalic areas. In 1951 Stephenson (83) reported on two cases of tumors, one extending beyond the sella turcica and pressing upward into the third ventricle and the other, a fibrillary astrocytoma, extending into the ependyma of the third ventricle. In 1960 Refsum et al. (73) mentioned two patients with positive spikes who had brain tumors. One tumor was a subependymal glioma in the fourth ventricle and the other was an astrocytoma invading subcortical regions. Glenn and Knuth (28) mentioned one case of craniopharyngioma. In 1961 Bevilacqua and Little (2) reported two cases of hypothalamic tumors showing the positive spike phenomenon. One of these cases was a teratoma of the hypophysis which compressed the ventral midbrain and hypothalamus (51).

Although the thalamic-hypothalamic locus has been the most popular, other areas have been suggested for the locus of positive spikes. Refsum et al. (73) and Niedermeyer and Knott (68) mentioned the possibility of a limbic involvement as the most likely site. Metcalf (57) has specified the hippocampus. Evidence for this locus includes the position of the posterior temporal scalp electrodes as the leads showing the highest amplitude of positive spikes, and the known hippocampal involvement with vegetative disturbances and with the integration of visceral sensations and affect. In addition, there is evidence that induced seizure activity may remain in the hippocampal system yet alter behavior. Also Metcalf mentioned one case (of E. Walker and C. Marshall) in whom depth recording revealed positive spikes, not from around the thalamic-hypotha-lamic region, but presumably from near the hippocampal area. In 1963 Metcalf (**58**) summarized that the positive spikes likely origi-nate in or close to the hippocampus and exert an impact on symptom formation by virtue of the induced or associated limbic system dis-turbance. As a possible locus Schwade and Geiger (**75, 76**) merely mentioned the amygdala and Shimoda (**80**) mentioned the medulla oblongata.

One last possibility for the locus of positive bursts deserves serious consideration. In 1952 Grossman (**29**) pointed out that spindles, originally biphasic, may be converted into monophasic positive bursts by the depressive action of various drugs locally applied to the cortex and by the resulting spreading depression. The conver-sion to positivity was viewed as a release phenomenon due to the transient depression of cortical structures. In 1953 Grossman (**30**) again emphasized the conversion of biphasic waves into positive bursts by the transient blocking of the superficial cortex by depres-sant drugs. This author also mentioned the ease with which positive bursts are produced in younger animals and suggested a greater susceptibility of the immature cortex to this transient blocking. It may be more than coincidental that patients with positive spikes tend to be adolescents with "immature" brains. In 1954 Grossman (**31**) summarized his conclusions by stating that the clinical mani-festations of rage attacks seen in many patients with positive spikes are due to a release phenomenon related to transient laminar block-ing of inhibitory mechanisms in the superficial layers of the asso-ciative cortex. With an idea that combines the salient features of the proposals of both Gibbs and Gibbs (**16**) and Grossman (**31**), Little (**50**) has suggested that hypothalamic activity might result in a negative DC shift of the cortex with the result that 14/sec sleep spindles would show a conversion to positive bursts.

TREATMENT AND PROGNOSIS

Anticonvulsants have been featured in the reports dealing with the treatment of cases with positive spikes. In their original report Gibbs and Gibbs (16) reported that the combination of Dilantin and phenobarbital produced a good response in patients with this abnormality. The same combination of drugs showed an appreciable improvement in asthmatics with positive bursts, both with regard to their wheezing and to their aggressive behavior (4). Kellaway et al. (43) and Druckman (11), summarizing their extensive experience with pediatric patients showing positive spikes, claimed that Dilantin alone or with phenobarbital is most effective in the majority of cases. In children and adolescents, Metcalf (57) also claimed that the drug of choice was Dilantin, which Sheeby et al. (78) claimed was especially effective in cases with abdominal pain and positive spikes. The combination of Dilantin and Mesantoin has also been mentioned by Gibbs and Gibbs (16, 20, 26) while Dilantin, phenobarbital, or Mesantoin has shown an improvement in 50 per cent of patients studied by Refsum et al. (77). Chieffi and Fois (9) have effectively used the combination of barbiturates, Dilantin, and high dosages of asparagine. Winfield (89) stated that the best response to anticonvulsants for paroxysmal attacks is seen with Dilantin or Diamox. Diamox has also been suggested by Chao and Plumb (8), who claimed that patients with positive spikes showed a good response to this drug in 80 per cent of cases, second in efficacy only to patients with 3/sec spike and wave.

General statements regarding the efficacy of anticonvulsants in the positive spike phenomenon have emphasized that these drugs are most effective in patients with paroxysmal attacks, especially with autonomic symptomatology. Anticonvulsants have not been found as effective with the chronic or more continuous type of disorder, especially in behavior disorders. Schwade and Geiger (75) specifically pointed out that anticonvulsants were less effective in the case of behavior disorder. Other investigators (43, 57, 66, 89) have concluded that anticonvulsants were most effective in patients with paroxysmal autonomic symptomatology and rarely showed a good response in cases with chronic behavior disorder. However, Poser and Ziegler (72) and Shimoda (80) have indicated that anticonvulsants often produced a dramatic disappearance of episodic disturbances and, in addition, showed improvement of chronic behavior disorders.

The use of tranquilizers has been featured in the reports dealing with severe behavior disorders. Schwade and Geiger (75) claimed that Serpasil alone or in combination with phenobarbital was most effective in the treatment of behavior disorders showing positive spikes. These authors also claimed that Thorazine, with or without Serpasil, produced beneficial effects on the disordered behavior. Winfield (89) agreed that for patients with the continuous or chronic type of behavior disorder the drugs of choice were Serpasil and Thorazine, mentioned also by Chieffi and Fois (9). In addition, Winfield and Aivazian (90) claimed that Librium may be of value, 74 per cent of their patients showing EEG improvement, 68 per cent clinical improvement, and 63 per cent both clinical and EEG improvement. The combination of Librium and anticonvulsants showed an EEG improvement in six out of seven cases but clinical improvement was seen in only four out of these seven cases. In problem children in school Weir and Anderson (87) found behavioral improvement in 91.3 per cent with Raudixin, in 74.5 per cent with Serpasil, and in 59.1 per cent with anticonvulsants.

Since the positive spike phenomenon has been extensively studied for only a relatively few number of years, the question regarding the prognosis in cases showing this electrographic entity cannot be fully answered. In 1958 Gibbs (24) claimed that this phenomenon was the most benign epileptiform disorder, and in 1959 Kellaway et al. (43) pointed out that this abnormality tends to disappear within one to two years regardless of the age of onset, although the authors had seen this phenomenon for as long as seven years in one patient. In 1958 Kellaway and his colleagues (42) had indicated that if positive spikes were present during childhood both the EEG pattern and the clinical symptoms generally disappear before or during adolescence. In the former report the authors pointed out that they had seen 21 cases of head injury who had developed positive spikes without symptomatology, but later tended to develop the symptoms with which the pattern was associated. Ontogenetic views of Gibbs and Gibbs (17, 27, 71) would suggest that patients with positive spikes during their teens may possibly develop anterior temporal spikes later in adulthood if they continue to show some type of epileptiform EEG discharge. It seems to the reviewer that this possibility dictates that more than casual attention should be directed toward patients showing positive spikes in the early years. It is well known that many temporal-lobe epileptics with anterior temporal foci show a poor response to anticonvulsants and frequently have grand mal seizures in addition to other relatively incapacitating symptomatology. Any conservative step that could be taken during the teens in patients with positive spikes would seem to be justified if the development of anterior temporal discharges might, therefore, be avoided. Theoretically, the suppression of positive spikes by anticonvulsants would seem to lower the probability that other spike discharges might later develop. Careful longitudinal studies are required to determine whether this theoretical point is also a significant practical measure.

SUMMARY

The positive spike phenomenon refers to an electrographic pattern that appears in bursts of spikes, positive in polarity and maximal on the posterior temporal area. The frequencies of the bursts can be divided into the slow form (6–8/sec) and the harmonically related fast form (14–16/sec), with mean frequencies at approximately 7/sec and 15/sec. Transmission from one side to the other can occur and bilateral synchrony can also be noted. Positive spikes usually appear from both the posterior temporal areas during a light-sleep state, but with a right-sided predominance. Related abnormalities are posterior slow activity, excessive hyperventilation response, and single, isolated epileptiform discharges.

The general symptomatology seen in patients with positive spikes includes autonomic dysfunction, behavior disorder, and convulsive attacks. Autonomic symptoms feature headaches, abdominal pain, vertigo, and syncope. Patients with severe behavior disorders usually have an emotionally traumatized past and show impulsive, destructive, uncontrolled behavior with a lack of appropriate remorse or guilt for their acts. These cases usually represent an example of the complicated interplay between organic and psychiatric factors. An experiment with patients with behavior disorders who show positive spikes suggests that they not only react prominently to anxiety-producing stimuli, but do not recover easily from their exaggerated response. Convulsive activity is frequently noted, mainly grand mal seizures. The possible epileptiform character of the symptoms seen in cases with positive spikes, especially the autonomic symptoms, has been considered by some investigators.

The incidence of positive spikes is approximately 10 per cent with pediatric referrals and 30 per cent with psychiatric referrals. Judging from the few reports, the incidence in "normals" appears to be 1.5–3 per cent, but more recent reports suggest a higher incidence. Positive spikes appear especially in teen-age males with head injury a major presumed etiology. The actual locus of these spikes is possibly from the thalamic-hypothalamic region, but the hippocampus and superficial cortex on the posterior temporal area must also be considered. The treatment of cases with positive spikes has featured anticonvulsants for paroxysmal symptoms and tranquilizers for the chronic types of behavior disorders.

The introduction emphasized the controversial nature of the positive polarity of the spikes, the apparent lack of the expected harmonic relationship between the frequencies of the bursts, the varying clinical symptomatology, and the relatively few electroencephalographers who have observed this phenomenon. The question of the possible artifactual nature of positive spikes is no longer reasonable. The frequencies of the burst are actually harmonically related; and the symptoms, similar to those seen in temporal-lobe epilepsy, can easily be categorized into behavior disorder, autonomic dysfunction, and convulsive phenomena. Recently, more laboratories have been looking for positive spikes and finding them. Therefore, the major reasons for most of the needless controversy regarding the positive spike phenomenon have vanished. Although the precise significance of positive spikes has not been fully determined, definite progress has been made by the many investigators whose contributions supply the data for this review.

BIBLIOGRAPHY

1. Albernaz, J. G. Aspectos electroencefalograficos dos espiculas positivas a 14 e 6 por segundo. *Arq. Neuropsiquiat.* **18**: 3–18, 1960.
2. Bevilacqua, A. R., and Little, S. C. Fourteen and six per second dysrhythmia with proven hypothalamic disease. *Electroenceph. clin. Neurophysiol.* **13**: 314, 1961.
3. Bishop, G. A critique of Gibbs' law with an experimental commentary. *Electroenceph. clin. Neurophysiol.* **2**: 91–92, 1950.
4. Blatman, S., and Metcalf, D. R. Abnormal electroencephalograms in asthmatic children. *Amer. J. Dis. Child.* **102**: 531, 1961.
5. Brandt, S. Electroencephalographic findings in 200 children with mental retardation. *Electroenceph. clin. Neurophysiol.* **9**: 735, 1957.
6. Brown, I. H. Clinical correlates of 14 and 6/sec positive spike discharges. *Electroenceph. clin. Neurophysiol.* **14**: 286, 1962.
7. Chao, D. H., Druckman, R., and Kellaway, P. *Convulsive Disorders of Children.* W. B. Saunders Co., Philadelphia, 1958.
8. Chao, D. H., and Plumb, R. L. Diamox in epilepsy. A critical review of 178 cases. *J. Pediat.* **58**: 211–218, 1961.
9. Chieffi, A., and Fois, A. Le disritmie vegetative parossistiche. In: A. Chieffi and G. Bellieni (Editors), *Atti del Symposium Nazionale di Pediatria sulle Cardiopatie Congenite Operabili.* La Galluzza, Siena, pp. 369–376, 1956.
10. Condon, J. V., Becka, D. R., and Gibbs, F. A. Electroencephalographic abnormalities in hyperthyroidism. *J. clin. Endocr.* **14**: 1511–1518, 1954.
11. Druckman, R. Pain and autonomic disturbances in convulsive equivalent states. In: P. Kellaway and H. F. Conn (Editors), *Med. Clin. N. Amer.* W. B. Saunders Company, Philadelphia, pp. 475–479, March, 1958.

12. Fois, A., Rosenberg, C., and Gibbs, F. A. The electroencephalogram in phenylpyruvic oligophrenia. *Electroenceph. clin. Neurophysiol.* 7: 569–572, 1955.
13. Garneski, T. M. Increased 6 and/or 14 per second spike dysrhythmia in juvenile behavior problems. *Electroenceph. clin. Neurophysiol.* 10: 358, 1958.
14. Garneski, T. M. Six and fourteen per second spikes in juvenile behavior disorders. *Electroenceph. clin. Neurophysiol.* 12: 505, 1960.
15. Garneski, T. M., and Green, J. R. Recording the fourteen and six-per second spike phenomenon. *Electroenceph. clin. Neurophysiol.* 8: 501–505, 1956.
16. Gibbs, E. L., and Gibbs, F. A. Electroencephalographic evidence of thalamic and hypothalamic epilepsy. *Neurology.* 1: 136–144, 1951.
17. Gibbs, E. L., Gillen, H. W., and Gibbs, F. A. Disappearance and migration of epileptic foci in childhood. *Amer. J. Dis. Child.* 88: 596–603, 1954.
18. Gibbs, E. L., Rich, C. L., Fois, A., and Gibbs, F. A. Electroencephalographic study of mentally retarded persons. *Amer. J. ment. Defic.* 65: 236–247, 1960.
19. Gibbs, E. L., Rich, C., Perlstein, M., and Gibbs, F. A. The predictive value of EEG as regards epilepsy in cerebral palsy. *Electroenceph. clin. Neurophysiol.* 12: 756, 1960.
20. Gibbs, F. A. Value of electroencephalography. *Mod. Med.* pp. 75–82, 1954.
21. Gibbs, F. A. Subjective complaints and behavior disturbances associated with fourteen and six per second positive spikes. *Electroenceph. clin. Neurophysiol.* 7: 315, 1955.
22. Gibbs, F. A. Clinical correlates of 14 and 6 per second positive spikes (1865 cases). *Electroenceph. clin. Neurophysiol.* 8: 148, 1956.
23. Gibbs, F. A. Abnormal electrical activity in the temporal regions and its relationship to abnormalities of behavior. *Res. Publ. Ass. Res. Nerv. Ment. Dis.* 36: 278–294, 1958.
24. Gibbs, F. A. Differentiation of mid-temporal, anterior temporal and diencephalic epilepsy. In: M. Baldwin and P. Bailey (Editors), *Temporal Lobe Epilepsy.* Charles C. Thomas, Springfield, Illinois, pp. 109–117, 1958.
25. Gibbs, F. A. Unpublished data presented at the Amer. EEG Soc., Atlantic City, June, 1962. See Gibbs, F. A., and Gibbs, E. L. Fourteen and six per second positive spikes. *Electroenceph. clin. Neurophysiol.* 15: 553–558, 1963.
26. Gibbs, F. A., and Gibbs, E. L. Thalamic and hypothalamic epilepsy. In: *Atlas of Electroencephalography.* Addison-Wesley Press, Inc., Cambridge, Mass. 2: 329–345, 1952.
27. Gibbs, F. A., and Gibbs, E. L. Changes in epileptic foci with age. *Electroenceph. clin. Neurophysiol.* Suppl. 4: 233–234, 1953.
28. Glenn, C. G., and Knuth, R. Incidence of fourteen and six per second positive spike discharges in routine sleeping EEGs. *Dis. nerv. Syst.* 20: 340–341, 1959.
29. Grossman, C. The relationship of "positive spikes" to "spontaneous" activity and cortical excitability. *Electroenceph. clin. Neurophysiol.* 4: 381, 1952.
30. Grossman, C. The role of "cortical laminar blocking" in the origin of evoked and spontaneous "positive bursts." *Electroenceph. clin. Neurophysiol.* Suppl. 3: 61, 1953.
31. Grossman, C. Laminar cortical blocking and its relation to episodic aggressive outbursts. *Arch. Neurol. Psychiat.* 71: 576–587, 1954.
32. Henry, C. E. Discussion. *IVth Int. Cong. EEG Clin. Neurophysiol.* pp. 29–30, 1957.
33. Henry, C. E. Positive spike discharges in the EEG and behavior abnormality. In: G. H. Glaser (Editor), *EEG and Behavior.* Basic Books, New York, pp. 315–344, 1963.
34. Hughes, J. R. The 14 and 7 per second positive spikes—a reappraisal following a frequency count. *Electroenceph. clin. Neurophysiol.* 12: 495–496, 1960.
35. Hughes, J. R. Oscilloscopic analysis of the temporal relationships in the positive spike phenomenon. *Proc. Amer. EEG Soc.* pp. 99–100, 1962.
36. Hughes, J. R. Unpublished data, 1962.
37. Hughes, J. R., Gianturco, D., and Stein, W. Electro-clinical correlations in the positive spike phenomenon. *Electroenceph. clin. Neurophysiol.* 13: 599–605, 1961.
38. Hughes, J. R., Jacobs, I., Baumel, L., Carboy, D., and Sobocinski, L. Autonomic changes from experimentally induced "anxiety" in cases with the positive spike phenomenon. *Electroenceph. clin. Neurophysiol.* 15: 163, 1963.
39. Hughes, J. R., and Schlagenhauff, R. E. Electro-clinical correlations in temporal lobe epilepsy with emphasis on interareal analysis of the temporal lobe. *Electroenceph. clin. Neurophysiol.* 13: 333–339, 1961.
40. Kellaway, P. Convulsive equivalent disorders. *Electroenceph. clin. Neurophysiol.* 5: 130, 1953.
41. Kellaway, P. Head injury in children. *Electroenceph. clin. Neurophysiol.* 7: 497–502, 1955.
42. Kellaway, P., and Conn, H. F. Electroencephalography in the diagnosis and management of the epilepsies. In: P. Kellaway and H. F. Conn (Editors), *Med. Clin. N. Amer.* W. B. Saunders Company, Philadelphia, pp. 439–460, March, 1958.

43. Kellaway, P., Crawley, J. W., and Kagawa, N. A specific electroencephalographic correlate of convulsive equivalent disorders in children. *J. Pediat.* **55**: 582–592, 1959.
44. Kellaway, P., Crawley, J. W., and Kagawa, N. Paroxysmal pain and autonomic disturbances of cerebral origin: A specific electro-clinical syndrome. *Epilepsia.* **1**: 466–483, 1960.
45. Kellaway, P., Moore, F. J., and Kagawa, N. The "14 and 6 per second positive spike" pattern of Gibbs and Gibbs. *Electroenceph. clin. Neurophysiol.* **9**: 165–166, 1957.
46. Kirschbaum, W. R., and Stehle, N. C. Electroencephalographic studies of patients with peptic ulcer and functional gastric disorders. *Electroenceph. clin. Neurophysiol.* **4**: 380, 1952.
47. Kirschbaum, W. R., and Stehle, H. C. Electroencephalographic studies of patients with peptic ulcer and functional gastric disorders. *Electroenceph. clin. Neurophysiol.* **5**: 513–524, 1953.
48. Koegler, R. R., Colbert, E. G., and Walter, R. D. Problems in the correlation of psychopathology with electroencephalographic abnormalities. *Amer. J. Psychiat.* **117**: 822–824, 1961.
49. Koizumi, A., Yamamasu, T., Morishita, T., Iwai, H., and Shimoda, Y. A statistic observation of 14 and 6 cps positive spikes. *Electroenceph. clin. Neurophysiol.* Suppl. **12**: 29, 1958.
50. Little, S. C. The fourteen and six per sec. dysrhythmia: Relationship to atypical sleep patterns. *Electroenceph. clin. Neurophysiol.* **15**: 162, 1963.
51. Little, S. C., and Bevilacqua, A. R. Dysrhythmia associated with proved hypothalamic disease, fourteen and six per second dysrhythmia. *Arch. Neurol.* **6**: 324–330, 1962.
52. Low, N. L., Bosma, J. F., and Armstrong, M. D. Electroencephalographic findings in phenylketonuria. *Electroenceph. clin. Neurophysiol.* **9**: 159–160, 1957.
53. Low, N. L., and Dawson, S. P. Electroencephalographic findings in juvenile delinquency. *Pediatrics.* **28**: 452–457, 1961.
54. Low, N. L., Gibbs, E. L., and Gibbs, F. A. Electroencephalographic findings in breath holding spells. *Pediatrics.* **15**: 595–599, 1955.
55. Lubchenco, L., and Metcalf, D. R. Follow-up study of children born prematurely in 1949 and 1950. *Amer. J. Dis. Child.* **106**: 101–115, 1963.
56. Metcalf, D. R. On the development of 6 and 14 per sec. spikes. *Electroenceph. clin. Neurophysiol.* **11**: 616–617, 1959.
57. Metcalf, D. R. Behavioral and physiologic implications of six and fourteen per second spikes on the EEG. *Proc. Eleventh Western Institute on Epilepsy*, Milwaukee, Wisconsin, 1959.
58. Metcalf, D. R. Controlled studies of the incidence and significance of 6 and 14 per sec. positive spiking. *Electroenceph. clin. Neurophysiol.* **15**: 161, 1963.
59. Metrakos, J. D., and Metrakos, K. Genetics of convulsive disorders: I. Introduction, problems, methods and base lines. *Neurology.* **10**: 228–240, 1960.
60. Millen, F. J. A study of fourteen and six per second dysrhythmia in children. *Electroenceph. clin. Neurophysiol.* **5**: 128, 1953.
61. Millen, F. J. Abdominal epilepsy. *Arch. Neurol.* **4**: 107–109, 1961.
62. Millen, F. J., and White, B. Fourteen and six per second positive spike activity in children. *Neurology.* **4**: 541–549, 1954.
63. Millen, F. J., and Winters, K. Fourteen and six per second positive spike activity in the EEG of identical twins and family. *Electroenceph. clin. Neurophysiol.* **11**: 845, 1959.
64. Millichap, J. G., Madsen, J. A., and Aledort, L. M. Studies in febrile seizures: V. Clinical and electroencephalographic study in unselected patients. *Neurology.* **10**: 643–653, 1960.
65. Mills, W. B. Paroxysmal 14 and 6/sec spike discharges and clinical cases, including a teenage murderer. *Electroenceph. clin. Neurophysiol.* **8**: 344, 1956.
66. Naoi, T., Shinozaki, T., and Hirosawa, M. On "14 and 6/sec positive spikes." *Electroenceph. clin. Neurophysiol.* Suppl. **9**: 59, 1957.
67. Nicholson, J. M., and Knott, J. R. Sleep EEGs in psychiatric patients. *Electroenceph. clin. Neurophysiol.* **9**: 375–376, 1957.
68. Niedermeyer, E., and Knott, J. R. Über die Bedeutung der 14 and 6/sec-positiven Spitzen in EEG. *Arch. Psychiat. Nervenkr.* **202**: 266–280, 1961.
69. Niedermeyer, E., and Knott, J. R. The incidence of 14 and 6/sec positive spikes in psychiatric material. *Electroenceph. clin. Neurophysiol.* **14**: 285–286, 1962.
70. Penfield, W., and Jasper, H. H. *Epilepsy and the Functional Anatomy of the Human Brain.* Little, Brown and Company, Boston, 1954.
71. Perlstein, M. A., Gibbs, E. L., and Gibbs, F. A. The electroencephalogram in infantile cerebral palsy. *Amer. J. phys. Med.* **34**: 477–496, 1955.

72. Poser, C. M., and Ziegler, D. K. Clinical significance of 14 and 6 per second positive spike complexes. *Neurology*. **8**: 903–912, 1958.
73. Refsum, S., Presthus, J., Skulstad, A., and Östensjö, S. Clinical correlates of the 14 and 6 per second positive spikes. An electroencephalographic and clinical study. *Acta psychiat. scand.* **35**: 330–344, 1960.
74. Schwade, E. D., and Geiger, S. C. Matricide with electroencephalographic evidence of thalamic or hypothalamic disorder. *Dis. nerv. Syst.* **14**: 18–20, 1953.
75. Schwade, E. D., and Geiger, S. G. Abnormal electroencephalographic findings in severe behavior disorders. *Dis. nerv. Syst.* **17**: 307–317, 1956.
76. Schwade, E. D., and Geiger, S. G. Severe behavior disorders with abnormal electroencephalograms. *Dis. nerv. Syst.* **21**: 616–620, 1960.
77. Schwade, E. D., and Otto, O. Homicide as a manifestation of thalamic or hypothalamic disorder with abnormal electroencephalographic findings. *Wisconsin med. J.* **52**: 171–174, 1953.
78. Sheeby, B. N., Little, S. C., Stone, J. J., McAvoy, M., and Rhea, E. Abdominal epilepsy. *J. Pediat.* **56**: 355–363, 1960.
79. Shimoda, Y. On primary thalamic and hypothalamic epilepsy. *IVth Int. Cong. EEG Clin. Neurophysiol.* p. 194, 1957.
80. Shimoda, Y. The clinical and electroencephalographic study of the primary diencephalic epilepsy or epilepsy of brain stem. *Acta neuroveg.* **23**: 181–191, 1961.
81. Shimoda, Y., Koizumi, A., Yamamasu, T., Yoskino, Y., Nanba, M., and Tanaka, K. Statistical observation of six and fourteen per second positive spikes. *Yonago Acta med.* **5**: 102–108, 1961.
82. Stehle, H. C. Thalamic dysfunction involved in destructive-aggressive behavior directed against persons and property. *Electroenceph. clin. Neurophysiol.* **12**: 264–265, 1960.
83. Stephenson, W. A. Intracranial neoplasm associated with fourteen and six per second positive spikes. *Neurology*. **1**: 372–376, 1951.
84. Walker, A. E. Murder or epilepsy? *J. nerv. ment. Dis.* **133**: 430–437, 1961.
85. Walter, R. D. Some clinical correlation of 14 and 6 per sec. spiking activity. *Electroenceph. clin. Neurophysiol.* **9**: 377, 1957.
86. Walter, R. D., Colbert, E. G., Koegler, R. R., Palmer, J. O., and Bond, P. M. A controlled study of the fourteen and six per second EEG pattern. *Arch. gen. Psychiat.* **2**: 559–566, 1960.
87. Weir, H. F., and Anderson, R. L. Organic and organizational aspects of school adjustment problems. *J. Amer. Med. Ass.* **166**: 1708–1710, 1958.
88. Williams, D. A study of thalamic and cortical rhythms in petit mal. *Brain*. **76**: 50–69, 1953.
89. Winfield, D. L. Emotional disturbances of the brain damaged child with reference to the electroencephalogram. *Memphis med. J.* **36**: 403–406, 1961.
90. Winfield, D. L., and Aivazian, G. H. Librium therapy and electro-encephalographic correlates. *J. nerv. ment. Dis.* **133**: 240–246, 1961.
91. Winfield, D. L., Britt, L. P., and Raskind, R. EEG findings in pseudo-hypertrophic muscular dystrophy. *Southern med. J.* **51**: 1251–1259, 1958.
92. Winfield, D. L., and Ozturk, O. Electroencephalographic findings in matricide (a case report). *Dis. nerv. Syst.* **20**: 176–178, 1959.
93. Woods, S. M. Adolescent violence and homicide: Ego disruption and the 6 and 14 dysrhythmia. *Arch. gen. Psychiat.* **5**: 528–534, 1961.

The author wishes to express his appreciation to Dr. Charles Henry for his aid in preparing the bibliography.

THE ELECTROENCEPHALOGRAM
IN ENDOCRINE DISORDERS

W. P. Wilson, M.D.

In lower animals the influence of endocrines on behavior has been described as clear cut. In spite of this seemingly clear-cut relationship in animals, there have been contradictory descriptions of presenting psychiatric symptomatology and behavioral disturbances in patients with endocrine disease. Because of the lack of a one-to-one relationship between excesses and deficiencies of hormones and behavioral change, questions have arisen as to the exact role that endocrines play in the determination of the behavioral concomitants of these disorders. Recent experimental studies have, however, begun to demonstrate specific alterations of function in specific systems of the brain. It seems possible, therefore, that in the future the role of endocrines in the regulation of the more complex behavior of man may be better understood.

Few practitioners of psychiatry have not been called upon to examine or manage the psychiatric complications of endocrine disease. Too, endocrine disorders must always be considered in the differential diagnosis of some psychiatric illnesses. In this last instance, electroencephalography has proved to be a useful tool, for many studies have demonstrated abnormal electroencephalographic patterns in endocrine disorders. It seems desirable, therefore, to summarize our current knowledge in this area in the hope that it will prove useful in the practice of EEG in psychiatry. As many of the effects of endocrine disease may be metabolic, this summary has been extended to include other metabolic diseases of non-endocrine origin that are also of importance.

PITUITARY

1. Pan-hypopituitarism

A decrease in the function of the anterior pituitary always results

102

in psychiatric symptomatology. The symptoms were first described by Simmonds and later clarified by Sheehan and Summers. The symptoms referable to the central nervous system that are most commonly encountered consist of torpor, loss of interest and energy, and a general state described as "placid inertia." If psychotic changes occur, these may consist of "depression or melancholia." Many cases of the syndrome may die in coma, as a result of hypoglycemia, electrolyte imbalance, or hypothermia.

Until recently, EEG studies of this syndrome had been few in number and for the most part consisted of isolated case reports of one or two patients (11). In 1956, however, Hughes and Summers (9) reported 14 cases of post-partum pituitary necrosis. All of the cases met the criteria for the syndrome described by Sheehan and the diagnosis had been confirmed by him. They reported a general slowing of the alpha rhythm to the theta frequency in the more severe cases, and a mixture of alpha and theta in those with less severe endocrine dysfunction. Hyperventilation responses were increased. They concluded that the severity of the endocrine disturbance was correlated with the degree of abnormality in the EEG.

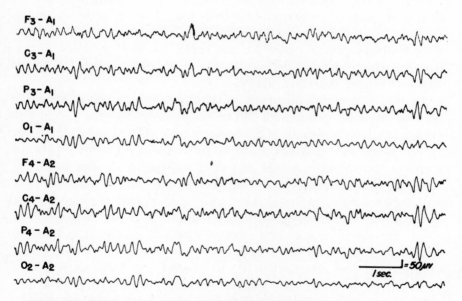

Figure 1. EEG of a 47-year-old patient with panhypopituitarism secondary to a chromophobe adenoma. There was marked reduction of thyroid and adrenal and gonadal function.

Although coma is a concomitant of hypopituitarism, relevant electroencephalographic studies are few. Kennedy *et al.* (**10**) have reported five patients who had one or more attacks of coma. Of the five patients, two who had suffered only a single attack of coma showed normal EEGs after endocrine replacement therapy. The three others with repeated attacks of coma had abnormal EEGs. The abnormalities consisted of generalized slowing in the theta and delta frequencies. Two treated patients with hypopituitarism who had not been in coma had normal EEGs. Salmon (**13**) followed one patient from a comatose state to restitution and observed a slow improvement of the cerebral rhythms with treatment. Epileptic spiking was described in one patient by Cloche and Stuhl (**7**).

Pituitary insufficiency associated with chromophobe adenomas and with Rathke's pouch cysts produce EEG abnormalities which can also be correlated with the severity of the endocrine change. The abnormalities in these cases are essentially similar to those seen in patients with post-partum necrosis. Boselli and Jefferson (**6**) reported the electroencephalographic findings in 59 patients with chromophobe adenomas and 17 patients with Rathke's pouch cysts. In both instances the EEG changes again correlated well with the degree of endocrine change. Abnormal records were, however, more frequent in patients with the adenomas (61 per cent) than those with Rathke's pouch cysts (17 per cent). In another series of 44 patients with pituitary tumors, Tonnis *et al.* (**14**) reported findings similar to those described above.

In the differential diagnosis of pituitary insufficiency, anorexia nervosa must be considered. However, in reviewing the recent literature on this subject (**8, 12**), we were able to find only two cases of this syndrome in which EEGs were obtained. The two patients reported were near terminal and died subsequent to the EEG recordings. Both tracings were abnormal, one with diffuse slowing and subharmonic responses to photic stimulation, the other with dysrhythmic slowing with hyperventilation. To these two reported cases, the author can add two others who had sustained less severe weight loss and who were ambulatory at the time the EEG was obtained. In one case the EEG was normal, but focal slowing was observed in the other. The patient was congenitally deaf and had other congenital anomalies which may have contributed to the abnormal EEG.

One may summarize the findings in pituitary insufficiency as generalized slow wave abnormalities which may be correlated with the degree of endocrine deficiency. The slow waves seen in the record may present as a replacement of normal rhythms by theta rhythms or a mixture of normal and slow rhythms. Delta rhythms usually are paroxysmal and mixed with the alpha or theta rhythms. Hyperventilation usually increases the degree of abnormality. Replacement therapy results in a slow return of the EEG to normal unless the patient has had recurrent bouts of hypopituitary coma. If these have occurred, the EEG may remain abnormally and diffusely slow. On the other hand, if anorexia nervosa is considered in the differential diagnosis, one can expect an abnormal EEG even if the patient's illness has not resulted in cachexia of such a severe degree that he is near terminal status.

2. Pituitary Hyperfunction

Basophilic adenomas of the pituitary are small and produce a Cushing's syndrome. The EEG findings in this syndrome are discussed elsewhere.

Acidophilic adenomas of the pituitary produce the syndrome of acromegaly. Although the number of reported cases is small, the incidence of EEG abnormalities would indicate that the procedure may be useful in this disease. Austt and Mussio-Fournier (5) reported abnormal EEGs in three of seven cases. Two had irregular 2-to-4-cycles-per-second slowing and all three had increased fast activity. They concluded that the changes were probably metabolic. Thiebaut *et al.* (3, 4) stated that the "EEG was often valuable in assessing the extent and rate of progression of the pituitary adenoma."

ADRENALS

Addison's disease, Cushing's syndrome, and those states that result from the administration of ACTH and cortisone are frequently accompanied by psychiatric symptoms that range from mild to those of psychotic proportions. In Addison's disease, apathy, indifference, negativism, irritability, and emotional liability are common symptoms of the untreated milder forms. In the more severe forms depression, hallucinations, delusions, and asthenia may complicate the picture. In Cushing's syndrome, depression is again one of the most frequently encountered symptoms. Irritability, anxiety, and negativism may occur. Again the range of severity of the symptoms is great. With the administration of ACTH and cortisone, patients may have symptoms consisting of euphoria and well-being early in the course of treatment, whereas prolonged administration can result in symptoms of depression, irritability, and restlessness. Severe symptoms are deliroid reactions, often with hallucinations and delusions or manic behavior.

When one compares the clinical psychiatric syndromes associated with adrenal hyper- or hypofunction, there are striking similarities and dissimilarities. The same may be said for the EEG findings. In Addison's disease the EEG patterns are characterized by spontaneous bursts of slow waves (16, 18–22, 24, 26, 28, 29). These slow rhythms are bilaterally synchronous and in the theta and delta frequency range. The slowing, interestingly enough, does not correlate with blood glucose, sodium, or potassium levels. Sensitivity to hyperventilation is marked. Epileptic discharge does not occur. Normal EEGs are seen in 30 to 50 per cent of the cases. Glucocorticoids are more effective in restoring normal rhythms than are mineral corticoids.

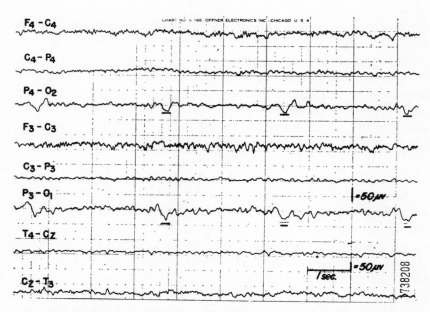

Figure 2. EEG of a 54-year-old patient with Addison's disease. Patient has severe hiccoughs producing rhythmic artifact (undetermined).

The findings in the few reported cases of Cushing's disease (**15, 24, 31, 32**) are more variable than those of Addison's disease. In a study of three patients Austt reported fast records in all. Trethowan and Cobb, on the other hand, observed normal records in two patients, but found intermittently slow and normal records in another patient, whose record was abnormal when mental symptoms were apparent. A fourth patient had slowing in all records. Glaser reported slowing as a concomitant of adrenal hyperfunction.

The administration of cortisone and ACTH has usually produced few changes in EEG patterns (**23, 25, 37, 30, 33, 34**). There is general agreement that if the EEG was normal before treatment, changes were not observed. On the other hand, if abnormal EEGs were seen before treatment, the effect of treatment was to improve the record, make it worse, or to produce no change. Pine *et al.* (**30**) reported normal EEGs in two patients who developed psychoses with treatment. Only Hoefer and Glaser (**27**) have reported a high incidence of abnormalities with ACTH, finding an increase or appearance of abnormalities in 13 of 15 patients. One patient with a psychosis had generalized slowing in the EEG.

To summarize, the usual EEG concomitants seen with alteration

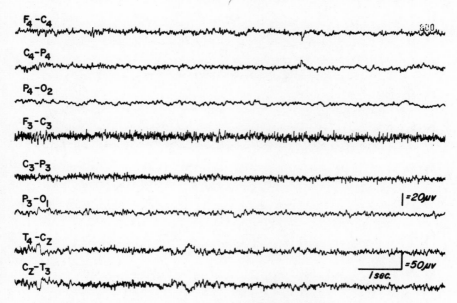

Figure 3. Low-voltage fast and slow EEG patterns in a patient with Cushing's syndrome.

of levels of adrenal hormones are bilaterally synchronous slow waves or the presence of normal rhythms. Patients with adrenal hypofunction are sensitive to hyperventilation. Epileptic discharge is seldom described. Focal abnormalities do not occur.

THYROID

Hyper- and hypothyroidism are frequently associated with psychiatric symptomatology. For the most part, these symptoms are determined by a change in affect. Depression is most commonly described, although elation may occur in hyperthyroidism. Loss of energy, apathy, irritability, psychomotor retardation, and easy fatiguability may occur in both myxedema and Grave's disease. On the other hand, many hyperthyroids have increased motor movements and hyperkinesis. Occasional cases may be elated and exhibit classical manic symptomatology. In severe and prolonged illnesses, patients may become delirious with both hyper- and hypofunction of the thyroid.

The electroencephalographic changes in myxedema (**2, 35, 36, 40, 43, 45**) are essentially those that are described for many endocrine diseases. Parieto-occipital rhythms are usually slow, often to

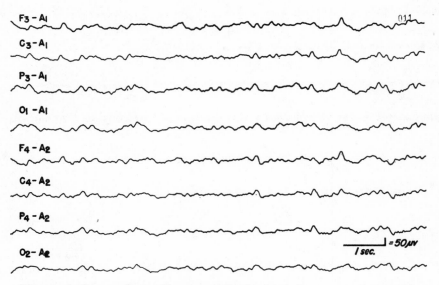

Figure 4. Low-voltage slow record obtained from a patient with myxedema coma.

the theta frequencies. Responses to hyperventilation are not marked, and all cerebral rhythms tend to be low voltage. In myxedema coma (4) the record may be that of low-voltage or moderate-voltage slow activity with delta and theta rhythms predominating. Thiebaut *et al.* (3), in a report of 13 adult cases of hypothyroidism, found some differences between the "adult congenital" and acquired forms of myxedema. Fast rhythms and central rhythms in the alpha frequency, the major differentiating findings, were more common in the acquired forms.

In hyperthyroidism (2, 38, 42, 46, 48, 50, 52) a number of reports have described slow rhythms as the major abnormalities seen. However, the EEG patterns may be quite variable, ranging from a predominantly low-voltage fast to a diffusely slow record. Vague (50) noted that the EEG was more likely to be characterized by slow rhythms if the patient was a young female. This impression was corroborated by Wilson and Johnson (51, 52), who demonstrated an increase in all abnormalities in young females. Males tended to have fewer and less severe abnormalities than young females, but post-menopausal females had the lowest incidence of abnormalities. Treatment with reserpine increased the degree of

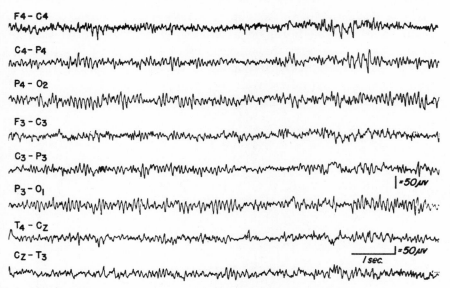

Figure 5. EEG of a patient with severe hyperthyroidism. Note diffuse slowing with increase in voltage and percent-time of beta activity. (RAI 55% in 24 hours and PBI > 20.)

abnormality in the EEG. Follow-up studies in patients treated with surgery or radioactive iodine have demonstrated a return of the EEG to normal usually within a period of three months. In an experimental study Milco (**42**) has reported that the EEGs of patients with hyperthyroidism become more abnormal rather promptly if the patient is given thyroxine.

Epileptic discharge has seldom been reported in hyperthyroidism. Skanse and Nyman (**47**) reported three patients with these abnormalities, and Milco (**42**) mentions its occurrence.

Congenital hypothyroidism (**37, 39, 41, 44, 49**) is accompanied by abnormal EEG records. The EEG patterns for the most part tend to be slow sinusoidal rhythms, usually of low voltage. With treatment, the EEG will return to a normal pattern, particularly if the mental development improves. In those instances where mental deficiency persists, however, the EEG most frequently remains abnormal. This point is graphically illustrated in a study by D'Avignon and Melin (**39**), who observed 22 cases that were diagnosed in the first three years of life. Four of seven patients with low I.Q.'s had abnormal records. Only three patients with normal intelligence had abnormal EEGs.

As a result of these observations we may summarize the EEG findings occurring in those clinical syndromes associated with deficiencies of thyroid hormone as consisting primarily of a slowing of the parieto-occipital frequencies, usually to the theta range, as well as an increase in the frequency of occurrence of delta rhythms with increasing central nervous system depression. Voltages of all rhythms tend to be low, and epileptic discharge is rare. Treatment of both myxedema and cretinism results in improvement or normalization of the EEG. Hyperthyroidism may also be accompanied by EEG slowing, but the slow rhythms are mixed with normal frequencies and normal EEG records may occur in a high percentage of patients. Abnormal records occur more frequently in young females than in older females or males. Photic responses are frequently potentiated. Epileptic discharges are seldom seen. Treatment results in restoration of normal EEG patterns.

PARATHYROID

Although diseases of the parathyroid gland rarely come under the care of the psychiatrist, they are worthy of mention, for mental deficiency is a common concomitant of long-standing hypoparathyroidism. Early cases may simulate anxiety reactions with hyperventilation attacks. The most common symptoms in hyperparathyroidism are weakness, poor appetite, loss of weight, fatigue, and apathy.

Most reports of electroencephalographic studies in parathyroid disease have been concerned with hypoparathyroidism. Indeed, the author was unable to find a single case of hyperparathyroidism reported in the literature. We will, therefore, review the literature relative to hypoparathyroidism, and in addition report two cases of hyperfunction of this gland.

In hypoparathyroidism the EEG is usually diffusely slow (**3, 53, 57, 59, 61**). In cases where tetany is manifest, the records are always slow. In adults the slow activity tends to be paroxysmal, whereas in children the background rhythms tend to be slowed. The EEGs in the chronic form of the disease have been reported to be abnormal in 80 per cent of the patients, even if tetany was not manifest at the time of the recording. Most authors comment on the sensitivity to hyperventilation, and sensitivity to photic stimulation has been reported. Epileptic discharges consisting of

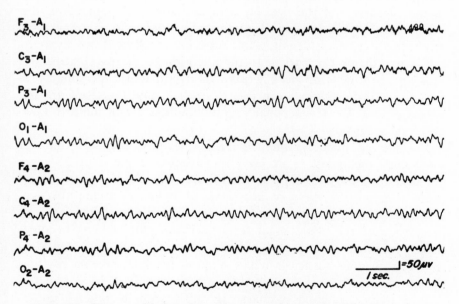

Figure 6. 67-year-old female with severe hyperparathyroidism secondary to a parathyroid adenoma. This record was obtained preoperatively.

spike and waves, spikes, and sharp waves have been observed in patients with hypocalcemia. In patients with normocalcemic tetany (58) the EEG is most often normal.

The EEG in hyperparathyroidism may also be abnormal. As there were no immediate available references, we have included observations on some cases seen in our laboratory. Both of the two patients reported here had abnormal EEGs, the background rhythms being slowed to the lower limit of normal in one and to the theta frequency in the other. In both cases there was bilaterally synchronous slowing. The one patient with a parathyroid adenoma had improvement of the EEG after operation. The alpha rhythm increased in frequency, and the bilaterally synchronous activity disappeared.

HYPOGLYCEMIA, INSULIN-SHOCK THERAPY, AND DIABETES

Reduction of the blood sugar levels to a value below 30 mgm per cent will almost always produce changes in the function of the central nervous system. The outstanding change that takes place is in the sensorium of the patient, with alterations of perception, disorientation, delirium, stupor, and finally coma. In some clinical syndromes, gross disturbances of behavior resulting from hypoglycemia may bring the patient to the attention of the psychiatrist.

Although much has been written in regard to the personality of the diabetic, the findings are poorly defined, and therefore are not included here. Electroencephalographic findings are of interest, however, and are reviewed.

In induced hypoglycemia, the EEG usually becomes diffusely slow when the blood sugar level drops below a mean of 35 mgm per cent (66, 67, 69, 73, 75, 79, 83, 86, 87). At the critical level the first abnormalities seen are those of bursts of bilaterally synchronous slowing in the theta frequency. The alpha rhythm may be preserved. As the blood sugar level decreases, the slowing becomes more prominent with a higher index of occurrence and a gradual shift to slower frequencies. When coma is reached, normal rhythms are absent, and the cerebral rhythms are characterized by continuous delta activity. Epileptic discharge is rarely seen in patients undergoing insulin-coma therapy, although it has been described in patients with islet cell tumors and in functional hypoglycemic attacks (66,

74). Erwin and Wilson (**70**) have recently reported small epileptic spikes on the lateral surfaces of the temporal lobe in some patients undergoing insulin-coma therapy. No epileptic discharge was seen in recordings from the nasopharyngeal electrodes.

Repeated episodes of induced hypoglycemia (insulin coma) rarely gave rise to changes in the EEG after treatment had been terminated (**86**. Patients with protracted coma have been observed with serial EEGs. The patterns are usually markedly slow in spite of high blood sugar levels. The delta and theta activity gradually disappears in three or more days (**80, 82**).

The EEGs of patients with islet cell adenomas of the pancreas are often abnormal (**62, 77, 85**). This is particularly true when the patient is hypoglycemic, although the record may remain abnormal even when blood sugar levels are returned to normal. Hoefer (**77**), in his report of 27 cases, observed diffuse slowing and "suggestive" convulsive spike-and-wave bursts.

In functional hypoglycemic attacks associated with "dumping syndromes" the EEG may be abnormal (**63**). The hypoglycemia usually follows ingestion of food. During the hypoglycemia psychiatric symptoms and diffusely abnormal EEGs are observed. Oper-

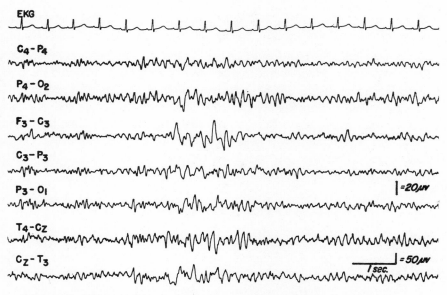

Figure 7. EEG obtained from patient with induced hypoglycemia. Blood glucose level was 19.1 mgm%.

ative revision of the gastrojejeunostomy may result in a relief of symptoms. Idiopathic functional hypoglycemia may also be associated with diffusely abnormal EEG records (**65**, **81**).

The EEGs of patients with diabetes are frequently observed to be abnormal (**68**, **76**). Izzo *et al.* (**78**) have reported abnormal EEGs in their series of 81 patients. Twenty-one per cent had slow records, 14 per cent had records which were both fast and slow, and another 26 per cent unusually had fast records. Thus, 61 per cent of the series had abnormal EEGs. Fabrykant (**71**) has reported a high incidence of abnormal EEGs in "brittle" diabetics and observed improvement in the EEG and control of patient's hypoglycemic attacks when Dilantin was administered. Wilson (**84**) corroborated these findings.

PHEOCHROMOCYTOMA

Hyperfunction of the adrenal medulla as a result of tumor of the chromaffin cells may give rise to symptoms of anxiety difficult to differentiate from the anxiety of psychiatric disease. The patient may have paroxysmal attacks of palpitation, precordial pain, severe headache, dizziness, sweating, weakness, vomiting, and an increase in blood pressure.

The EEG findings in the six patients in the literature indicate that the patterns are usually slow (**88**, **92**, **94**). Two patients have had unequivocally abnormal records with diffuse delta waves, two have had slight slowing, and two have been reported to have normal records. As a result of the relatively few observations reported, it was of interest that Rothballer (**93**) has recently reviewed the literature relative to the effect of epinephrine and norepinephrine on the EEG when this was administered to a normal subject. His review indicated that no specific changes are observed, either with intramuscular or intravenous injection of the two drugs.

THE TESTES AND THE OVARIES

Although there are a few animal studies in which the effects of testosterone on the electrical activity of the brain have been investigated, the author has been unable to find any references to studies of the influence of this hormone on the human EEG.

The influence of gonadotrophic, androgenic, and ovarian hormones have been reported. In a series of reports of pathologic and normal endocrine states Faure *et al.* (**96, 98**) described the following changes: (1) rhythmic discharges in bursts as a result of increase secretion of FSH, (2) bursts of rhythmical waves with increased 17-ketosteroids, (3) disorganization of the EEG patterns with 11-oxysteroid increases, and (4) fast patterns with increases of progesterone. They concluded that the EEG changes correlate well with the hormonal imbalance rather than the clinical syndrome.

Normal hormonal changes occurring during the menstrual cycle have been correlated with the EEG by Dusser de Barenne and Gibbs (**95**). In 11 normal women they reported shifts in the frequency of the order of 1/4 to 1 cycle per second in all cases over a 24-hour period. The timing and magnitude of the shifts suggested a relationship to the menstrual cycle in 7 of 11 cases. The onset of menstruation was followed by slowing in 9 of the 11 cases, while shifts in frequency possibly related to ovulation occurred in the mid-menstrual period in 8 of the 11 cases. They concluded that a simple rigid relationship between the menstrual cycle and the electrical activity of the cortex did not exist. Ulett (**99**), in a study of premenstrual tension, was unable to demonstrate a correlation of the EEG with symptoms. Lindsley (**100**) reported a variability of the EEG during a period of one to two weeks in the middle of the menstrual cycle.

Loiseau *et al.* (**102**) have reported dysrhythmic EEGs in the menopause. The disturbances were usually seen in the basal and temporal areas.

Although not pertinent to this discussion, it is of interest that progesterone seems to have an inhibiting effect on epileptic discharge, while estrogens have an excitatory effect (**101**). The effects of an estrogenic substance (Premarin) were independent of metabolic changes.

In hypothalamic amenorrhea the EEG was abnormal in 14 of 26 cases (**103**). Four of the patients were observed to have atypical spike-and-wave discharges.

METABOLIC DISEASE

Since many diseases in general medicine are accompanied by disturbances of metabolism, we have restricted our discussion to a few diseases that may be of interest to the psychiatrist. These are:

1. Hepato-lenticular degeneration.
2. Phenylpyruvic acid oligophrenia.
3. Familial periodic paralysis.
4. Porphyria.
5. Infantile Tay-Sach's disease.
6. Cerebral lipidosis.

In hepato-lenticular degeneration the EEG may be abnormal (117). The EEG findings were reported in nine patients, five with normal EEGs, two having borderline records with irregular runs of intermediate slow activity in the frontal and central regions, and two having grossly abnormal records with slow waves in the occipital region at one cycle per second. In one case a generalized slow wave abnormality occurred at 3 to 6 cycles per second. This seemed to be lateralized.

In phenylpyruvic acid oligophrenia the EEG is most often abnormal. In a survey of 19 patients Fois *et al.* (107) reported that the waking record was usually abnormal, being either slightly fast or slightly slow, or a mixture of the two. Eighteen of the 19 patients were observed to have epileptic discharge while asleep. Three-per-second spike-and-wave discharges were the most common abnormalities seen.

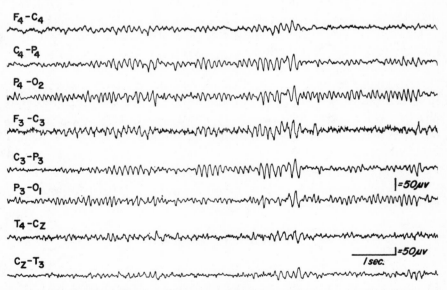

Figure 8. Mild abnormalities occurring in patient recovering from the acute symptoms of porphyria.

Several cases of familial periodic paralysis have been reported (**108, 112, 114, 115, 118**). In general, the EEG is little changed during an attack. Slow waves of 6 to 7 per second are observed mostly in the temporal region during the attack. These are not present after the attack.

The EEG in porphyria is often abnormal. In a recent report of two cases Sikes (**116**) observed generalized slowing in one case in the theta frequencies. These were of increased voltage and were accentuated by hyperventilation. A second case that was remitting showed similar but less severe changes. Sikes reviewed the literature and found six other cases in which the EEG changes consisted of generalized slowing with occasional localized abnormalities. In those reports where patients were studied in remission, the EEG often was normal. Olmstead (**111**) reported one case with generalized slowing. Since the review of Dow (**105**) three other cases have been reported. The findings were again similar to those reported by others.

In Tay-Sachs disease the EEG is abnormal (**113**). The usual changes consist of a mixed fast and slow dysrhythmia with high-voltage triphasic waves, occasionally of spike form.

Patients with cerebral lipidosis (**104**) have been reported to have generalized, irregular, recurring transients, usually triphasic, appearing on a background of generalized high-voltage slow waves. The two components bear no constant relationship.

SUMMARY

It appears that slow waves are the most common abnormalities seen in endocrinopathies and metabolic disorders. In endocrinopathies they occur both with hypo- and hypersecretion of the various glands affected. Epileptic discharges are not usually seen with endocrinopathies. In metabolic disease epileptic discharge is frequent in phenylpyruvic acid oligophrenia.

The dearth of information available relative to EEG findings in some endocrinopathies and metabolic diseases indicates a great need for further clinical investigative effort.

BIBLIOGRAPHY

General

1. Condon, J. V., Becka, D. R., and Gibbs, F. A. Electroencephalographic abnormalities in endocrine disease. *New Engl. J. Med.* **251**: 638–641, 1954.

2. Rohmer, F., Wackenheim, A., and Kurtz, D. L'E.E.G. dans les syndromes endo-crininiens: Hypophysaires, thyroidiens, surrénaux et dans la tétanie de l'adulte. *Rev. neurol.* **100**: 297–314, 1959.
3. Thiebaut, F., Rohmer, F., and Wackenheim, A. Contribution a l'étude électroencé-phalographique des syndromes endocriniens. *Electroenceph. clin. Neurophysiol.* **10**: 1–30, 1958.
4. Thiebaut, F., Rohmer, F., and Wackenheim, A. Contribution to the electroence-phalographic study of endocrine syndromes. *Electroenceph. clin. Neurophysiol.* **8**: 173, 1956.

Pituitary

5. Austt, E. G., and Mussio Fournier, J.-C. Étude encéphalographique de l'acromégalie. *Presse Med.* **59**: 645, 1951.
6. Boselli, F., and Jefferson, A. A. Electroencephalogram with chromophobe adenomata and Rathke pouch cysts: Modification by associated metabolic disorder. *Electro-enceph. clin. Neurophysiol.* **9**: 275–290, 1957.
7. Cloche, R., and Stuhl, L. EEG aspects in some cases of global anterior hypophyseal insufficiency. *Electroenceph. clin. Neurophysiol.* **10**: 759, 1958.
8. Heidrich, R., and Schmidt-Matthias, H. Encephalographische Befunde bei Anorexia Nervosa. *Arch. Psychiat. Nervenkr.* **202**: 183–201, 1961.
9. Hughes, R. R., and Summers, V. K. Changes in the electroencephalogram associated with hypopituitarism due to post-partum necrosis. *Electroenceph. clin. Neurophysiol.* **8**: 87–96, 1956.
10. Kennedy, J. M., Thomson, A. P., and Whitfield, I. C. Coma and electroencephalo-graphic changes in hypopituitarism. *Lancet.* **269**: 907–908, 1955.
11. Krump, J. E. Die klinische und differential-diagnostische Bedeutung des elektro-encephalogramms beim Sheehansyndrom. *Symposium der deutschen Gesellschaft für Endocrinologia.* **4**: 111–133, 1957.
12. Martin, F. Pathologie des aspects neurologiques et psychiatriques dans quelques manifestations carentielles avec troubles digestifs et neuro-endocriniens: II. Études des altérations du système nerveux central dans deux cas d'anorexie survenue chez la jeune fille (dite anorexie mentale). *Helv. Med. Acta.* **22**: 522–529, 1955.
13. Salmon, H. A. Case of hypopituitary coma with serial electroencephalography. *Brit. med. J.* **1**: 1397–1399, 1956.
14. Tonnis, W., Steinmann, H-W., and Krenkel, W. Elektroencephalographische Befunde bei 44 Tumoren der Sellagegend. *Acta Neuroveg.* **5**: 291–305, 1953.

Adrenals

15. Austt, E. G. (Jr.), Torrents, E., and Mussio Fournier, J.-C. The electroencephalo-gram in Cushing's syndrome. *Electroenceph. clin. Neurophysiol.* **2**: 103, 1950.
16. Azerad, E., and Cloche, R. L'électro-encéphalographie des Addisonniens. *Sem. Hop. Paris.* **26**: 3150–3151, 1950.
17. Bricaire, H., Misès, R., Dreyfus-Brisac, C., and Fischgold, H. Initiation a l'électro-encéphalographie E.E.G. d'un cas de maladie d'Addison. *Presse Med.* **61**: 750–751, 1953.
18. Cleghorn, R. A. Adrenal cortical insufficiency: Psychological and neurological observations. *Canad. Med. Ass. J.* **65**: 449–454, 1951.
19. DeCastro, P., Sacristan, J. M., and Van T'Hoff, R. G. Some aspects of the EEG in Addison's disease in connection with a possible mesodiencephalic involvement. *Electroenceph. clin. Neurophysiol.* **6**: 530, 1954.
20. Dreyfus-Brisac, C., and Misès, R. Étude E.E.G. de 28 addisoniens. *Rev. neurol.* **87**: 468–470, 1952.
21. Engel, G. L., and Margolin, S. G. Neuropsychiatric disturbances in Addison's disease and role of impaired carbohydrate metabolism in production of abnormal cerebral function. *Arch. Neurol. Psychiat.* **45**: 881–884, 1941.
22. Engel, G. L., and Margolin, S. G. Neuropsychiatric disturbances in internal disease: Metabolic factors and electroencephalographic correlations. *Arch. intern. Med.* **70**: 236–259, 1942.
23. Freidlander, W. J., and Rottger, E. The effect of cortisone on the electroencephalo-gram. *Electroenceph. clin. Neurophysiol.* **3**: 311–313, 1951.
24. Glaser, G. H. EEG activity and adrenal-cortical dysfunction. *Electroenceph. clin. Neurophysiol.* **10**: 366, 1958.

25. Glaser, G. H., Kornfeld, D. S., and Knight, R. P. Intravenous hydrocortisone, corticotropin and the electroencephalogram. *Arch. Neurol. Psychiat.* **73**: 338–344, 1955.
26. Hernandex Peniche, J. El electroencefalograma en la enfermedad de Addison. *Rev. Invest. Clin.* **5**: 439–444, 1953.
27. Hoefer, P. F. A., and Glaser, G. H. Effects of pituitary adrenocorticotrophic hormone (ACTH) therapy. *J. Amer. Med. Ass.* **143**: 620–624, 1950.
28. Hoffman, W. C., Lewis, R. A., and Thorn, G. W. The electroencephalogram in Addison's disease. *Bull. Johns Hopkins Hosp.* **70**: 335–361, 1942.
29. Jefferson, A. A clinical correlation between encephalopathy and papilloedema in Addison's disease. *J. Neurol. Neurosurg. Psychiat.* **19**: 21–27, 1956.
30. Pine, I., Engel, F. L., and Schwartz, T. B. The electroencephalogram in ACTH and cortisone treated patients. *Electroenceph. clin. Neurophysiol.* **3**: 301–310, 1951.
31. Sanabra, F. R. Aspectos electroencefalográficos del síndrome de Cushing. *Bol. Inst. Patol. Med.* **10**: 211–215, 1955.
32. Trethowan, W. H., and Cobb, S. Neuropsychiatric aspects of Cushing's syndrome. *Arch. Neurol. Psychiat.* **67**: 283–309, 1952.
33. Wayne, H. L. Convulsive seizures complicating cortisone and ACTH therapy: Clinical and electroencephalographic observations. *J. clin. Endocr.* **14**: 1039–1045, 1954.
34. Wayne, H. L., and Boyle, J. Electroencephalographic observations on patients undergoing cortisone and ACTH therapy. *J. clin. Endocr.* **13**: 1070–1081, 1953.

Thyroid

35. Bertrand, I., Delay, J., and Guillain, J. L'électroencéphalogramme dans le myxodème. *C. R. Soc. Biol.* **129**: 395–398, 1938.
36. Browning, T. B., Atkins, R. W., and Weiner, H. Cerebral metabolic disturbances in hypothyroidism: Clinical and electroencephalographic studies of the psychosis of myxedema and hypothyroidism. *Arch. intern. Med.* **93**: 938–950, 1954.
37. Chaptal, J., Passouant, P., Jean, R., Cadilhac, J., and Carli, N. La souffrance cérébrale dans le myxoedème de l'enfant: Étude électro-encephalographique. *Presse Med.* **64**: 2257–2258, 1956.
38. Condon, J. V., Becka, D. R., and Gibbs, F. A. Electroencephalographic abnormalities in hyperthyroidism. *J. clin. Endocr.* **14**: 1511–1518, 1954.
39. D'Avignon, M., and Melin, K.-A. The electroencephalogram in congenital hypothyreosis. *Acta Paediat.* (Stockholm). **38**: 37–44, 1949.
40. Guillain, G., Bertrand, I., Delay, J., and Guillain, J. Les anomalies de l'électroencéphalogramme dans le myxoedème. *Bull. Soc. Med. Hop. Paris.* **54**: 1610–1617, 1938.
41. Mai, V. H., and Schaper, G. Beitrag zur Klinik der Hypothyreose. Studie über die nach langdauernder Thyreoidinbehandlung erreichte Intelligenz und über das Verhalten des Hirnstrombildes. *Ann. Paediat.* (Basel). **180**: 65–97, 1953.
42. Milco, M., Brosteano, E., Nicolesco-Catargi, A., and Ionesco, B. Electroencephalographic studies in Grave's disease. *Electroenceph. clin. Neurophysiol.* **8**: 731, 1956.
43. Nieman, E. A. The electroencephalogram in congenital hypothyroidism: A study of 10 cases. *J. Neurol. Neurosurg. Psychiat.* **24**: 50–57, 1961.
44. Nieman, E. A. The electroencephalogram in myxoedema coma: Clinical and electroencephalographic study of three cases. *Brit. med. J.* **1**: 1204–1208, 1959.
45. Passouant, P., Cadilhac, J., and Jean, R. The differences in electroencephalographic abnormalities of two forms of myxoedema in childhood, one due to thyroid insufficiency, the other to a cerebral disorder. *Electroenceph. clin. Neurophysiol.* **9**: 368–369, 1957.
46. Ross, D. A., and Schwab, R. S. The cortical alpha rhythm in thyroid disorders. *Endocrinology.* **25**: 75–79, 1939.
47. Skanse, B., and Nyman, G. E. Thyrotoxicosis as a cause of cerebral dysrhythmia and convulsive seizures. *Acta Endocr.* **22**: 246–263, 1956.
48. Theibaut, F., Rohmer, F., Wackenheim, A., and Kurtz, D. Les données E.E.G. dans les hyperthyroidies secondaires. *Presse Med.* **66**: 1323–1326, 1958.
49. Topper, A. Mental achievement of congenitally hypothyroid children: A follow-up study of twenty cases. *Amer. J. Dis. Child.* **81**: 233–249, 1951.
50. Vague, J., Gastaut, H., Codaccioni, J. L., and Roger, A. L'électroencéphalographie des maladies thyroidiennes. *Ann. Endocr.* **18**: 996–1009, 1957.
51. Wilson, W. P., and Johnson, J. E. Clinical laboratory and electroencephalographic correlations in hyperthyroidism. *South. med. J.* **53**: 606–610, 1960.
52. Wilson, W. P., and Johnson, J. E. Thyroid hormone and brain function. I. The EEG

in hyperthyroidism with observations on the effect of age, sex, and reserpine in the production of abnormalities. *Electroenceph. clin. Neurophysiol.* **16**: 321–328, 1964.

Parathyroid

53. Dickson, L. G., Morita, Y., Cowsert, E. J., Graves, J., and Meyer, J. S. Neurological electroencephalographic, and heredo-familial aspects of pseudohypoparathyroidism and pseudo-pseudohypoparathyroidism. *J. Neurol. Neurosurg. Psychiat.* **23**: 33–39, 1960.
54. Glaser, G. W., and Levy, L. Seizures and idiopathic hypoparathyroidism. A clinical-electroencephalographic study. *Epilepsia.* **1**: 454–465, 1960.
55. Gotta, H., and Odoriz, J. B. The electroencephalogram in hypoparathyroidism with tetany and epilepsy. *J. clin. Endocr.* **8**: 674–686, 1948.
56. Hanstead, C., and Brandt, S. Electroencephalographic changes in siblings with hypocalcemia due to hypoparathyroidism. *Electroenceph. clin. Neurophysiol.* **5**: 101–104, 1953.
57. Klotz, H.-P. Épilepsie et tétanie chroniques. *Rev. neurol.* **92**: 254–269, 1955.
58. Nevsimal, O., and Roth, B. EEG studies of 89 cases of normocalcemic tetany. *Electroenceph. clin. Neurophysiol.* **11**: 181, 1959.
59. Odoriz, J. B., del Castillo, E. B., Manfredi, J. F., and de la Balze, F. A. Parathyroid insufficiency and the human electroencephalogram. *J. clin. Endocr.* **4**: 493–499, 1944.
60. Roth, B., and Nevsimal, O. EEG study of 42 cases of hypocalcemic tetany. *Electroenceph. clin. Neurophysiol.* **11**: 181, 1959.
61. Solomon, S., and Fine, D. The precipitation of seizures by photic stimulation in a patient with hypoparathyroidism. *J. nerv. ment. Dis.* **130**: 253–260, 1960.

Hypoglycemia, Pancreas, and Diabetes

62. Alajouanine, T., Nehlil, J., Contamin, F., Cathala, H.-P., and Cloarec. Encéphalopathie hypoglycémique par adénome Langerhansien probable disparition des troubles sous l'effet de la corticothérapie. *Rev. neurol.* **100**: 3–13, 1959.
63. Belding, W. L., and Freedman, D. A. Postprandial hypoglycemia presenting as a neurologic problem. *Neurology.* **10**: 613–618, 1960.
64. Boudin, G., Lauras, A., and Labet, R. Les encéphalopathies des hypoglycémies spontanées (Revue analytique de 37 cas à propos d'une observation personnelle): I. Étude clinique. *Presse Med.* **68**: 270–272, 1960.
65. Boudin, G., Lauras, A., and Labet, R. Les encéphalopathies des hypoglycémies spontanées: II. Étude électroéncephalographique. *Presse Med.* **68**: 321–324, 1960.
66. Brandt, S. Epilepsy and spontaneous hypoglycemia in children. *Electroenceph. clin. Neurophysiol.* **9**: 735, 1957.
67. Chamberlain, G. A. A., and Lyketaos, G. Relationship between insulin coma threshold of schizophrenic patients and their resting E.E.G.s. *J. ment. Sci.* **98**: 122–129, 1952.
68. Ellenberg, M., and Pollack, H. Convulsive states in diabetes. *Amer. J. med. Sci.* **214**: 503–506, 1947.
69. Engel, R., Halberg, F., Tichy, F. Y., and Dow, R. Electrocerebral activity and epileptic attacks at various blood sugar levels (with a case report). *Acta Neuroveg.* **9**: 147–167, 1954.
70. Erwin, C. W., and Wilson, W. P. Unpublished observations.
71. Fabrykant, M. Further studies on electrocerebral dysfunction and the use of anticonvulsants in labile diabetes. *Ann. intern. Med.* **38**: 814–823, 1953.
72. Fister, W. P. Serial EEG and clinical follow-up studies of a prolonged coma insulin reaction. *Electroenceph. clin. Neurophysiol.* **5**: 474, 1953.
73. Funderburk, W. H., and Bauman, J. C. The effect of repeated insulin coma on the electroencephalogram. *Electroenceph. clin. Neurophysiol.* **4**: 116–117, 1952.
74. Gibbs, F. A., and Murray, E. L. Hypoglycemic convulsions (Three case reports). *Electroenceph. clin. Neurophysiol.* **6**: 674–678, 1954.
75. Goldring, S., Ulett, G., O'Leary, J., and Greditzer, A. Initial survey of slow potential changes obtained under resting conditions and incident to convulsive therapy. *Electroenceph. clin. Neurophysiol.* **2**: 297–308, 1950.
76. Greenblatt, M., Murray, J., and Root, H. F. Electroencephalographic studies in diabetes mellitus. *New Engl. J. Med.* **234**: 119–121, 1946.
77. Hoefer, P. F. A. Neurological and EEG manifestations in hyperinsulinism. *Electroenceph. clin. Neurophysiol.* **10**: 366, 1958.
78. Izzo, J. L., Schuster, D. B., and Engel, G. L. The electroencephalogram of patients with diabetes mellitus. *Electroenceph. clin. Neurophysiol.* **4**: 380, 1952.

79. Regan, P. F., and Browne-Mayers, A. N. Electroencephalography, frequency analysis, and consciousness. A correlation during insulin-induced hypoglycemia. *J. nerv. ment. Dis.* **124**: 142–147, 1956.
80. Revitch, E. Observations on organic brain damage and clinical improvement following protracted insulin coma. *Psychiat. Quart.* **28**: 72–92, 1954.
81. Ross, I. S., and Loeser, L. H. Electroencephalographic findings in essential hypoglycemia. *Electroenceph. clin. Neurophysiol.* **3**: 141–148, 1951.
82. Shagass, C., and Rowsell, P. W. Serial electroencephalographic and clinical studies in a case of prolonged insulin coma. *Arch. Neurol. Psychiat.* **72**: 705–711, 1954.
83. Tchondnovski, V. S. Dynamics of bioelectric modifications of cerebral activity in schizophrenic patients undergoing insulin therapy. *Neuropat. Psikhiat.* (Moskva). **58**: 1079–1089, 1958.
84. Wilson, D. R. Electroencephalographic studies in diabetes mellitus. *Canad. Med. Ass. J.* **65**: 462–465, 1951.
85. Wyke, B. D. Brain function and blood sugar: Observations based on a case of islet cell adenoma of the pancreas. *Electroenceph. clin. Neurophysiol.* **4**: 339–350, 1952.
86. Yeager, C. L., Simon, A., Margolis, L. H., and Burch, N. R. Electroencephalographic studies in post-hypoglycemic coma. *J. nerv. ment. Dis.* **118**: 435–441, 1953.
87. Ziegler, D. K., and Presthus, J. Normal electroencephalogram at deep levels of hypoglycemia. *Electroenceph. clin. Neurophysiol.* **9**: 523–526, 1957.

Pheochromocytoma

88. Apter, N. S., Halstead, W. C., Alving, A. S., Talso, P. J., and Case, T. J. Alterations of cerebral functions in pheochromocytoma. *Neurology.* **1**: 283–292, 1951.
89. Bruce, G. M. Ocular fundus in pheochromocytoma of adrenal gland; report of 3 cases. *Trans. Amer. Ophthal. Soc.* **45**: 201–228, 1947.
90. Guarneri, V., and Evans, J. A. Pheochromocytoma: Report of a case, with a new diagnostic test. *Amer. J. Med.* **4**: 806–813, 1948.
91. Mortell, E. J., and Whittle, J. P. Pheochromocytoma: Case report with certain observations on the pathologic physiology. *J. clin. Endocr.* **5**: 396–402, 1945.
92. Raab, W., and Smithwick, R. H. Pheochromocytoma with hypothalamic manifestations and excessive hypermetabolism: A case report. *J. clin. Endocr.* **9**: 782–790, 1949.
93. Rothballer, A. B. The effects of catecholamines on the central nervous system. *Pharm. Rev.* **11**: 494–547, 1959.
94. Spatt, S. D., and Grayzel, D. M. Pheochromocytoma of the adrenal medulla: A clinico-pathological study of five cases. *Amer. J. med. Sci.* **216**: 39–50, 1948.

Testes and Ovaries

95. DeBarenne, D. D., and Gibbs, F. A. Variations in the electroencephalogram during the menstrual cycle. *Amer. J. Obstet. Gynec.* **44**: 687–690, 1942.
96. Faure, J., Guérin, A., Loiseau, P., Dutertre, F., Got, M., and Pressy, J. Critical EEG study in women suffering from gynecological disorders. *Electroenceph. clin. Neurophysiol.* **10**: 760, 1958.
97. Faure, J., and Loiseau, P. The electroencephalogram in menstrual disturbances. *Electroenceph. clin. Neurophysiol.* **9**: 364, 1957.
98. Faure, J., Magendie, J., Boussemart, E., and Masquelier, M. A comparison of the EEG with hormonal changes in female patients. *Electroenceph. clin. Neurophysiol.* **8**: 172–173, 1956.
99. Lamb, W. M., Ulett, G. A., Masters, W. H., and Robinson, D. W. Premenstrual tension: EEG, hormonal, and psychiatric evaluation. *Amer. J. Psychiat.* **109**: 840–848, 1953.
100. Lindsley, D. B., and Rubenstein, B. B. Relationship between brain potentials and some other physiological variables. *Proc. Soc. Exp. Biol. Med.* **35**: 558–563, 1937.
101. Logothetis, J., Harner, R., Morrelli, F., and Torres, F. The role of estrogens in catamenial exacerbation of epilepsy. *Neurology.* **9**: 352–360, 1959.
102. Loiseau, P., Dutertre, F., Guérin, A., des Termes, H. and Faure, J. Epilepsy and menopause. *Electroenceph. clin. Neurophysiol.* **10**: 759–760, 1958.
103. Rohmer, F., Gandar, R., Wackenheim, A., and Hollaender, A. Electroencephalographic study of hypothalamic amenorrhea. *Electroenceph. clin. Neurophysiol.* **8**: 730–731, 1956.

Metabolic Diseases

104. Cobb, W. A., Martin, F., and Pampiglione, G. The EEG in cerebral lipidosis. *Electroenceph. clin. Neurophysiol.* **4**: 110, 1952.
105. Dow, R. S. The electroencephalographic findings in acute intermittent porphyria. *Electroenceph. clin. Neurophysiol.* **13**: 425–437, 1961.
106. Duran, P., Vailke, J., Judeau, P., Juillet, P., Bernot, J., and Gilbert, J. Alterations importantes du tracé électroencéphalographique dans un cas de porphyrie aiguë traité par la chlorpromazine. *Rev. neurol.* **92**: 624–627, 1955.
107. Fois, A., Rosenberg, C., and Gibbs, F. A. The electroencephalogram in phenylpyruvic oligophrenia. *Electroenceph. clin. Neurophysiol.* **7**: 569–572, 1955.
108. Hammes, E. M. Periodic paralysis: A report of three cases. *J. Amer. Med. Ass.* **146**: 1401–1405, 1951.
109. Jung, R. Physiologische Untersuchungen bei der familiaren paroxysmalen Lahmung. III *Congr. Neurol. Int.*, Copenhagen, p. 291, 1939.
110. Livingston, S. Correlation of EEG changes with clinical results observed in the treatment of epilepsy with the ketogenic diet. *Electroenceph. clin. Neurophysiol.* **3**: 371–372, 1951.
111. Olmstead, E. G. The neuropsychiatric aspects of abnormal porphyrin metabolism: A clinical study. *J. nerv. ment. Dis.* **117**: 300–309, 1953.
112. Pudenz, R. H., McIntosh, J. F., and McEachern, D. The role of potassium in familial periodic paralysis. *J. Amer. Med. Ass.* **111**: 2253–2258, 1938.
113. Rosenbaum, H. E., and Stein, J. M. EEG findings in infantile Tay-Sachs disease. *Electroenceph. clin. Neurophysiol.* **5**: 603–605, 1953.
114. Saunders, M. G. Electroencephalographic findings in a case of familial periodic paralysis with hypopotassemia. *Electroenceph. clin. Neurophysiol.* **6**: 499–501, 1954.
115. Schwartz, W. B., and Relman, A. S. Metabolic and renal studies in chronic potassium depletion resulting from overuse of laxatives. *J. clin. Invest.* **32**: 258–271, 1953.
116. Sikes, Z. S. Electroencephalographic abnormalities and psychiatric manifestations in intermittent porphyria. *Dis. nerv. Syst.* **21**: 226–229, 1960.
117. Stephens, J. W. The EEG in hepato-lenticular degeneration. *Electroenceph. clin. Neurophysiol.* **3**: 524, 1951.
118. Watson, C. W. Familial periodic paralysis: Report of a case showing no changes in serum potassium level with a description of electroencephalographic findings. *Yale J. biol. Med.* **19**: 127–135, 1946.

THE ELECTROENCEPHALOGRAM IN ALCOHOLISM, TOXIC PSYCHOSES, AND INFECTION

Robert L. Green, Jr., M.D.

Next to brain injuries, the most frequent causes of cerebral dysrhythmia are alcohol, drugs, and infection. A review of articles published during the last three decades indicates that electroencephalographic studies have already proved valuable in increasing our knowledge of these conditions, and hold promise of becoming still greater aids to diagnosis, prognosis, and therapy.

ALCOHOLISM

According to John A. Lewis (35), the annual expenditure for alcoholic beverages in this country exceeds the entire national expenditure for education. Yet the economic impact of this type of spending is minor when compared with the total cost of maintaining medical facilities, social agencies, and judicial bodies to deal with the large segment of our population who tend to abuse this ancient medicinal. Twelve thousand deaths each year are attributed to chronic alcoholism and its related complications. It has been stated that there are in this country approximately five million chronic alcoholics. Among the nations of the world, however, the United States is ranked *fourth* in the rate of alcoholism by the Committee on Alcoholism of the World Health Organization.

The problem is not a modern one. Noah was the first known inebriate, and the drinking of wine is mentioned numerous times in the Bible, sometimes with approval and sometimes with disapproval.

There is no common agreement concerning the etiology of alcoholism, and modern neuropsychiatric therapy is relatively ineffective in treating the alcoholic in the community. The best hope for this group of patients lies in Alcoholics Anonymous, an organization

123

made up of approximately 160,000 alcoholics throughout the world, most of them in the United States. The success of this mode of treatment depends on the understanding one alcoholic has for another, and on the earnest desire of the patient to obtain help.

Psychiatry still has a role to play, however, in the management of the acute and chronic syndromes secondary to the excessive use of alcohol. The most common of these are: (1) acute intoxication; (2) delirium tremens; (3) seizures; (4) hallucinosis; (5) pathologic intoxication; (6) emotional disturbances, characterized primarily by severe anxiety or depression; and (7) metabolic alterations with and without physical debility. The unusual sensitivity of the nerve cell to alcohol indicates that the nervous system is involved in these syndromes, and suggests the desirability of electroencephalographic investigation. The following is an attempt to summarize the EEG findings in alcoholism and its most frequent complicating syndromes.

Acute Intoxication

Victor and Adams (50) have devised a table of toxic symptoms which correlate with specific levels of alcohol in the blood. At 10 mg per 100 cc (10 mg per cent) the subject has a feeling that his mind is clearing. At 20 mg per cent, he experiences dizziness, a general feeling of physical well-being, and a feeling tone of pleasantness. At 30 mg per cent the feeling tone changes to mild euphoria, worries disappear, and time passes quickly. At 40 mg per cent energy increases, and the subject becomes boisterous and loquacious. At 50 mg per cent normal inhibitions are lost, feelings of omnipotence are common, and the individual begins to show incoordination. At 70 mg per cent there is increasing lack of coordination and a feeling of remoteness. At 100 mg per cent gross incoordination leads to a staggering gait, and feelings of drowsiness are noted. At 200 mg per cent the subject needs help to walk, frequently has amnesia, and is easily angered. A level of 300 mg per cent is associated with stupor, and 400 mg per cent with coma. This correlation is valid only for non-alcoholic subjects whose blood alcohol level rises steadily over a period of approximately two hours.

Although Victor and Adams did not attempt to correlate electroencephalographic changes with the toxic symptoms of alcohol ingestion, the observations of Davis et al. (9) and of Engel and Rosenbaum (13) suggest that a correlation could be established. In 13 subjects studied by these two groups of investigators, the induction of acute alcoholic intoxication was associated with progressive slowing of the brain waves. The degree of slowing proved to be a more reliable index of intoxication than the development of any particular wave frequency. A change of 2 to 3 cycles per second in mean frequency was a sign of gross intoxication. Engel and Rosenbaum also observed that subjects with a fast or fast normal preintoxication record had a frequency distribution within the normal range during gross intoxication. With recovery, the EEG returned to the preintoxication status. The EEG correlated closely with the level of consciousness, but not with the behavior pattern. In the subjects studied by Davis *et al.* blood alcohol levels did not exceed 140 mg per 100 cc. Engel and Rosenbaum did not report blood alcohol levels.

Although this review is concerned primarily with studies on human subjects, the observations made on cats by Horsey and Akert (**28, 29**) are worthy of inclusion. These investigators recorded the electrical activity of the brain in 47 cats in which blood levels of ethyl alcohol were raised as high as 900 mg per 100 cc. Recordings were obtained from the cortex, thalamus, and striatum of unrestrained, restrained, and immobilized cats. At blood alcohol levels below 50 mg per 100 cc, changes in the EEG patterns were very slight. At 100 mg per cent drowsy patterns appeared with spindles and slow waves. At 200 mg per cent delta activity occurred, and the spindles decreased in frequency. At 400 mg per cent bilateral generalized delta activity predominated. At 500 mg per cent bursts of spindles on a cycle of 5 to 6 per second alternated with intervals of 5 to 10 seconds during which the record was almost flat. At 800 to 900 mg per 100 cc all cortical activity disappeared. Subcortical activity was similar to the cortical activity. If the blood alcohol level rose above 500 mg per 100 cc, the EEG did not return to normal.

Chronic Alcoholism

Except when it has led to complications, the chronic ingestion of alcohol rarely produces alterations in the resting EEG pattern. Greenblatt, Levin, and di Cori (**26**) reported the EEG findings in 157 patients with chronic alcoholism, with and without complications. They observed no significant changes in the EEG of chronic alcoholics without psychosis, regardless of the duration of drinking. The incidence of EEG abnormalities in chronic alcoholics increases

with age. In alcoholics with psychosis or confusion the incidence of
EEG abnormalities was higher than that found in the normal population. The highest incidence of EEG abnormalities, however, was
found among patients with mental deterioration or Korsakoff's
syndrome.

In a similar study of 189 alcoholics, Funkhouser and his co-
workers (18) observed poor alpha and increased beta rhythms, but
predominantly normal EEGs even in alcoholics with psychoses. The
incidence of abnormalities was increased in patients who had
convulsions.

Little and McAvoy (37, 38) have reported a detailed study of the
alpha activity in 34 chronic alcoholics and 55 normal controls. The
alpha index of the alcoholics (.46) was significantly lower than that
of the normal controls (.71). Although they observed no significant
differences in the alpha amplitude, good amplitude modulation was
seen in 86 per cent of the controls (including patients with anxiety reaction) and in only 50 per cent of the alcoholics. This difference was also significant.

In an attempt to corroborate the findings of Little and McAvoy,
we have analyzed the electroencephalograms of 37 alcoholic patients
and 30 patients with anxiety reaction hospitalized at the Durham
VA Hospital during the years 1961 and 1962. The 37 alcoholic
patients had been drinking continuously or periodically for a col-
lective total of almost six centuries. The EEG findings on the two
groups of patients are summarized in Table I. These data corroborate
in part the findings of Little and McAvoy.

Table I. Comparison of the EEG Changes in 37 Alcoholics and 30
Patients with Anxiety Reactions

	Alcoholic patients	Patients with anxiety
Mean alpha index	.55	.51
Mean alpha frequency	9.8	
Hyperventilation responses	not unusual	not unusual
Abnormalities	2 cases	
Low-voltage fast records	3 cases	

Seizures (Rum Fits)

The reported incidence of abnormal electroencephalograms in patients with convulsions secondary to chronic alcoholism is variable.

Greenblatt and his associates (**26**) reported an incidence of 17 per cent in 24 patients with "rum fits." In the series reported by Giroire *et al.* (**23**) the incidence of abnormal EEGs was 25 per cent. The incidence of normal EEGs in the series of convulsive alcoholics studied by Funkhauser (**17**) was 59 per cent, very close to the figure of 54 per cent reported by Gibbs (**22**) in sleep EEGs of patients with grand mal epilepsy. Vercellette (**49**) studied 80 alcoholics whose first seizures occurred after the age of 25. In 10 of these cases tracings were normal except for paroxysmal activity in the temporal regions on six occasions. The remaining 70 cases showed alterations in the rhythm of the basal activity with the appearance of paroxysmal bursts.

Rosenbaum and his associates (**45**) studied 305 patients with active delirium tremens, 29 (9 per cent) of whom had convulsions as a part of their illness. In all but one of these 29 patients, the fits began after many years of alcoholism, the average age at the onset of the seizures being 39 years. These investigators believe that four factors may contribute to the occurrence of seizures in patients with delirium tremens: (1) a constitutional predisposition to epilepsy; (2) cerebral lesions, such as head injury or alcoholic damage to the brain, that may tend to lower the convulsive threshold; (3) acute cerebral lesions, such as severe metabolic strain resulting from delirium tremens; and (4) the exaggeration of existing abnormalities in the brain waves as a result of alcohol. They point out that the incidence of seizures in their patients with delirium tremens (9 per cent) is almost identical with the incidence of cerebral dysrhythmia in the general population, reported by Lennox and his associates (**33**) as 10 per cent. Such cerebral dysrhythmia may indicate a predisposition to convulsions.

The relationship between alcohol intoxication and the activation of latent epilepsy was re-examined in 1953 by Courjon and Perrin (**8**), who also concluded that the chronic alcoholic showed no specific EEG anomalies.

Laennec's Cirrhosis

The EEG in metabolic disorders will be covered in more detail by another participant in the symposium. One such disorder, however, is so intimately related to the subject of alcoholism and toxic psychosis that at least a portion of the literature should be included in this review. While chronic alcoholism does not always precede

Laennec's cirrhosis, or portal cirrhosis, the incidence of this disease is approximately seven times as great in alcoholics as in the general population. As the cirrhotic process involves more and more of the liver, it produces a clinical syndrome referred to as "impending" hepatic coma, hepatic coma, or hyperammoniemic encephalopathy. From the numerous reports on the clinical features of hepatic coma, it is apparent that the mental disturbance may be minimal to severe, varying with the functional state of the liver, the nitrogenous load, the portal-caval communications, the use of antibiotics, and other factors.

The principal substance responsible for the precipitation of hepatic coma is believed to be ammonia, one of the end products of protein metabolism. The increased concentration of ammonia in the blood acts as a toxic agent, depressing the function of the brain by decreasing the oxidation of neuronal cells and tissues. The resulting syndrome is a good example of a toxic coma without gross structural damage to the brain, and thus is particularly suitable for experimental study.

Bickford and Butt (2, 3) obtained electroencephalograms from 12 patients in various stages of hepatic coma. Three distinct EEG patterns, which they designated as "stages," were obtained at different levels of coma. The *theta stage,* observed during the precoma phase of mental clouding, was characterized by diffuse rhythms at frequencies of 4 to 7 cycles per second. The *triphasic stage* was associated with a slightly deeper level of coma and characterized by diffuse, bilaterally synchronous triphasic waves somewhat resembling the eye-blink artifact. The maximal deflection was surface positive, and the authors suggested that this rhythm may represent "conducted cortical disturbance." In the last stage, referred to as the *delta stage,* the triphasic waves disappeared and random arrhythmic waves with little bilateral synchrony tended to dominate the record. Most patients in the theta stage were moderately confused, while those in the triphasic and delta stages were usually semicomatose or completely unresponsive. The type of cirrhosis responsible for coma did not appear to influence the EEG pattern.

Parsons-Smith and his co-workers (41) reported 157 electroencephalograms obtained in 62 patients with liver disease and various degrees of mental disturbance. The electroencephalograms, graded from A to E, showed a high degree of correlation with the severity of neuropsychiatric or mental disturbances preceding hepatic coma.

Correlation with the level of ammonia in the blood or cerebrospinal fluid was less well defined. These authors stated their belief that the slow, high-voltage delta discharges originally described by Foley and others (**15**) in 1950, represent the same level as their advanced grade E. Although their grades C and D correspond with the "theta stage" reported by Bickford and Butt (**2, 3**), the triphasic waves emphasized by those workers were rarely a feature of the records in this study.

Between 1956 and 1958, Abbott (**1**), Friedlander (**16**), Cloche (**7**) and Poser (**42**) all reported progressive slowing of EEG rhythms in association with increasing blood levels of ammonia. In reporting "Some Observations on the Electroencephalogram in Hepatic Coma," Silverman (**47**) referred to the triphasic wave of Bickford and Butt as "pseudoparoxysmal." In his patients, progressive changes in the EEG were associated with increasing depth of coma. He described these changes as a continuum ranging from normal, through theta and pseudoparoxysmal, to delta.

In two additional studies carried out at the Durham VA Hospital (**25**), serial EEGs and serial blood ammonia levels were recorded in 10 patients with chronic disease of the portal system. These patients were examined regularly for periods of time varying from 14 to 38 months, and their EEGs were graded according to a modification of the system used by Parsons-Smith (**41**). When the EEG grades were plotted against the blood ammonia levels obtained on the same dates, a reasonable correlation was demonstrable in only one-third of the patients. These were the patients with the highest ammonia levels, the most abnormal EEG tracings, and the most noticeable variations from one examination to the next.

DELIRIUM

This clinical entity, considered by many to be the most common acute psychiatric disorder, is characterized by a disturbance of sensorium in which orientation is impaired. For the purpose of this review it is further defined as an organic brain syndrome or toxic psychosis from which the patient usually recovers. In clinical practice delirium is most frequently encountered in the chronic alcoholic whose alcohol intake has been abruptly reduced or discontinued, but it may be caused by any serious illness capable of disturbing the sensitive metabolic needs of cerebral tissue.

Romano and Engel (**43, 44**) made repeated mental and electro-encephalographic examinations of 53 delirious patients. Among the diseases responsible for the delirium in this group of patients were cardiac decompensation, pulmonary decompensation, structural cerebral disease, malnutrition, chronic alcoholism, and toxic states due to infection, severe anemia, acidosis, glomerular nephritis, and Addison's disease. Electroencephalographic abnormalities were observed in all the patients during delirium. Changes were diffuse, and a significant relationship was found between the EEG changes and the intensity, duration, and reversibility of the noxious factors. These changes were reversible to the extent that the clinical delirium was reversible. The EEG abnormalities, in order of intensity, included: (1) decrease in frequency, (2) disorganization, and (3) reorganization at a lower energy level—that is, at a slower frequency with higher amplitude. The authors emphasized the nonspecificity of these EEG changes, stating that they were essentially the same as changes previously reported by independent observers in association with cerebral trauma, encephalitis, neurosyphilis, increased intracranial pressure, hypoglycemia, and the administration of certain drugs which influence consciousness.

In another study of delirious patients, Engel and Romano (**10**) used experimental procedures in an attempt to reverse the major physiologic derangements accompanying the underlying disease. Where these procedures were successful, the EEG rhythms tended to return to normal. These studies support the belief that the danger of permanent cortical damage rises as the duration of the noxious factors increases.

In a study of 71 alcoholic patients, 59 of whom had delirium tremens, Kennard, Bueding, and Wortis (**31**) observed a relatively high incidence of fast (16 to 30 cycles per second), low-voltage activity. The incidence of such rhythms decreased during recovery, which took place more slowly in the patients with the greatest amount of fast activity and the lowest amplitude at the onset of the disorder. The patients who had delirium tremens showed a low alpha index in addition to the increased fast activity. These changes were not seen in the 12 alcoholics without delirium tremens, who were either in an acute stage of intoxication, were markedly deteriorated, or had polyneuropathy.

It is well known that the excessive use of certain drugs can produce intoxication which takes the form of delirium. Gibbs and

Lennox (21) were the first to study the effects of bromides and barbiturates on the electroencephalograms of normal and epileptic subjects. Greenblatt, Levin, and Schegloff (27) later studied 39 cases of bromide intoxication and reported a high incidence of EEG abnormalities during the intoxicated state, with progressive improvement in the EEG tracings as the patient's sensorium cleared. They found that the EEG changes are definitely related to the blood-bromide level and the clinical picture. When the blood-bromide level is over 200 mg per 100 cc, the EEG tends to show diffuse slow activity and the patient is usually confused and dysarthric. With falling blood-bromide levels, a mixture of the slow and fast activity is observed in the EEG, and when the bromide concentration returns to normal levels EEG abnormalities usually disappear.

In a case of bromide intoxication reported by Rubin and Cohen (46) an attempt was made to correlate the percent-time alpha and alterations in the alpha frequency with the blood-bromide levels. In this study the authors attributed the alteration in alpha frequency accompanying the decrease in the bromide levels of the blood to changes in the metabolic rate of the cortical neurons. They suggested that the EEG may be of use in ascertaining the presence or absence of physiologic bromide intoxication.

Engel, Romano, and Goldman (11) reported on EEG studies on a patient with acute arsenical encephalopathy. They described alterations in the mean frequency, and emphasized that the degree of change in the electroencephalogram was more important than the appearance of any particular wave frequency.

INFECTIONS

In the Gibbses' *Atlas of Electroencephalography* (22), infection in the form of encephalitis, meningitis, or brain abscess is listed as a possible cause of many diverse epileptic patterns, including hypsarrhythmia, petit mal, petit mal variant, myoclonic seizures, grand mal seizures, psychomotor seizures, Jacksonian seizures, focal seizures, thalamic or hypothalamic epilepsy, and various mixed types. These abnormalities, however, are usually residua of the infection. This review will deal chiefly with the electroencephalographic findings in relation to the acute and subacute infectious process—specifically, encephalitis and neurosyphilis.

Acute Encephalitis

The literature contains many individual articles describing altera-tions in the cerebral electrical activity in relation to encephalitis of various types. In 1945 Ross (98) described gross disturbances in the EEGs of four children during the acute stage of encephalitis and meningo-encephalitis. The abnormalities consisted of generalized, bilateral synchronous slow waves of high amplitude. The author com-mented that the EEG disturbance accompanying encephalitis is non-specific and not related to the severity of the clinical picture.

Glaser and Hoefer (72) studied 50 cases of encephalitis, and reported that during the acute stage all patients showed EEG ab-normalities of varying intensity, wave form, and distribution. These included diffuse slowing, spike-and-wave discharges, larval spike and wave patterns, and focal asymmetries. Follow-up studies were performed on 25 patients after intervals ranging from five months to nine years. In most cases the EEG and clinical pictures showed gradual improvement, but postencephalitic epilepsy developed in 11 cases. Disturbances in personality and behavior developed in 9 pa-tients, 8 of whom had lasting generalized abnormalities in their electroencephalograms.

The progressive EEG changes in a child recovering from en-cephalitis were described by Lindsley and Cutts (86). Abnormalities consisting of diffuse slow waves (2 to 3 per second), plus focal short bursts in the right occipital region, gradually disappeared over a period of 17 months.

In the supplementary bibliography printed at the end of this article are listed numerous other articles on this subject containing observa-tions which do not differ significantly from those reported by Gibbs and Gibbs (71) following their study of 240 cases of encephalitis. These authors believe that there is a direct correlation between the severity of symptoms during the acute and subacute phases of illness and the degree of electroencephalographic abnormality. The abnor-malities were frequently focal, 3-per-second activity of the classic petit mal type being common. In the postencephalitic syndrome, EEG abnormalities persisted only in cases in which seizures continued.

Postencephalitic convulsions occur more commonly in children than in adults. Abnormal EEGs were observed in 87 per cent of the patients with seizures following encephalitis due to infections other than syphilis. In 58 per cent of these cases the abnormality consisted of paroxysmal patterns. Of the postencephalitic patients without seizures, 18 per cent had abnormal EEGs, but only 1 per cent of these were paroxysmal. Gibbs concluded that the electroencephalogram is of diagnostic value in acute encephalitis and of prognostic value in postencephalitic epilepsy.

Subacute Encephalitis

Two pathologic types of sporadic, subacute encephalitis have so far been recognized. One of these was described by Van Bogaert (**106**) and the other by Dawson (**66**). Among the many writers who have published their observations on this disease are Anderman (**52**), Brierly (**58**), Gozzano (**73**), Maleci (**87, 88**), and Levin (**84**). The serial EEG changes in this type of encephalitis have been described by Radermacker (**94**) and by Cobb and Hill (**64, 65**). Clinically, this illness is usually characterized by progressive dementia, leading to stupor and associated with episodic involuntary movements. Serial EEGs reveal progressive disappearance of normal rhythms. As the disease progresses, outbursts of single "sharp waves" and other epileptic-like disturbances may be seen in the frontal or temporal regions, and repetitive paroxysmal high-voltage slow waves with a tendency toward periodicity are noted. Later each slow wave complex is preceded by irregular slow activity, and still later each complex appears in the record as a group of approximately three slow waves of great amplitude followed by a few seconds of relative inactivity. These complexes tend to become periodic, being repeated at intervals of 7 to 10 seconds. Cobb and Hill (**64, 65**) feel that the periodic outbursts of electrical activity associated with the involuntary movements are so characteristic that their occurrence suggests the diagnosis.

Measles Encephalitis

Several interesting studies have been made on the incidence, clinical features, and EEG changes of measles encephalitis. While most such reports are based on populations of children, Mitchell and Pampiglione (**91**) described the clinical and EEG changes in a 45-year-old businessman with measles encephalitis. The rubella apparently affected his brain stem and spinal cord, and probably the frontal lobes as well. Gross mental disturbances were associated with abnormal brain waves. The EEG was characterized by excessive slowing and paroxysmal prolonged runs of 2-to-4-per-second waves occurring predominantly in the frontal regions and easily activated by sudden noises. Severe mental and electroencephalographic disturbances persisted for two months, but gradually cleared over a period of six months.

As in other types of encephalitis, the dysrhythmia associated with measles encephalitis is usually severe in the acute stages and may be focal, scattered, or generalized.

Hodes and Livingston (78) reported that detectable evidence of encephalitis develops in at least 1 out of 1,200 cases of measles in children. In 31 cases of measles encephalitis studied by Spragins *et al.* (102), convulsive activity occurred in more than half the patients. In these cases the abnormalities in the initial EEG, which was made before the onset of convulsions, were usually much greater than would be suspected from the clinical picture. In follow-up tracings a direct correlation was observed between clinical severity and EEG changes. The authors concluded that persistent EEG changes following encephalitis, even in the absence of demonstrable clinical abnormalities, would call for a guarded prognosis as to the patient's future ability to adjust to the complexities of life. Such changes are associated with a high incidence of severe residua—most often disturbances of personality, concentration, and memory.

Neurosyphilis

This survey would not be complete without at least a brief mention of the electroencephalographic changes observed in cases of neurosyphilis. In 1942 Finley, Rose, and Solomon (69) obtained a series of EEGs on 175 patients over a period of two and a half years. Included in this group were 124 patients with dementia paralytica, 20 with tabes, 11 with juvenile dementia, 12 with meningovascular neurosyphilis, and 8 with atrophy of the optic nerve. A comparison of the electroencephalograms obtained in these patients with the records from 215 normal control subjects is shown in Table II. The patterns observed in the neurosyphilitic patients were not

Table II. The Incidence of EEG Abnormalities in 175 Patients with Neurosyphilis: Comparison with 215 Normal Controls*

	EEG Patterns		
	Normal	Borderline	Abnormal
Neurosyphilitic patients	19	28	53
Controls	70	23	7

*Statistics given by Finley, Rose, and Solomon (69).

consistent, but most of the abnormal activity occurred in the frontal and precentral regions. Although slow, high-voltage activity usually indicates a severe alteration in cerebral function, it is not necessarily irreversible.

The authors concluded that the diagnosis of neurosyphilis cannot be made on the basis of the EEG findings, but that electroencephalography is a useful tool in assessing the severity of the disease prior to treatment, as well as the response to treatment. With the advent of more effective methods of treatment, several investigators have reported a correlation between the EEG picture and clinical improvement.

The report of Arentsen and Voldby (53) on 110 cases of neurosyphilis, in which 241 EEGs were obtained, is slightly at variance with that of Seeley and Dille (100) and Finley and his associates (69). Their series of patients consisted of 35 with dementia paralytica, 24 with taboparalysis, 19 with tabes dorsalis, and 32 with other varieties of neurosyphilis. The EEG records on these 110 patients were divided as follows: 38 normal, 13 borderline, 23 slightly abnormal, 30 moderately abnormal, and 6 severely abnormal. Of the 59 abnormal EEGs, 53 showed marked constancy, but no correlation with the spinal fluid findings. The incidence of abnormalities was found to be much higher in young patients than in older ones.

CONCLUSION

The ultimate goal of investigators in the fields of neurology and electroencephalography is to correlate electroencephalographic patterns with neurophysiologic processes. Although such correlations are rather gross at present, studies in human beings and experimental animals are steadily increasing our knowledge of brain function. This research, combined with further refinement of recording techniques, offers exciting possibilities for the future.

BIBLIOGRAPHY

PART I

1. Abbott, J. A. Blood ammonia levels, electroencephalograms and states of consciousness. *Electroenceph. clin. Neurophysiol.* **8:** 525–526, 1956. (Abstract)
2. Bickford, R. G., and Butt, H. R. EEG findings in hepatic coma, *Electroenceph. clin. Neurophysiol.* **5:** 480, 1953. (Abstract)
3. Bickford, R. G., and Butt, H. R. Hepatic coma: The electroencephalographic pattern. *J. clin. Invest.* **34:** 790–799, 1955.

4. Bochnik, H. J., and Wullstein, O. The EEG and the antabuse-alcohol test. *Electroenceph. clin. Neurophysiol.* **5**: 122, 1953.
5. Busse, E. W., and Barnes, R. H. The effects of antabuse on the electroencephalogram. *Electroenceph. clin. Neurophysiol.* **3**: 381, 1951.
6. Busse, E. W., Barnes, R. H., and Ebaugh, F. G. The effect of antabuse on the electroencephalogram. *Amer. J. med. Sci.* **223**: 126–130, 1952.
7. Cloche, R. Étude Électroencéphalographique de quelque cas de coma hépatique. *Presse Med.* **65**: 135–137, 1957.
8. Courjon, J., and Perrin, J. Intérêt du controls électroencéphalographique des alcoholiques chroniques. *Electroenceph. clin. Neurophysiol.* **4**: 248, 1952.
9. Davis, P. A., Gibbs, F. A., Davis, H., Jetter, W. W., and Trowbridge, L. S. The effects of alcohol upon the electroencephalogram. *Quart. J. Stud. Alcohol.* **1**: 626–637, 1951.
10. Engel, G. L., and Romano, J. Delirium: II. Reversibility of the electroencephalogram with experimental procedures. *Arch. Neurol. Psychiat.* **51**: 378–392, 1944.
11. Engel, G. L., Romano, J., and Goldman, L. Delirium: IV. Quantitative electroencephalographic study of a case of acute arsenical encephalopathy. *Arch. Neurol. Psychiat.* **56**: 659–664, 1946.
12. Engel, G. L., and Rosenbaum, M. Studies of the electroencephalogram in acute alcoholic intoxication. *Proc. Centr. Soc. Clin. Res.* **17**: 62–63, 1944.
13. Engel, G. L., and Rosenbaum, M. Delirium: III. Electroencephalographic changes associated with acute alcoholic intoxication. *Arch. Neurol. Psychiat.* **53**: 44–50, 1945.
14. Engel, G. L., Webb, J. P., and Ferris, E. B. Quantitative electroencephalographic studies of anoxia in humans; comparison with acute alcoholic intoxication and hypoglycemia. *J. clin. Invest.* **24**: 691–697, 1945.
15. Foley, J. M., Watson, C. W., and Adams, R. W. Significance of EEG changes in hepatic coma. *Trans. Amer. Neurol. Ass.* **75**: 161–165, 1950.
16. Friedlander, W. J. Electroencephalographic changes in hyperammonemia. *Electroenceph. clin. Neurophysiol.* **8**: 513–516, 1956.
17. Funkhauser, J. B. Electroencephalographic studies in alcoholism. *Electroenceph. clin. Neurophysiol.* **5**: 130, 1953.
18. Funkhauser, J. B., Nagler, B., and Walke, N. D. The electroencephalogram of chronic alcoholism. *Southern med. J.* **46**: 423–428, 1953.
19. Gibbs, E. L., and Gibbs, F. A. Diagnostic and localizing value of electroencephalographic studies in sleep. *Proc. Ass. Res. Nerv. Ment. Dis.* **26**: 366–376, 1946.
20. Gibbs, E. L., and Lennox, W. E. Cerebral dysrhythmias of epilepsy; measures for their control. *Arch. Neurol. Psychiat.* **39**: 298–314, 1938.
21. Gibbs, F. A., Gibbs, E. L., and Lennox, W. G. Effect on the electroencephalogram of certain drugs which influence nervous activity. *Arch. intern. Med. (Chic.).* **60**: 154–166, 1937.
22. Gibbs, F. A., and Gibbs, E. L. *Atlas of Electroencephalography.* Vol. 2, Addison-Wesley Press, Inc., 1952.
23. Giroire, H., Charbonnel, A., Vercellette, P., and Trichet. Considerations concerning electroencephalograms in 200 cases of generalized epileptic seizures which started late in life. *Electroenceph. clin. Neurophysiol.* **8**: 733–734, 1956.
24. Gorman, W. F., Stearns, E., and Wortis, S. B. The electroencephalogram in Korsakoff syndrome. *Amer. J. Psychiat.* **107**: 20–24, 1950.
25. Green, R. L. Serial EEG studies in patients with chronic hyperammonemia. Presented to Annual Meeting South, EEG Society, December, 1961.
26. Greenblatt, M., Levin, S., and di Corti, F. The electroencephalogram associated with chronic alcoholism, alcoholic psychosis and alcoholic convulsions. *Arch. Neurol. Psychiat.* **52**: 290–295, 1944.
27. Greenblatt, M., Levin, S., and Schegloff, B. Electroencephalographic findings in cases of bromide intoxication. *Arch. Neurol. Psychiat.* **53**: 431–436, 1945.
28. Horsey, W. J., and Akert, K. Influence of ethyl alcohol on the electroencephalogram of the cat. *Electroenceph. clin. Neurophysiol.* **5**: 318, 1953.
29. Horsey, W. J., and Akert, K. The influence of ethyl alcohol on the spontaneous electrical activity of the cerebral cortex and subcortical structures of the cat. *Quart. J. Stud. Alcohol.* **14**: 363–377, 1953.
30. Johnson, J. H., Green, R. L., Owen, E. E., and Tyor, M. P. Chronic portal systemic encephalopathy. *J. South. Med. Ass.* **53**: 1537–1542, 1960.
31. Kennard, M. A., Bueding, E., and Wortis, S. B. Some biochemical and electroencephalographic changes in delirium tremens. *Quart. J. Stud. Alcohol.* **6**: 4–14, 1945.
32. Lennox, M. Effects of sedative drugs on the electroencephalogram. *Amer. J. Psychiat.* **102**: 799–804, 1946.

33. Lennox, W. G., Gibbs, F. A., and Gibbs, E. L. Effect on the electroencephalogram of drugs and conditions which influence seizures. *Arch. Neurol. Psychiat.* **36**: 1236–1245, 1936.

34. Lennox, W. G., and Lennox, M. A. *Epilepsy and Related Disorders.* 2 vols. Little, Brown and Co., Boston, 1960.

35. Lewis, John A. The scope of alcoholism. Presented to Mississippi State Nurses Assoc., Jackson, Miss., Nov. 18, 1955.

36. Little, S. C. The use of electroencephalography in clinical medicine. *J. Med. Ass. Alabama.* **19**: 231–237, 1950.

37. Little, S. C., and McAvoy, M. Electroencephalographic findings in chronic alcoholism. *Electroenceph. clin. Neurophysiol.* **4**: 245–246, 1952.

38. Little, S. C., and McAvoy, M. Electroencephalographic studies in alcoholism. *Quart. J. Stud. Alcohol.* **13**: 9–15, 1952.

39. Loomis, A. L., Harvey, E. N., and Hobart, G. Electrical potentials of the human brain. *J. exp. Psychol.* **19**: 249–279, 1936.

40. Mirsky, I. A., Piker, P., Rosenbaum, M., and Lederer, H. "Adaptation" of the central nervous system to varying concentrations of alcohol in the blood. *Quart. J. Stud. Alcohol.* **2**: 35–45, 1941.

41. Parsons-Smith, B. G., Summerskill, W. H. J., Dawson, A. M., and Sherlock, S. The electroencephalograph in liver disease. *Lancet.* **2**: 867–871, Nov., 1957.

42. Poser, C. M. Electroencephalographic changes and hyperammonemia. *Electroenceph. clin. Neurophysiol.* **10**: 51–62, 1958.

43. Romano, J., and Engel, G. L. Delirium: I. Electroencephalographic data. *Arch. Neurol. Psychiat.* **51**: 356–377, 1944.

44. Romano, J., and Engel, G. L. Physiologic and psychologic considerations of delirium. *Med. Clin. N. Amer.* **28**: 629–638, May, 1944.

45. Rosenbaum, M., Lewis, M., Piker, P., and Goldman, D. Convulsive seizures in delirium tremens. *Arch. Neurol. Psychiat.* **45**: 486–493, 1951.

46. Rubin, M. A., and Cohen, L. H. The electroencephalogram in bromide intoxication. *Arch. Neurol. Psychiat.* **40**: 922–927, 1938.

47. Silverman, D. Some observations on the EEG in hepatic coma. *Electroenceph. clin. Neurophysiol.* **14**: 53–59, 1962.

48. Strauss, H. Clinical and electroencephalographic studies: The electroencephalogram in psychoneurotics. *J. nerv. ment. Dis.* **101**: 19–26, 1945.

49. Vercellette, P. Épilepsie pubertaire et comitialité tardive apparue chez des ethyliques. *Electroenceph. clin. Neurophysiol.* **4**: 249, 1952.

50. Victor, M., and Adams, R. A. The effect of alcohol on the nervous system. *Proc. Ass. Res. Nerv. Ment. Dis.* **32**: Chapter 28, 1953.

51. Williams, D., and Gibbs, F. A. Electroencephalography in clinical neurology: Its value in routine diagnosis. *Arch. Neurol. Psychiat.* **41**: 519–534, 1939.

PART II

52. Anderman, F., Cosgrove, J. B. R., and Gloor, P. Subacute encephalitis involving primarily temporal and subcortical structures. *Electroenceph. clin. Neurophysiol.* **13**: 776–780, 1961.

53. Arentsen, K., and Voldby, H. Electroencephalographic changes in neurosyphilis. *Electroenceph. clin. Neurophysiol.* **4**: 331–337, 1952.

54. Bental, E., and Liebowitz, U. Flat electroencephalograms during 28 days in a case of "encephalitis." *Electroenceph. clin. Neurophysiol.* **13**: 457–460, 1961.

55. Bercel, N. A. Infectious mononucleosis, encephalitis, epilepsy. *Amer. J. med. Sci.* **224**: 667–672 1952.

56. Berger, H. Über das Elektrenkephalogramm des Menschen: III. *Arch. Psychiat. Nervenkr.* **94**: 16–60, 1931.

57. Berger, H. Über das Elektrenkephalogramm des Menschen: VI. *Arch. Psychiat. Nervenkr.* **99**: 555–574, 1933.

58. Brierly, J. B., Corsellis, J. A. N., Hierons, R., and Nevin, S. Subacute encephalitis of later life. Mainly affecting the limbic areas. *Brain.* **83**: 357–368, 1960.

59. Brissaud, Lefèbvre, J., Lérique-Koechlin, and Nekhorocheff, I. L'Électroencéphalogramme dans les méningites aiguës, subaiguës ou chroniques de l'enfance. *Electroenceph. clin. Neurophysiol.* **2**: 104, 1950.

60. Busse, E. W., and Robinson, A. M. Electroencephalographic changes associated with tuberculous meningitis. *Electroenceph. clin. Neurophysiol.* **4**: 384, 1952.

61. Callaway, J. L., Lowenbach, H., Noojin, R. O., Kuhn, B. H., and Riley, K. A.

Electroencephalographic findings in central nervous system syphilis. *J. Amer. Med. Ass.* **129**: 938–939, 1945.

62. Cazzullo, C. L., and Pacella, B. L. Electroencephalographic studies on experimental allergic encephalomelitis in rhesus monkeys. *Arch. Neurol. Psychiat.* **63**: 125–132, 1950.

63. Clearkin, K. B., and Miller, J. H. D. A case of subacute encephalitis. *Electroenceph. clin. Neurophysiol.* **4**: 105–106, 1952.

64. Cobb, W., and Hill, D. Electroencephalogram in subacute progressive encephalitis. *Brain.* **73**: 392–404, 1950.

65. Cobb, W., and Hill, D. Periodic EEG abnormality in cases of subacute progressive encephalitis. *Electroenceph. clin. Neurophysiol.* **2**: 104–105, 1950.

66. Dawson, J. R. Cellular inclusions in cerebral lesions. *Arch. Neurol. Psychiat.* **31**: 685, 1934.

67. Dow, R. S. Toxoplasmic encephalitis—clinical findings in two patients from Pacific Northwest. *Northwest Med.* **44**: 382–387, 1945.

68. Euzière, J., Passouant, P., and Latour, H. La souffrance basale provoquée par la méningite tuberculeuse. *Electroenceph. clin. Neurophysiol.* **2**: 348, 1950.

69. Finley, K. H., Rose, A. S., and Solomon, H. C. Electroencephalographic studies on neurosyphilis. *Arch. Neurol. Psychiat.* **47**: 718–736, 1942.

70. Freedman, M. J., Odland, L., and Cleve, E. A. Infectious mononucleosis with diffuse involvement of nervous system. *Arch. Neurol. Psychiat.* **69**: 49–54, 1953.

71. Gibbs, F. A., and Gibbs, E. L. The electroencephalogram in encephalitis. *Arch. Neurol. Psychiat.* **58**: 184–192, 1947.

72. Glaser, G. H., and Hoefer, P. F. A. Electroencephalographic changes during and after encephalitis. *Electroenceph. clin. Neurophysiol.* **2**: 361, 1950.

73. Gozzano, M., Mengoli, G., and Schiavi, E. Studio electroencefalografico' di un caso di leucoencefalite subacute sclerosante (EEG study of a case of subacute leucoencephalitis). *Electroenceph. clin. Neurophysiol.* **3**: 369, 1951.

74. Greenblatt, M., and Levin, S. Factors affecting the electroencephalogram of patients with neurosyphilis. *Amer. J. Psychiat.* **102**: 40–48, 1945.

75. Greenblatt, M., and Levin, S. Neurosyphilis, convulsions and electroencephalography. *Urol. Cut. Rev.* **I**: 331–334, 1946.

76. Grossi-Bianchi, M. L., and Durand, P. Contribution to the study of children with basal meningitis by EEG and cisternography. *Electroenceph. clin. Neurophysiol.* **4**: 234, 1952.

77. Harrell, G. T. Rickettsial involvement of the nervous system. *Med. Clin. N. Amer.* **37**: 395–422, March, 1953.

78. Hodes, H. L., and Livingston, S. Electroencephalographic findings in measles encephalitis. *J. Pediat.* **36**: 577–582, 1950.

79. Holmgren, E. B. EEG i nagra meningo-encephalitifall. *Nord. Med.* **40**: 1810–1812, 1948.

80. Laget, P., and Colat, J. Épisode encéphalitique avec photophobie découvert au cours d'une activation par stimulation lumineuse intermittente. *Electroenceph. clin. Neurophysiol.* **4**: 247, 1952.

81. Landau, W. M., and Gitt, J. J. Subacute encephalitis: Three year survival with long-term remission. *Neurology.* **2**: 488–495, 1952.

82. Lerique, A. L'EEG dans la méningite tuberculeuse de l'enfant. *Electroenceph. clin. Neurophysiol.* **3**: 110, 1951.

83. Lerique-Koechlin, A. Aspect de trois EEG successifs dans un cas d'encéphalite subaiguë (type Van Boogaert). *Electroenceph. clin. Neurophysiol.* **4**: 240, 1952.

84. Levin, P. M. Epilepsy and "Progressive Encephalitis": A study in epileptic degeneration. *Electroenceph. clin. Neurophysiol.* **4**: 242, 1952.

85. Lichtenstein, A., and Melin, K. A. The electroencephalogram in cases of tuberculous meningitis. *Acta Paediat. (Stockholm).* Suppl. **75**: 75–82, 1949.

86. Lindsley, D. B., and Cutts, K. K. Clinical and electroencephalographic changes in a child during recovery from encephalitis. *Arch. Neurol. Psychiat.* **45**: 156–161, 1941.

87. Maleci, O. EEG in a case of subacute sclerosant leuco-encephalitis. *Electroenceph. clin. Neurophysiol.* **4**: 229, 1952.

88. Maleci, O., and Baggio, G. O. The EEG in tuberculous meningitis of the child. *Electroenceph. clin. Neurophysiol.* **5**: 617, 1953.

89. Marsh, C. The electroencephalographic findings in measles encephalitis. *Bull. Los Angeles Neurol. Soc.* **13**: 15–18, 1948.

90. Miller, H. G. Acute disseminated encephalomyelitis treated with ACTH. *Brit. Med. J.* **1**: 177–183, 1953.

91. Mitchell, W., and Pampiglione, G. Neurological and mental complications of rubella. *Lancet.* **2**: 1250–1253, 1959.

92. Oldfelt, V. Sequelae of mumps-meningoencephalitis. *Acta med. scand.* **134:** 405–414, 1949.ǀ
93. Pacella, B. L., Jungeblut, C. W., Kopeloff, N., and Kopeloff, L. M. The electroencephalogram in poliomyelitis. *Arch. Neurol. Psychiat.* **58:** 447–451, 1947.
94. Radermacker, J. Aspects clinique et électroencéphalographique de la leuco-encéphalite sclérosante subaiguë. *Electroenceph. clin. Neurophysiol.* **4:** 240, 1952.
95. Radtke, H. EEG changes in lesions of the central nervous system due to typhus fever. *Electroenceph. clin. Neurophysiol.* **7:** 662, 1955.
96. Roger, J., and Roger, A. Manifestations électroencéphalographiques de la meningoencéphalite myoclonique hérédosyphilitique. *Electroenceph. clin. Neurophysiol.* **2:** 344, 1950.
97. Rose, F. C., and Symonds, C. P. Persistent memory defect following encephalitis. *Brain.* **83:** 195–212, 1960.
98. Ross, I. S. Electroencephalographic findings during and after acute encephalitis and meningo-encephalitis. *J. nerv. ment. Dis.* **102:** 172–182, 1945.
99. Schmidt, R. P., Levy, L. L., Turrell, R. C., Hopkins, W. E., Bloor, B. M., and Roseman, E. Diagnostic and therapeutic clues in the study of tetanus. *Arch. Neurol. Psychiat.* **69:** 55–63, 1953.
100. Seeley, L. J., and Dille, R. S. Variation of EEG patterns in a case of neurosyphilis. *Dis. nerv. Syst.* **14:** 138–140, 1953.
101. Shinners, B. M., Krauss, R. F., and Rochester, B. Encephalitis in children with electroencephalographic changes. *New York J. Med.* **49:** 2140–2144, 1949.
102. Spragins, M., Shinners, B. M., and Rochester, B. Measles encephalitis: Clinical and electroencephalographic study. *Pediatrics.* **5:** 599–616, 1950.
103. Tsung-Yi, Lin, Healey, M. M., Finn, M. F., and Greenblatt, M. EEG changes during fever produced by inductothermy (fever cabinet) in patients with neurosyphilis. *Electroenceph. clin. Neurophysiol.* **5:** 217–224, 1953.
104. Turner, M., Vigouroux, R., Roger, A., and Taury, M. Electroencephalography in the course of bacillar meningitis in children. *Electroenceph. clin. Neurophysiol.* **5:** 468–469, 1953.
105. Turrell, R. C., Shaw, W., Schmidt, R. P., Levy, L. L., and Roseman, E. Electroencephalographic studies of the encephalopathies: II. Serial studies in tuberculous meningitis. *Electroenceph. clin. Neurophysiol.* **5:** 53–63, 1953.
106. Van Bogaert, L. Une Leuco-encéphalite sclérosante subaiguë. *J. Neurol. Neurosurg. Psychiat.* **8:** 101, 1945.
107. Van Straaten, J. J. EEG in patients with intracranial inflammatory processes. *Electroenceph. clin. Neurophysiol.* **5:** 125, 1953.
108. Vigouroux, M., Gallais, P., and Gastaut, H. Développement électroencéphalographique de deux épilepsies temporales post encéphalatiques. *Electroenceph. clin. Neurophysiol.* **5:** 477, 1953.

THE NEUROSES AND EEG

W. P. Wilson, M.D., and M. J. Short, M.D.

It was not incongruous that electroencephalography was developed by a psychiatrist who hoped it would be of value in his specialty. His hopes were shared by other workers in the fields of psychiatry, psychology, neurology, and neurophysiology, many of whom immediately addressed themselves to the study of the electroencephalograms of normal subjects as well as psychoneurotic and psychotic patients. Although in the psychoses the definition of patient groups was not difficult, the problem of nosology proved a serious impediment when attempts were made to define and classify psychoneurotic illnesses. It was particularly difficult to define what was meant by anxiety. Even today a perusal of the literature affords a variety of definitions as to the characteristics and symptoms of anxiety. The term anxiety reaction (or anxiety neurosis) has fewer but equally diverse definitions. The problem is just as great when one attempts to define conversion reaction (hysteria), dissociative reaction (hysterical fugue states), or to a lesser extent obsessive-compulsive reactions. Unfortunately, a new classification of psychiatric disease was introduced after the advent of electroencephalography, so that today there is the problem of translating older nosological concepts into our current formulations. It is quite possible that this lack of clear definitions served as a deterrent to the continued use of the electroencephalogram in the investigation of the clinical neurophysiology of psychoneurosis. In order to minimize confusion in this review, the definitions of the psychoneurotic reaction types will be those currently described in the American Psychiatric Association's *Diagnostic and Statistical Manual of Mental Disorders*. When necessary the patient material in the various reports is reclassified to fit this nomenclature.

In early research efforts an attempt was made to correlate personality types with the percent-time incidence of Berger's alpha rhythm. Thus, Lemere (9) found a high alpha index present in

140

schizoid personalities. A distinction between introversion and extraversion was interpreted as passivity versus activity by Saul, Davis,
and Davis (**15**) in their analysis of the recordings obtained from 70
individuals undergoing psychoanalysis. They were impressed that the
individuals with the greatest alpha activity seemed to demonstrate
more obvious passive-receptive (introverted) trends, while those with
little or no alpha rhythm showed more active (extraverted) tendencies. Later Gottlober (**5**) correlated a high alpha index with
extraversion, but was unable to correlate a low alpha index with
introversion. Henry and Knott (**6**) subsequently combined their
patient data with that of Gottlober because of the latter's relatively
high proportion (72 per cent) of high alpha index subjects. When
equal proportions of high and low alpha groups were thus compared, it was demonstrated that there were an equal number of in-
troverts and extraverts in both the high and the low alpha index
range.

The results obtained in the above and other studies failed to
establish conclusive bases for a correlation of personality characteristics and electroencephalographic patterns. However, they did
establish that there was a meaningful change in the electroencephalographic pattern during anxiety (tension).

A consistent feature in the EEG of anxious or tense patients has
been the presence of low-voltage fast activity. This has been interpreted to be manifestation of the altered brain metabolism which is
the substrate of anxiety (**3**). An early experimental design to evaluate the influence of anxiety on the electroencephalogram was
conducted by Williams in 1937 (**22**). In a group of normal individuals he recorded the EEG while producing anxiety by unexpected questioning of the subject, sudden signals, and forced task
completion. This situational anxiety increased the amount of beta
and delta activity in his 38 male subjects. Finley (**4**) subsequently
found an increased incidence of high-voltage fast activity in psychoneurotic reactions as well as in other psychiatric and neurological
patients with manic-depressive psychosis, involutional melancholia,
and neurosyphilis. In an extensive study of 500 normal adults and
100 psychoneurotic patients, Brazier, Finesinger, and Cobb (**1**)
found that normal subjects (aviation cadets) had dominant parieto-
occipital frequency at 10 cps while the psychoneurotic group showed
a bimodal distribution with peaks at 9 and 10.5 cps. In addition,
the psychoneurotic group demonstrated a further peak in the beta

frequencies in the range of 13.5 to 17.5 cps. Their conclusion was that the incidence of beta activity increased with the level of anxiety inherent in the three groups. The percent-time of beta rhythm was least in the "normal subjects" who were successful in completing their pilot training and was greatest in the psychoneurotic patients.

EEG examination of 300 patients with war neurosis (anxiety reactions) in World War II by Heppenstall, Hill, and Slater (7) demonstrated abnormally fast rhythms in 18 per cent of the records. In 58 per cent of the records there was an additional peak in the theta frequency (4 to 7 cps). They found that the prognosis for treatment was poorest when the abnormally fast activity was combined with theta activity. The quantity or quality of alpha rhythm had no relation to the prognosis.

In 1945 Strauss (19) reported his observations on EEG patterns of psychoneurotic patients at rest and during hyperventilation. It was his conclusion that the amount of continuity of alpha activity was less in psychoneurotics and particularly rare in persons with chronic anxiety and difficulties in adjustment. He also observed that the incidence of alpha during hyperventilation was decreased to a greater degree in neurotics than in normals. Faure (3) was not equally impressed by the variants of the EEGs of anxious individuals. However, he did feel that there was a disturbance in the regulatory brain mechanisms reflected in the dysrhythmic alpha and increased sensitivity to light and hyperventilation of these patients. Using automatic frequency analysis Ulett, Gleser, Winoker, and Lawler (21) compared the electroencephalographic responses to photic stimulation of 40 cases of anxiety-prone subjects with those who were not. The incidence of alpha rhythm was greatest in the non-anxiety-prone group, less in the anxiety-prone group, and least in the anxiety patients with anxiety reactions. The 40 patients suffering from anxiety reactions showed an additional feature of increased fast and slow activity in the resting EEG. No differences in response to photic stimulation were observed.

Another early index of biological change with anxiety was the so-called delta index (D.I.). Hoagland, Cameron, and Rubin (8) recorded an enhanced delta index in a group of psychotic and normal persons when they were stimulated by emotionally charged comments or questions. However, no separation of the responses of the patient and control groups was made. Subsequently Thiesen (20) refuted this finding, stating that the delta index did not increase during emotional excitement and there was only an attended "flattening" of the record. Since this report there has been no further investigation of the delta index in mental illness.

Not all investigators have been initially impressed by electroencephalographic changes of persons suffering emotional ills. Oberman (11) noted no statistically significant difference in the index of alpha when subjects were challenged by pleasant or unpleasant words or when listening to emotional or unemotional statements. In an extensive summary article on the incidence of EEG abnormality among patients with mental disorders of non-organic origin, Ellingson (2) reported a high incidence of abnormality in the EEGs of psychopaths, but stated that the data on psychoneurotic reactions was conflicting and, therefore, inconclusive.

In 1954 Shagass (16) introduced the sedation threshold as an investigative tool in psychiatry. In this procedure amytal is slowly injected intravenously, producing an increased level of fast rhythm response in the EEG with a concomitant slurring of speech. When the amplitude of frontal fast rhythm is plotted against the amount of drug injected, a sigmoid curve with an inflection point is produced. This usually corresponds to the time when slurring of speech develops. The sedation threshold corresponds to the amount of drug needed to reach this inflection point. The threshold has been evaluated in different types of psychiatric conditions. The closest correlation occurred in relation to the level of anxiety present in the illness (16, 17, 18).

To summarize, current knowledge reveals no one-to-one relationship of EEG changes and anxiety. The percent-time beta activity tends to be increased in anxiety reactions. The alpha index tends to be decreased. Provocative techniques have not demonstrated any consistently different responses in normal subjects or patients with anxiety.

Surprisingly, the conversion reaction (hysteria) has attracted little electroencephalographic interest. Only a few reports of EEG studies of limited scope in conversion reactions are available. Romano and Engle (14) investigated syncope to differentiate hysterical faint from vasodepressor fainting. They found no change in the electroencephalogram, electrocardiogram, or blood pressure of patients with hysterical fainting. In an attempt to differentiate real and feigned amnesia, Lennox (10) studied the EEG patterns of amnestic individuals. He found that amnesia fell into three clinical groups: (1) those with inherent brain disorder (head injuries, fever, hyperglycemia, drug and alcohol intoxication, and amnesia associated with epileptic seizures; (2) neurosis or hysteria; and (3) feigned amnesia. Only in the first group is there abnormal electrical activity. This is not clear evidence for organic origin of amnesia, however, as 15 per cent of epileptics have normal EEGs and "15 per cent of the normal population" have abnormal records. Thus, only in cases of amnesia with objective electroencephalographic abnormality is there evidence of a pathophysiological basis for the amnestic episode. Investigations of the EEG patterns of patients with other forms of conversion are not available.

The electroencephalographic literature on obsessive-compulsive reactions is not abundant and the few reports available are conflicting. In a study of 26 psychoneurotic and 5 schizophrenic patients with this symptom complex, Pacella, Polantin, and Nagler (12) found normal EEGs in only 9 cases. Of the 20 abnormal records, 14 were classified "convulsive-type patterns" with runs of 2 to 4 cps high-voltage potentials. The remaining 6 had irregularities and disorganization of the electroencephalographic patterns. Two recordings were borderline, exhibiting mild irregularities. The greatest incidence of abnormal records was obtained from the age group below 30 years. In contrast, Rockwell and Simons (13) found that 9 of 11 patients with uncomplicated obsessive-compulsive illness had normal EEGs. One of the abnormal records was obtained following insulin therapy and showed excessive low-voltage fast activity. The eleventh had a heightened response to hyperventilation with a buildup of 5 to 7 cps at the end of one minute. This response was negated by the administration of dextrose prior to a repeat EEG with hyperventilation. In their second group of patients, whose obsessive-compulsive illness was complicated by disorganization of personality (sociopathic personality), they demonstrated the presence of excessive slow waves at 3 to 7 cps in the electroencephalogram.

EEG investigation of patients with other forms of psychoneurotic illnesses have not been conducted.

In conclusion, the pioneer electroencephalographers who studied patients with psychoneurosis were apparently discouraged when their efforts came to naught. No consistent changes have been observed in any neurotic reaction either in the resting EEG or when provocative techniques have been used. Since few investigative efforts have been made in recent years a careful evaluation of possible new approaches seems warranted. A reconsideration of the nosology of psychoneurosis as well as a more careful definition of the reaction type as a group seems indicated before further investigations will be meaningful.

BIBLIOGRAPHY

1. Brazier, M. A. B., Finesinger, J. E., and Cobb, S. A contrast between the electroencephalograms of 100 psychoneurotic patients and those of 500 normal adults. *Amer. J. Psychiat.* **101**: 443–448, 1945.
2. Ellingson, R. J. The incidence of EEG abnormality among patients with mental disorders of apparently non-organic origin: A critical review. *Amer. J. Psychiat.* **111**: 263–275, 1954.
3. Faure, J. Contribution a l'électroencéphalographie de l'anxiété, *Rev. neurol.* **80**: 648–649, 1948.
4. Finley, K. H. On the occurrence of rapid frequency potential changes in the human electroencephalogram. *Amer. J. Psychiat.* **101**: 194–200, 1944.
5. Gottlober, A. B. The relationship between brain potentials and personality. *J. exp. Psychol.* **22**: 67–74, 1938.
6. Henry, C. E., and Knott, J. R. A note on the relationship between "personality" and the alpha rhythm of the electroencephalogram. *J. exp. Psychol.* **28**: 362–366, 1941.
7. Heppenstall, M. E., Hill, D., and Slater, E. The EEG in the prognosis of war neurosis. *Brain.* **68**: 17–22, 1945.
8. Hoagland, H., Cameron, D. E., and Rubin, M. A. Emotion in man as tested by the delta index of the electroencephalogram: I. *J. gen. Psychol.* **19**: 227–245, 1938.
9. Lemere, F. The significance of individual differences in the Berger rhythm. *Brain.* **59**: 366–375, 1936.
10. Lennox, W. G. Amnesia, real and feigned. *Amer. J. Psychiat.* **99**: 732–743, 1943.
11. Oberman, C. E. The effect on the Berger rhythm of mild affective states. *J. abnorm. soc. Psychol.* **34**: 84–95, 1939.
12. Pacella, B. L., Polatin, P., and Nagler, S. H. Clinical and EEG studies in obsessive-compulsive states. *Amer. J. Psychiat.* **100**: 830–838, 1944.
13. Rockwell, F. V., and Simons, D. J. The electroencephalogram and personality organization in the obsessive-compulsive reactions. *Arch. Neurol. Psychiat.* **57**: 71–77, 1947.
14. Romano, J., and Engel, G. L. Studies of syncope: III. Differentiation between vasodepressor and hysterical fainting. *Psychosomat. Med.* **7**: 3–15, 1945.
15. Saul, L. J., Davis, H., and Davis, P. A. Correlations between electroencephalograms and the psychological organization of the individual. *Trans. Amer. Neurol. Ass.* **63**: 167–169, 1937.
16. Shagass, C. The sedation threshold. A method for estimating tension in psychiatric patients. *Electroenceph. clin. Neurophysiol.* **6**: 221–233, 1954.
17. Shagass, C., and Naiman, J. The sedation threshold, manifest anxiety, and some aspects of ego function. *Arch. Neurol. Psychiat.* **74**: 397–406, 1955.
18. Shagass, C., and Naiman, J. The sedation threshold as an objective index of manifest anxiety psychoneurosis. *J. psychosomat. Res.* **1**: 49–57, 1956.
19. Strauss, H. Clinical and electroencephalographic studies: The electroencephalogram in psychoneurotics. *J. nerv. ment. Dis.* **101**: 19–27, 1945.
20. Thiesen, J. W. Effects of certain forms of emotions on the normal electroencephalogram. *Arch. Psychol.* **40**: No. 285, 1943.
21. Ulett, G. A., Gleser, G., Winokur, G., and Lawler, A. The EEG and reaction to photic stimulation as an index of anxiety-proneness. *Electroenceph. clin. Neurophysiol.* **5**: 23–32, 1953.
22. Williams, A. C., Jr. Some psychological correlates of the electroencephalogram. *Arch. Psychol.* **34**: No. 240, 1939.

THE EEG IN AFFECTIVE PSYCHOSES

Charles Shagass, M.D.

The American Psychiatric Association diagnostic classification includes as affective reactions only the various forms of manic-depressive psychosis and psychotic depressive reaction (11). The involutional psychotic reactions in which depression is predominant are obviously closely allied. Two main affects are thus involved in the major affective psychoses: depression and elation. In addition, anxiety may play an important role (28). The EEG findings in relation to anxiety will be dealt with elsewhere in this symposium.

Absence of Specific EEG Abnormalities

Workers from Berger on have failed to find specific EEG abnormalities associated with the affective psychoses. On the contrary, the discovery of such abnormalities in patients presenting with depressive symptoms would lead one to a revision of the original diagnosis. For example, Strauss (62) reported four cases of intracranial neoplasm which had been diagnosed and treated as depressions and in which the EEG aided correct assessment. Weil (66) described six patients with paroxysmal depressive reactions, lasting for a duration of hours to weeks, which were associated with temporal-lobe discharges. While refractory to psychotherapy, the depressive episodes responded to energetic anticonvulsant medication. Williams (68) has reported five somewhat similar cases. It is noteworthy, however, that Daly (4), who reviewed a large series, found depression to be a relatively rare manifestation of ictal affect. Although the incidence is low, most electroencephalographers who study psychiatric populations have found abnormalities pointing to convulsive or neoplastic disease in patients with classical schizophrenic or neurotic syndromes. Consequently, there is no good evidence of a consistent association between specific EEG abnormality and clinical manifestations of depression or elation.

146

Quantitative Variations in Distribution of Normal EEG Characteristics

The absence of distinctive alterations in wave form led workers to compare the distributions of normal EEG characteristics in psychiatric and control populations.

Davis and Davis (5) reported their early findings in 100 normals and 70 patients in 1937. They found a normal distribution of alpha activity in manic-depressives. Two years later they described their results in 232 mental patients, of whom 64 were manic-depressive (9). Their patient group had a very low average alpha index compared to the non-patients. They also found that patients had a much higher incidence of irregular and abnormal records when rated on the five-point scale described by Pauline Davis (7).

Two subsequent reports by Pauline Davis dealt specifically with the EEG in manic-depressive psychosis and comparison with that found in schizophrenia (6, 8). Among 81 manic-depressive patients, 52 were depressed, 22 manic, and 7 mixed. Davis found very little change in the EEG when patients shifted from one phase of the illness (depressed or manic) to the other, except when level of consciousness was altered. She stated that those patients whose EEGs showed erratic slow wave disturbances were those whose behavior was unpredictable, regardless of diagnosis. The majority of the depressed group displayed a predominant alpha pattern or MS (mixed alpha and slow components) pattern, with alpha frequencies of 10 cps or slower. The manic group tended to have MF (mixed alpha and fast activity) patterns, with alpha frequencies of 10 cps or faster. Comparing the EEGs of this group with those of 126 schizophrenics, Davis (8) found A patterns more common in the manic-depressives (36 vs. 20 per cent) and B patterns (low-voltage fast records) less common (10 vs. 24 per cent). Alpha frequency was in the 10 to 10.5 cps range more often in the manic-depressives, and 11 cps or faster in more of the schizophrenics. Alpha voltage, assessed as low, average, or high, was about equally distributed in both groups. "Choppy" activity, which was the term Davis used for disorganized low-voltage fast activity, (26 to 50 cps) was much more common in schizophrenics (14 vs. 60 per cent). The different incidence of "choppy" activity was not attributable to age differences. Davis believed the "choppy" activity to be an indication of overstimulation or irritation of the cortex due to unsynchronized activity within the central nervous system. She cited experiments with mescaline in which this activity appeared and disappeared in conjunction with schizophrenic-like symptoms. The contribution of muscle activity to the "choppy" pattern remains in question, although Davis believed that the activity was cerebral in origin.

Davis did not report tests of statistical significance for her data. Calculation of chi square ratios for the data in her reports supports her conclusions.

Lemere (26) included 31 manic-depressive patients (19 depressed, 12 manic) in a study of psychiatric and normal populations. He found a greater incidence of high-voltage "strong" alpha rhythm in the manic-depressives than in normals, who in turn showed more than schizophrenics. He found no difference between manic and depressed patients. His interpretation of the data was that there was an overproduction of energy in the manic-depressive cases, a conclusion exactly opposite to that derived from similar data by P. Davis.

Greenblatt, Healey, and Jones (20) reviewed their EEG findings in 1,593 psychiatric patients. Their sample included 145 manic-depressive depressed type; 82 manic-depressive manic type; and 70 involutional psychoses. Their statistics were based on the incidence of records in which the predominant rhythm was outside the limits of 8 to 12 cps and/or there was a marked hyperventilation response. The percentage incidence of "abnormality" according to these criteria was as follows: manic-depressive depressed, 31; manic-depressive manic, 42; involutional psychosis, 51. The percentage in a young control group was 10, in schizophrenia 23, and in a group with senile and arteriosclerotic psychoses 54. There was a large amount of fast activity in the manic-depressive depressed type, and in the involutional psychoses. These authors recognized the importance of the age factor. Relating incidence of "abnormality" to age, they found a hyperbolic curve, with least "abnormality" in the middle years from 25 to 45. Slow activity was more common in young patients, fast activity in older ones. They concluded that the EEG findings in the various neuropsychiatric conditions were largely explained by changes associated with age.

Finley (15) has paid particular attention to fast activity in psychiatric disorders. He emphasized the need to use sufficient amplification in order adequately to record rapid rhythms, which are predominant in anterior derivations. Although noting that a single dominant fast frequency was usually present, he also pointed out that most recordings contained a fair range of frequencies. He tabulated the incidence of rapid activity in a large series of neuro-psychiatric patients, which included 89 manic-depressives and 53 involutional psychotics. He found the rapid patterns widely distributed throughout all types of disorder, and much more common than in a control group of 300 non-patients. The greatest incidence was in involutional psychoses (50 to 75 per cent), with manic-depressives also showing frequent rapid activity. Manic and depressive types were about equal at 25 to 40 per cent. Neurosyphilis ranked second to the involutional states (40 to 55 per cent). Finley was able to study some cases of manic-depressive psychosis in remission and found a decrease of rapid activity in these. He considered high-voltage rapid activity as a form of neurophysiological disturbance within the cerebrum.

Hurst, Mundy-Castle, and Beerstecher (**22**) had carried out the most exhaustive study of the EEG in manic-depressive psychosis, using frequency analysis in addition to standard EEG recording. They verified Pauline Davis' findings that mean alpha frequency was higher in the patients with predominantly manic phases of the disorder than those with predominantly depressed phases, and that this difference was present regardless of the clinical phase at the time of the test. They were unable to demonstrate a correlation between alpha frequency and clinically assessed degree of depression or mania. They attempted to apply Pauline Davis' "choppy" classification, but were forced to abandon it because of the small number of records which they were able to classify as such with certainty. They also found a higher incidence of low-voltage fast records in the psychotic group than in a group of 160 normals. Although the normals were younger, there was no significant difference in incidence between the psychotics below and above the age of 55. It should be noted, how-ever, that this is not a sufficient test for the age factor. Hurst *et al.* also found a higher incidence of abnormal EEGs in the total psycho-tic group (24 *vs.* 10 per cent). The influence of age on this finding must also be questioned.

Comparing a variety of EEG characteristics in the manic-depres-sives with those of a normal control group, Hurst *et al.* found that the psychotic group had significantly lower mean alpha fre-quency, significantly lower mean alpha amplitude, and significantly lower alpha index. The psychotic and normal groups showed no differences in the distribution of R (responsive), P (persistent), and M (minus) alpha types of Grey Walter. With respect to characteristics of beta activity, they found significantly higher mean beta frequency in the psychotic group and a trend toward somewhat higher beta amplitude. Theta amplitude was also significantly higher in the psychotic group. The incidence of beta rhythm was significantly higher and the theta rhythm significantly lower in the manic-depressives.

Table I. EEG Findings in Manic-Depressive Psychosis

Characteristic		
Alpha Frequency	Lower in depressives than manics	P. Davis Hurst, Mundy-Castle, and Beerstecher
	Less than in schizophrenics	P. Davis
	Lower than normal	Hurst *et al.*
Alpha Index	Lower than normal	Hurst *et al.*
Pattern	"Strong" alpha (more than normals or schizophrenics)	Lemere
	Predominantly A or MS in depression: MF in mania	P. Davis
	Low "choppy" incidence	P. Davis
	More low-voltage fast irregular than in normals	Hurst *et al.*

Beta Activity	Higher frequency and amplitude, more
	    prominent and common than in normals
		Hurst *et al.*
		Finley
		Greenblatt, Healey,
		    and Jones

Theta Activity	Amplitude higher and incidence less than normal	Hurst *et al.*
"Abnormality"	More common than in normal	Greenblatt *et al.* Hurst *et al.* Davis and Davis

Table I summarizes the various findings that have so far been reviewed. It would seem that manic-depressive patients, when depressed, show a tendency toward lower alpha frequency, fairly predominant alpha activity but with a low alpha index, prominent beta activity, and a higher incidence of abnormality than normal control populations in terms of accepted frequency standards. The alpha frequency of the depressives tends to be lower than that in manics, as does the relative predominance of alpha activity. The extent to which these findings represent significant deviations from normal is obscured by age differences between patient and control groups. This uncertainty is accentuated by the findings of Maggs and Turton (31). They studied 82 normal control patients over 60 years of age and compared these with 96 cases of depression. They found no difference in record type between the depressed patients and control subjects, but they did find more abnormalities in the patients whose illness began at the age of 60 or above. They found a considerable number of abnormal and borderline records in both controls and patients, and considered this to be an expression of a general aging process, not limited to any one specific symptom complex or disorder. There is thus considerable doubt that even the relatively consistent statistical findings of a deviant distribution of alpha and beta characteristics in the affective psychoses can be interpreted as more than a correlate of the age distribution in these disorders.

Responses to Activation Procedures

The possibility that procedures for eliciting changes in the EEG might reveal differential responsiveness in psychiatric disorders has engaged the attention of several workers. Liberson (29) used the term "functional electroencephalography" to designate this approach. Hyperventilation has been used as an activation procedure since the earliest days of electroencephalography. Greenblatt et al. (20) took an excessive response to hyperventilation as one of their criteria of "abnormality," but they do not indicate to what extent this contributed to their classification of abnormal findings in the affective psychoses. Liberson (29) reported the results obtained in 945 psychiatric patients under conditions of early-morning fasting with undisturbed recording to produce a drowsy state, and also visual stimulation with flashes of light at 2 per second. His population included 51 manic-depressive depressed patients, 49 manics, and 111 cases of involutional melancholia, together with 38 reactive depressions. He found drowsy patterns in 70 per cent of the manics; in 55 per cent of the manic-depressive depressed patients; and 50 per cent of the involutional melancholias. These drowsy patterns were most pronounced in patients with symptoms of insomnia. The drowsy patterns varied from one group to another with respect to locus, speed, and pattern of onset. In response to visual stimulation prolonged reduction of alpha activity was most prominent in involutional states, but was as common in psychopaths.

Diaz-Guerrero, Gottlieb, and Knott (12) compared the all-night sleep EEGs in six manic-depressive depressed patients with those in a normal sample. They found that the patients not only had greater difficulty in falling asleep and staying asleep, but that the EEGs showed a greater proportion of their sleep to be light and oscillating more frequently than in normal subjects from one level of sleep to another.

Hurst, Mundy-Castle, and Beerstecher (**22**) studied effects of rhythmic photic stimulation in their manic-depressive sample and compared these with their normal control group. They found greater flicker following in the psychotics over the 4 to 20 fps range but not in the 21 to 26 fps range. Harmonically related responses were not significantly different, nor were abnormal responses more common in the psychotic group. There was a tendency for the manic group to show a higher incidence of harmonics and to show more flicker following in the beta range than the depressed group. These authors found no differences between manic-depressives and normals with respect to hyperventilation responses.

Shagass (**47**) studied photic driving responses in relation to affect. He compared the amplitude of driving at flash rates of 10 and 15 per second in a non-patient group and in patients with anxiety and depression. The amplitude of driving responses was significantly higher in females, necessitating separate treatment of the sexes. The main finding was that the relative amount of driving to 15 fps compared with 10 fps (15:10 ratio) was highest in anxiety states, intermediate in controls, and lowest in depressive psychoses. This relationship was statistically significant for females, but not for males, although the trend was present in the latter. Longitudinal studies of driving responses in two female employees also seemed to support a relationship between the 15:10 ratio and current affective state (**46**). However, subsequent attempts to repeat these findings with photic driving yielded inconsistent results (**50**). Ulett, Gleser, Winokur, and Lawler (**64**) have also apparently found their initial correlations between photic driving and anxiety-proneness difficult to repeat. It seems probable that the driving response may be influenced by several unknown factors which vary from experiment to experiment.

Leiberman, Hoenig, and Hacker (**25**) applied Gastaut's method of Metrazol-flicker (**16**) in a group of psychiatric patients which included 36 cases of anxiety or depressive states, not further described. The mean Metrazol threshold in this group was not significantly different from that in the majority of other patients. Shagass (45) studied the photomyoclonic response in a group of 411 psychiatric patients, which included 143 depressions and 5 hypomanic states. The incidence of these responses was about the same in the affective psychoses as in most other patient groups and was not significantly greater than normal.

Goldman (18) has described a technique of Pentothal activation of the EEG. He found that this discriminated between schizophrenic patients and those with other psychiatric diagnoses. His technique was based upon assessment of EEG changes, primarily in the beta range, that occur within a five-minute period after the intravenous injection of 300 mgm of Pentothal. He devised a system for scoring the effects of Pentothal administration by this method. Sila, Mowrer, Ulett, and Johnson (61) attempted to verify Goldman's findings by means of frequency analysis. Comparing 39 schizophrenic patients with 19 psychotic depressives, they found no difference in the frequency analysis spectrum of the pre-injection EEG in these two groups. During the first minute after the Pentothal injection, the increase in activity over almost the entire frequency range was considerably greater in the schizophrenics than in the depressions. This finding seemed to verify Goldman's results, but when Sila *et al.* eliminated the patients with overlapping symptomotology, so that there were only 12 clear schizophrenics and 12 clear depressives left, no significant difference remained between the groups.

Sedation Threshold

Although bearing a superficial resemblance to Goldman's Pentothal activation procedure, the sedation threshold procedure devised by Shagass (44) is not truly an activation technique, insofar as it depends upon the *rate* of elicitation of the normal EEG response to amobarbital sodium. Injecting amobarbital at the rate of 0.5 mg/kg/40 sec., Shagass recorded and measured the EEG fast-frequency response to this drug. Administration was continued until well after the clinical sign of slurred speech was elicited. The mean amplitude of fast activity was plotted in relation to amount of drug given. The threshold point was the second of two adjacent points between which the greatest increase in fast-activity amplitude occurred. Shagass and Jones found that the mean sedation threshold in normal subjects was about 3 mg/kg. In patients with anxiety neurosis and/or neurotic depressive states the threshold approached 5 mg/kg, whereas in psychotic depressives the mean threshold was somewhat less than 3 mg/kg (**51**). Although the sedation threshold was therefore not really different in normals and in psychotic depressive states, this permitted differentiation between neurotic depressions and various forms of psychotic depression (**52**). Within the psychotic depressive group, the sedation threshold did not differentiate between manic-depressive or involutional states, nor was it related to the presence of retardation or agitation.

Attempts to duplicate Shagass' sedation threshold findings have met with varying success. Essentially similar results were obtained by Nymgaard (**35**) and Seager (**43**) in depressive states, whereas Ackner and Pampiglione reported inability to verify the correlation Shagass reported with level of anxiety (**1**). Important differences in method seem to be involved, since the mean threshold values reported vary widely. Recently, Giberti and Rossi (**17**) have devised a "stimulation threshold" based on blood pressure and pulse changes to injected methamphetamine. The "stimulation threshold" also discriminated between neurotic and psychotic depressions, but in the opposite direction; thresholds were low in neurotic depressions and high in psychotic depressions.

It should be emphasized that the sedation threshold procedure uses the EEG only as an indicator of a drug effect. There are numerous possible indicators of the effects of depressant and excitant drugs. Although the underlying concept involved in such drug threshold procedures is that they will reveal characteristics of cerebral responsiveness, these may not be manifested in the usual EEG tracings.

Personality Correlates

Several workers have attempted to relate the predominant pattern in the EEG with dimensions of personality, and have extended these concepts to the study of psychophysiological disorders. Important early findings in this area were those of Saul, Davis, and Davis (**40**), who studied patients in psychoanalysis. They found that high alpha indices were associated with a passive-dependent, receptive attitude toward other persons, provided this attitude was freely accepted and not thwarted or inhibited internally. Low alpha indices were associated with consistent, well-directed, freely indulged drive to activity. Davis (**6**) had found relatively slow, alpha-dominant

EEGs in the depressed type of manic-depressive psychosis, and fast low alpha index records in the manic type. These findings were considered by Rubin and Moses (**39**) to agree with the concept that depressed patients, as a group, appear passive-dependent, whereas manic patients are more likely to be described as active, energetic, and independent. Rubin and Bowman (**38**) studied 100 cases of proven peptic ulcer and compared these with a control group collected by H. Davis. High alpha index, greater than 75 per cent, was much more frequent in the peptic ulcer group. Rubin and Moses (**39**) also studied 54 cases of bronchial asthma and found that the asthmatics had about three times as many dominant alpha records as a normal control group. Moses (**33**) later studied 25 additional cases of duodenal ulcer and again found dominant alpha records in these subjects.

Introversion-extraversion is another personality dimension which has received study. Gottlober (**19**) found that subjects with alpha index above 50 per cent were more likely to be extraverts. The "typical" cyclothymic is, of course, extraverted. However, Gottlober's findings were not confirmed by Henry and Knott (**21**).

Hurst *et al.* (**22**) related their findings in manic-depressive psychoses to previous studies of the Heymans-Wiersma temperament variable, secondary function. Heymans and Wiersma maintain that the poles of the manic-depressive continuum are comparable to extremes of the primary-secondary function continuum and that the two are comparable. However, Hurst *et al.* pointed out that their findings did not support this contention, since they did not find a shift in alpha frequency when the phase of illness changed in individual manic-depressives. They felt the main finding to be that the dominant clinical phase was determined by a basic temperamental factor, i.e., degree of secondary function, and that swings toward the opposite phase were brought about by some extraneous factor.

It would seem there is a degree of correlation between some quantitative characteristics of the EEG and personality variables which many consider to be associated with the manic-depressive psychosis. Correlative trends of this kind leave one some distance from any precise statement of psychophysiologic relationships. Personality variables, such as passive-receptive, passive-aggressive, or primary-secondary function, are difficult to define with precision. It would be surprising indeed, therefore, if a high level of correlation were found between such loosely formulated variables and precisely measurable EEG characteristics, which in themselves may reflect quite primitive functional states. Furthermore, it may well be that the notion that depression is associated with passive-dependence and mania with aggressive attitudes is based more upon behavior during the illness than upon enduring personality characteristics. Certainly McAdam, Tait, and Orme (30) obtained completely negative results when they tested a number of hypotheses relating EEG variables to personality assessment, based upon both clinical and psychological test estimates, in a group of female involutional patients.

Convulsive Therapy

The EEG changes associated with convulsive therapy merit consideration here, as the affective psychoses are the clinical states most favorably influenced by this form of treatment. However, the voluminous literature in this area precludes any attempt at a comprehensive review. Electroconvulsive therapy (ECT) has been the most widely used form, although there has been considerable observation of convulsions induced by drugs, notably Metrazol.

Kiloh and Osselton (23) present a succinct and well-illustrated description of the EEG changes associated with a single major convulsion. The postictal phase is characterized by low-amplitude slow delta. The frequencies gradually become faster and, after a variable time, the record assumes its normal appearance. As successive treatments are administered, the generalized delta and theta activity following the fit becomes more persistent, often frontally predominant. In the average case, the slow activity fails to disappear completely after three or four treatments, spaced two or three days apart. Subsequent treatments result in the slow activity becoming more widespread, of higher amplitude, and of lower frequency. The alpha rhythm becomes disturbed and may disappear. Clinical evidence of confusion may appear along with the EEG changes, but there is no essential parallelism.

The sensitivity of the EEG to ECT shows much variation between individuals. Some show marked alterations after two or three treatments, others show little change after a dozen. Klotz (24) found that 82 per cent of 167 patients receiving a "standard" course of ECT showed changes. Changes are greater when treatments are given closer together. After the end of a course of ECT, the record gradually returns to its normal appearance, the frequencies increasing until the alpha rhythm is again present at usual frequency. The rate of return is also variable. Following 6 to 12 treatments given thrice weekly the changes usually disappear after one to three months. In Klotz's series 98 per cent returned to normal by the third month. However, Klotz noted seizure activity in seven patients and one of these had persistent clinical seizures and EEG abnormalities for at least one year after treatment. The occurrence of clinical convulsive disorder after ECT may be more frequent when large numbers of treatments are given. Blumenthal (2) reported 12 such cases, among whom 4 of 6 were known to have a normal pretreatment EEG.

With intensive ECT, consisting of four treatments daily for seven consecutive days, Callaway (3) found that slow wave activity actually increased for several days after cessation of treatment. It then diminished, and there was no residual EEG abnormality in any of his 23 cases after five months. Intensive treatment thus appears to alter the temporal course of slow wave development and regression.

Many workers have attempted to relate the EEG changes to therapeutic effects of convulsive therapy. In an early study, Levy, Serota, and Grinker (27) reported their findings in 11 patients treated with Metrazol and 12 patients given ECT. They found the characteristic EEG changes in half of their patients and concluded that recovery or improvement did not depend on such changes. Mosovitch and Katzenelbogen (34), with a larger series, concluded that greater EEG abnormality after ECT was more common in unimproved than in improved patients. Moriarty and Siemens (32) found no relationship between EEG change and recovery after ECT. More recently, Fink and Kahn (14) carried out a careful quantitative study of delta activity during a standard course of 12 ECT. They related various measures of delta to degree of improvement, concluding that early induction and persistence of high degree delta activity (frequency less than 4 cps, amplitude greater than 100 microvolts) was associated with a higher short-term remission rate. Fink and Kahn attributed divergent results of different workers to differences in method. They interpreted their findings as indicating that ECT induces non-specific, persistent states of altered cerebral function to provide a physiologic milieu in which changes in adaptive interpersonal behavior appear.

Roth (36) employed a special technique, involving injection of thiopentone (Pentothal) to elicit changes in the EEG at an earlier stage of treatment than found in routine recordings. The drug is given intravenously about three to four hours after ECT at an injection rate of 50 mgm every 20 seconds until consciousness is lost. Delta activity, maximal in frontal regions, appears and lasts up to 300 seconds, when it is replaced by barbiturate fast activity. Roth found that delta was usually increased after the third treatment and often after the second. The rate of return to normal depended upon the number of ECT administered, being five to seven weeks for 10 to 12 treatments. In cases of endogenous depression, the amount of delta response showed little relationship to initial outcome, most patients being improved. There was, however, some suggestion that the EEG changes were a necessary, if not sufficient, accompaniment of recovery.

In a subsequent report Roth *et al.* (37) related the thiopentone-induced delta response to prognosis in a series of 41 psychotic depressions, obtaining follow-up data for 12 months. They found that the relapse rate was significantly higher in patients whose peak delta activity was lower. Taking the percentage of time occupied by delta for the 300-second period following its commencement as an index, only 2 of 19 patients with indices greater than 40 per cent relapsed, while 13 of 22 with lower indices relapsed. Their data seem to be in general agreement with those of Fink and Kahn (14) in suggesting that a significant alteration in cerebral activity must be produced by ECT to exert favorable therapeutic effects.

If slow waves produced by ECT are a prerequisite for clinical benefit, what would happen if one blocked the appearance of slow activity? Ulett and Johnson (65) explored the effects of atropine and scopolamine as delta activity inhibitors in patients given ECT. They found that the delta activity was indeed blocked by these anticholinergic agents. However, if the drugs were discontinued at a time when slow activity would usually be present, delta waves reappeared. It thus appeared that the mechanism of ECT-induced delta activity was not affected, although the manifestation of this activity could be altered. Fink (13) studied a series of experimental anticholinergic compounds (diethazine, Win-2299, benactyzine, JB-318 and JB-336) and also found these to reduce ECT-induced delta activity. He concluded that an increase in CNS cholinergic activity is a concomitant of ECT.

The prognostic value of the pretreatment EEG has been considered by several workers. Although there seems to be some trend to indicate that an abnormal record indicates a lower probability of favorable outcome (**34, 63, 67**) agreement is not universal (**32**).

Shagass *et al.* (**52**) attempted to relate the sedation threshold to outcome of treatment by ECT. In accordance with the diagnostic correlates of this determination, it was found that relatively few depressed patients with high thresholds (neurotic depressions) were given ECT. Among those treated, a more favorable therapeutic outcome was associated with low than with high thresholds. A similar relationship was observed in schizophrenic patients treated with ECT (**49**). The sedation threshold thus seemed of value as a prognostic indicator of ECT effect. Shagass (**48**) also studied the changes in sedation threshold produced by ECT. Although there was a tendency for thresholds to increase after ECT, this seemed to depend upon the pretreatment level. Relatively large changes were found in cases with very low pretreatment thresholds, slight or no changes in cases with average values.

In general, then, the EEG has served to demonstrate that ECT affects brain function, producing changes that are usually reversible. It has also led to development of some suggestive indicators of prognosis with ECT. However, the mechanisms by which ECT acts, and the important clues which they would afford for understanding the neurophysiology of affective psychoses, are still almost unknown.

Studies of Evoked Potentials

The recent development of averaging instruments for extracting the cortical potentials evoked by sensory stimulation from the EEG has added a new dimension to human neurophysiological studies (**10**). These methods make it possible to study reactive characteristics of a sensory system directly at the level of the cortex, and to compare such characteristics in different populations. Employing the cortical response to electrical pulses administered over the skin at the ulnar nerve, Shagass and Schwartz have carried out a series of studies in psychiatric patients, comparing the responses in different diagnostic groups and in non-patients.

Shagass and Schwartz confined their measurements to the initial, or primary, negative-positive complex of the somato-sensory response (Fig. 1). The mean latencies of maximum negativity and positivity are about 20 and 25 msec, respectively. The first evidence of response occurs at a stimulus intensity corresponding to the sensory

160

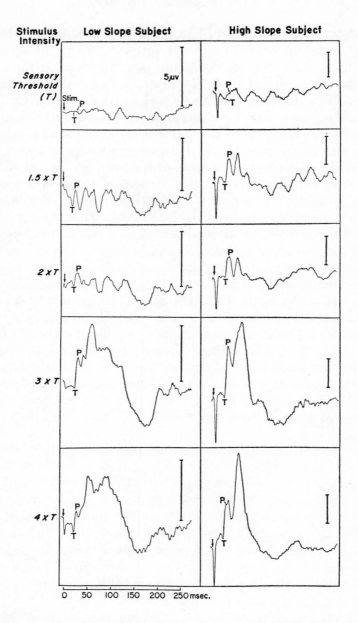

Figure 1. Effect of increasing intensities of electrical stimulation to the ulnar nerve on somatosensory evoked potentials in two subjects. Downward deflection under arrow is stimulus artifact. T—maximum negativity: P—maximum positivity of initial component. Amplitudes in later figures measured between T and P. Note increasing amplitude and changes in form with increasing stimulus intensity.

threshold (**53, 58**). The amplitude of the response then increases as a function of intensity. A comparison of the intensity-response curves in a heterogeneous psychiatric population with a non-patient sample revealed significant differences (**58, 60**). For any given intensity of stimulation, the mean amplitude of the primary component was greater in the patients (Fig. 2). Breaking down the patient group by psychiatric diagnosis, only one group was similar to non-patients: this group included psychoneurotics with anxiety, depressive, obsessive-compulsive reactions, and psychophysiologic reactions. They could be called "dysthymic." The psychotic depressive syndromes, although deviant from normal, were indistinguishable from schizophrenics and personality disorders. It is probable that the deviant intensity-response function in psychotic depressions is reversible by effective therapy. This is indicated by the findings that response amplitudes decreased appreciably in several patients who responded to either antidepressant drugs or ECT (**57**).

Shagass and Schwartz also measured the recovery function of the primary somatosensory response, using the method of paired "conditioning" and "test" stimuli (**54, 56**). In normal man the first 200 msec of the recovery function is biphasic, with an early peak of recovery occurring by 20 msec and a later one at about 100 msec. There is a period of subnormal responsiveness between these peaks (Fig. 3). A heterogeneous population of 167 psychiatric patients differed from 40 non-patients mainly with respect to the amount of

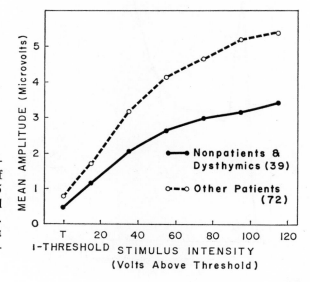

Figure 2. Mean intensity-response curves of 24 non-patients and 15 dysthymics compared with 72 other patients. Differences at all points were statistically significant (**60**).

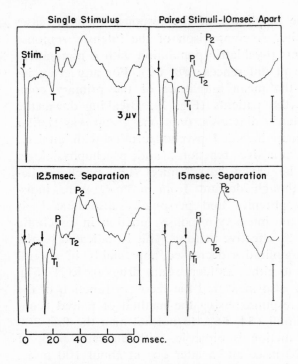

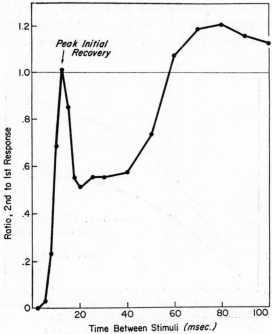

Figure 3. Sample tracings and recovery curve obtained by paired "conditioning" and "test" stimulus method. Symbols and polarity as in Fig. 1. Recovery ratio equals 1.0 when R2 = R1. Curve is arithmetically smoothed. Note its biphasic form.

recovery occurring during the early phase, i.e. by 20 msec (**59**). As with the intensity-response function, the "dysthymic" group of psychoneuroses gave recovery findings similar to the non-patients, whereas the functional psychoses and personality disorders differed significantly from normals and dysthymics. Figure 4 compares the mean recovery curves for initial samples of 13 non-patients and 21 patients with psychotic depressions (**55**). Effective treatment with ECT or antidepressant drugs returned the recovery curves to the normal pattern (Fig. 5). The results in three manic patients were inconsistent (**59**). It is also noteworthy that the intensity-response and recovery function measures were relatively independent of one another with respect to clinical differentiation.

It should be obvious that application of the evoked potential method to studies of psychiatric illness is in its early, exploratory stages. Although the positive findings so far obtained are relatively non-specific, it may be hoped that greater specificity of correlations will emerge with further development of the physiological tech-

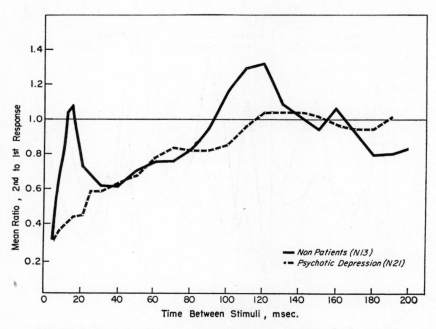

Figure 4. Mean recovery curves for 13 non-patients and 21 psychotic depressive patients (**55**). Note marked reduction of early recovery in patients.

nique and better definition of psychological variables. The results already obtained have provided a focus for animal studies aimed at clarifying relevant brain mechanisms (**41, 42**).

Conclusion

The material reviewed here leads to the inescapable conclusion that there are no specific findings, qualitative or quantitative, obtainable by currently known standard or special EEG procedures, which characterize the various affective psychoses. The available positive findings with standard recordings are of statistical nature and attributable to an uncertain, but important, degree to age differences. On all measures the findings in affective psychoses overlap considerably with those of other clinical groups. The results with special procedures such as the sedation threshold may have some value in differential diagnosis, but are also non-specific. Although the therapeutic effects of ECT in affective psychoses differ from those in other groups, the EEG effects do not show comparable differences. It seems as though the altered brain functions, which one

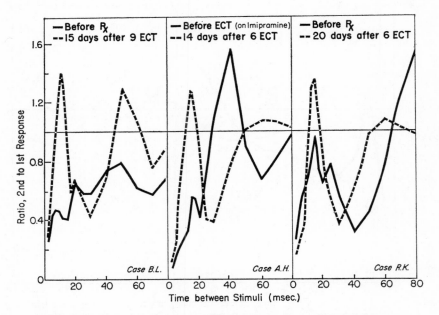

Figure 5. Recovery curves before and after successful treatment in three patients with depression (**55**). Note augmented early recovery after treatment.

would believe to underly the affective psychoses, are not directly reflected in anything electroencephalographers have so far been able to measure. One can only place hope in future studies aimed at exploring the mechanisms underlying such non-specific changes as have been found. It is likely that several mechanisms may lead to a similar end result. Definition of such mechanisms may point to those specifically involved in the affective psychoses.

BIBLIOGRAPHY

1. Ackner, B., and Pampiglione, G. An evaluation of the sedation threshold test. *J. psychosom. Res.* **3**: 271–281, 1959.
2. Blumenthal, I. J. Spontaneous seizures and related electroencephalographic findings following shock therapy. *J. nerv. ment. Dis.* **122**: 581–588, 1955.
3. Callaway, E. Slow wave phenomena in intensive electroshock. *Electroenceph. clin. Neurophysiol.* **2**: 157–162, 1950.
4. Daly, D. Ictal affect. *Amer. J. Psychiat.* **115**: 97–108, 1958.
5. Davis, H., and Davis, P. A. The human electroencephalogram in health and in certain mental disorders. *Arch. Neurol. Psychiat.* **37**: 1461–1462, 1937.
6. Davis, P. A. Electroencephalograms of manic-depressive patients. *Amer. J. Psychiat.* **98**: 430–433, 1941.
7. Davis, P. A. Technique and evaluation of the electroencephalogram. *J. Neurophysiol.* **4**: 92–114, 1941.
8. Davis, P. A. Comparative study of the EEGs of schizophrenic and manic-depressive patients. *Amer. J. Psychiat.* **99**: 210–217, 1942.
9. Davis, P. A., and Davis, H. The electroencephalograms of psychotic patients. *Amer. J. Psychiat.* **95**: 1007–1025, 1939.
10. Dawson, G. D. A summation technique for the detection of small evoked potentials. *Electroenceph. clin. Neurophysiol.* **6**: 65–84, 1954.
11. *Diagnostic and Statistical Manual: Mental Disorders*, prepared by the Committee on Nomenclature and Statistics of the American Psychiatric Association. American Psychiatric Association Mental Hospital Service, Washington, 1952.
12. Diaz-Guerrero, R., Gottlieb, J. S., and Knott, J. R. The sleep of patients with manic-depressive psychosis, depressive type; an electroencephalographic study. *Psychosom. Med.* **8**: 399–404, 1946.
13. Fink, M. Effect of anticholinergic compounds on post convulsive electroencephalogram and behavior of psychiatric patients. *Electroenceph. clin. Neurophysiol.* **12**: 359–369, 1960.
14. Fink, M., and Kahn, R. L. Relation of electroencephalographic delta activity to behavioral response in electro-shock. *Arch. Neurol. Psychiat.* **78**: 516–525, 1957.
15. Finley, K. H. On the occurrence of rapid frequency potential changes in the human electroencephalogram. *Amer. J. Psychiat.* **101**: 194–200, 1944.
16. Gastaut, H. Combined photic and metrazol activation of the brain. *Electroenceph. clin. Neurophysiol.* **2**: 249–261, 1950.
17. Giberti, F., and Rossi, R. Proposal of a psychopharmacological test ("stimulation threshold") for differentiating neurotic from psychotic depressions. Preliminary Report. *Psychopharmacologia.* **3**: 128–131, 1962.
18. Goldman, D. Specific electroencephalographic changes with Pentothal activation in psychotic states. *Electroenceph. clin. Neurophysiol.* **11**: 657–667, 1959.
19. Gottlober, A. B. The relationship between brain potentials and personality. *J. exp. Psychol.* **22**: 67–74, 1938.
20. Greenblatt, M., Healey, M. M., and Jones, G. A. Age and electroencephalographic abnormality in neuropsychiatric patients: A study of 1593 cases. *Amer. J. Psychiat.* **101**: 82–90, 1944.
21. Henry, C. E., and Knott, J. R. A note on the relationship between personality and the alpha rhythm of the electroencephalogram. *J. exp. Psychol.* **28**: 362–366, 1941.
22. Hurst, L. A., Mundy-Castle, A. C., and Beerstecher, D. M. The electroencephalogram in manic-depressive psychosis. *J. ment. Sci.* **100**: 220–240, 1954.
23. Kiloh, L. G., and Osselton, J. W. *Clinical Electroencephalography*. Butterworths, London, p. 31, 1961.

24. Klotz, M. Serial electroencephalographic changes due to electrotherapy. *Dis. nerv. Syst.* **16**: 120–121, 1955.
25. Leiberman, D. M., Hoenig, J., and Hacker, M. The metrazol-flicker threshold in neuro-psychiatric patients. *Electroenceph. clin. Neurophysiol.* **6**: 9–18, 1954.
26. Lemere, F. Cortical energy production in the psychoses. *Psychosom. Med.* **3**: 152–156, 1941.
27. Levy, N. A., Serota, H. M., and Grinker, R. R. Disturbances in brain function following convulsive shock therapy. *Arch. Neurol. Psychiat.* **47**: 1009–1029, 1942.
28. Lewis, A. J. Melancholia: A clinical survey of depressive states. *J. ment. Sci.* **80**: 277–378, 1934.
29. Liberson, W. T. Functional electroencephalography in mental disorders. *Dis. nerv. Syst.* **5**: 357–364, 1944.
30. McAdam, W., Tait, A. C., and Orme, J. E. Initial psychiatric illness in involutional women. III. Electroencephalographic findings. *J. ment. Sci.* **103**: 824–829, 1957.
31. Maggs, R., and Turton, E. C. Some EEG findings in old age and their relationship to affective disorder. *J. ment. Sci.* **102**: 812–818, 1956.
32. Moriarty, J. D., and Siemens, J. C. Electroencephalographic study of electric shock therapy: Psychotic patients treated in a United States Naval Hospital. *Arch. Neurol. Psychiat.* **57**: 712–718, 1947.
33. Moses, L. Psychodynamic and electroencephalographic factors in duodenal ulcer. *Psychosom. Med.* **8**: 405–409, 1946.
34. Mosovich, A., and Katzenelbogen, S. Electro-shock therapy, clinical and electroencephalographic studies. *J. nerv. ment. Dis.* **107**: 517–530, 1948.
35. Nymgaard, K. Studies on the sedation threshold. *Arch. gen. Psychiat.* **1**: 530–536, 1959.
36. Roth, M. Changes in the EEG under barbiturate anaesthesia produced by electroconvulsive treatment and their significance for the theory of ECT action. *Electroenceph. clin. Neurophysiol.* **3**: 261–280, 1951.
37. Roth, M., Kay, D. W. K., Shaw, J., and Green, J. Prognosis and Pentothal induced electroencephalographic changes in electro-convulsive treatment: An approach to the problem of regulation of convulsive therapy. *Electroenceph. clin. Neurophysiol.* **9**: 225–237, 1957.
38. Rubin, S., and Bowman, K. M. Electroencephalographic and personality correlates in peptic ulcer. *Psychosom. Med.* **4**: 31–39, 1944.
39. Rubin, S., and Moses, L. Electroencephalographic studies in asthma with some personality correlates. *Psychosom. Med.* **6**: 31–39, 1944.
40. Saul, L. J., Davis, H., and Davis, P. A. Correlations between electroencephalograms and the psychological organization of the individual. *Trans. Amer. Neurol. Ass.* **63**: 167–169, 1937.
41. Schwartz, M., and Shagass, C. Effect of different states of alertness on somatosensory and auditory recovery cycles. *Electroenceph. clin. Neurophysiol.* **14**: 11–20, 1962.
42. Schwartz, M., and Shagass, C. Reticular modification of somatosensory cortical recovery function. *Electroenceph. clin. Neurophysiol.* **15**: 265–271, 1963.
43. Seager, C. P. A clinical evaluation of the sedation threshold in psychiatry. M. D. Thesis, University of Wales, Nov., 1960.
44. Shagass, C. The sedation threshold. A method for estimating tension in psychiatric patients. *Electroenceph. clin. Neurophysiol.* **6**: 221–233, 1954.
45. Shagass, C. Clinical significance of the photomyoclonic response in psychiatric patients. *Electroenceph. clin. Neurophysiol.* **6**: 445–453, 1954.
46. Shagass, C. Anxiety, depression, and the photically driven electroencephalogram. *Arch. Neurol. Psychiat.* **74**: 3–10, 1955.
47. Shagass, C. Differentiation between anxiety and depression by the photically activated electroencephalogram. *Amer. J. Psychiat.* **112**: 41–46, 1955.
48. Shagass, C. Neurophysiological studies of anxiety and depression. *Psychiat. Res. Rep. Amer. Psychiat. Ass.* **8**: 100–117, 1957.
49. Shagass, C. A neurophysiological study of schizophrenia. *Report, 2nd International Congress for Psychiatry*, **2**: 248–254, 1959.
50. Shagass, C. Unpublished observations.
51. Shagass, C., and Jones, A. L. A neurophysiological test for psychiatric diagnosis: Results in 750 patients. *Amer. J. Psychiat.* **114**: 1002–1010, 1958.
52. Shagass, C., Naiman, J., and Mihalik, J. An objective test which differentiates between neurotic and psychotic depression. *Arch. Neurol. Psychiat.* **75**: 461–471, 1956.
53. Shagass, C., and Schwartz, M. Evoked cortical potentials and sensation in man. *J. Neuropsychiat.* **2**: 262–270, 1961.
54. Shagass, C., and Schwartz, M. Reactivity cycle of somatosensory cortex in humans with and without psychiatric disorder. *Science.* **134**: 1757–1759, 1961.

55. Shagass, C., and Schwartz, M. Cerebral cortical reactivity in psychotic depressions. *Arch. gen. Psychiat.* **6**: 235–242, 1962.
56. Shagass, C., and Schwartz, M. Excitability of the cerebral cortex in psychiatric disorders. In: R. Roessler and N. S. Greenfield (Editors), *Physiological Correlates of Psychological Disorder.* University of Wisconsin Press, Madison, pp. 45–60, 1962.
57. Shagass, C., Schwartz, M., and Amadeo, M. Some drug effects on evoked cerebral potentials in man. *J. Neuropsychiat.* **3**: Suppl. 1, 849–858, 1962.
58. Shagass, C., and Schwartz, M. Cerebral responsiveness in psychiatric patients. *Arch. gen. Psychiat.* **8**: 177–189, 1963.
59. Shagass, C., and Schwartz, M. Psychiatric correlates of evoked cerebral cortical potentials. *Amer. J. Psychiat.* **119**: 1055–1061, 1963.
60. Shagass, C., and Schwartz, M. Psychiatric disorder and deviant cerebral responsiveness to sensory stimulation. *Recent Advances Biol. Psychiat.* **5**: 321–330, 1963.
61. Sila, B., Mowrer, M., Ulett, G., and Johnson, M. The differentiation of psychiatric patients by EEG changes after sodium pentothal. *Recent Advances Biol. Psychiat.* **4**: 191–203, 1961.
62. Strauss, H. Intracranial neoplasms masked as depressions and diagnosed with the aid of electroencephalography. *J. nerv. ment. Dis.* **122**: 185–189, 1955.
63. Turner, W. J., Lowinger, L., and Huddleson, J. H. The correlation of pre-electroshock electroencephalogram and therapeutic result in schizophrenia. *Amer. J. Psychiat.* **102**: 299–300, 1945.
64. Ulett, G. A., Gleser, G., Winokur, G., and Lawler, A. The EEG and reaction to photic stimulation as an index of anxiety-proneness. *Electroenceph. clin. Neurophysiol.* **5**: 23–32, 1953.
65. Ulett, G. A., and Johnson, M. W. Effect of atropine and scopolamine upon electroencephalographic changes induced by electro-convulsive-therapy. *Electroenceph. clin. Neurophysiol.* **9**: 217–224, 1957.
66. Weil, A. A. Depressive reactions associated with temporal lobe-uncinate seizures. *J. nerv. ment. Dis.* **121**: 505–510, 1955.
67. Weil, A. A., and Brinegar, W. C. Electroencephalographic studies following electric shock therapy: Observations on fifty-one patients treated with unidirectional current. *Arch. Neurol. Psychiat.* **57**: 719–729, 1947.
68. Williams, D. The electroencephalogram in affective disorders. *Proc. Roy. Soc. Med.* **47**: 779–782, 1954.

THE EEG IN SCHIZOPHRENIA

Margaret A. Kennard, M.D.

Historically, the interest in psychological relationships to the EEG pattern must have started with Berger, the originator of the EEG, who noted what we used to call the "Berger Rhythm," which is now known as alpha activity. His clinical correlations, however, were limited to the study of epilepsy and of the normal EEG. In 1936 Pauline Davis reported, in a series of three papers, EEG studies of patients with psychiatric disorders. She and her associates reported that the EEGs of schizophrenics were "less stable" than those of the normal individuals (12), that longitudinal study showed no changes (12), and that EEG instability was related to anxiety and tension. Little change appeared after frontal lobotomy (11). Later Saul, Davis, and Davis (71) studied the EEGs of patients undergoing treatment over a five-year period, finding "no appreciable changes which could be attributed either to lapse of time or to emotional changes during or following psychoanalysis occurred in the EEG of any individual." They related EEG patterns to personality types.

A second area of correlation between schizophrenia and the EEG pattern appeared first in the publications of Gibbs and Gibbs. In 1935 (21) Gibbs and Davis discussed changes in the human EEG in relation to changes of consciousness. In 1938 (22) the similarities between the cortical dysrhythmias of schizophrenia and a psychomotor epilepsy were discussed by Gibbs, Gibbs, and Lennox, who compared the similarities in pattern between the EEGs of individuals with psychomotor seizures, those with schizophrenia, and those of "psychopathic" children. From then on, the tendency of schizophrenics to have seizures and the similarities of the other two clinical syndromes have been discussed many times.

There were many very early inquiries into psychopathology and the EEG. The matter has been reviewed elsewhere (36) in more detail. One of the earliest investigations was that of A. C. Williams,

168

who in 1939 (87) analyzed "some psychological correlates of the electroencephalogram." In a careful study he examined the effect on beta and delta potentials of attention and tension. In 1941 Denis Williams (88) decided that "an abnormal EEG in an otherwise normal subject is strong evidence of an inborn constitutional abnormality involving the central nervous system." It may "manifest itself in the subject or his offspring as a behavior disturbance which may be psychoneurotic, psychopathic, psychotic or epileptic in nature."

In 1943 Thiesen (79) studied the effects of certain forms of emotion on the normal EEG. He felt that the cortical components of some emotional reactions are reflected in the EEG. His bibliography, containing 61 references, is excellent.

CORRELATION OF EEG PATTERN WITH CLINICAL TYPES OF SCHIZOPHRENIA

There have been many reports on the frequency of abnormality in the EEGs of schizophrenics. In 1938 (60) and again in 1952 (61) Newman examined the EEG in schizophrenia. He found an increased number of abnormalities in patients with "functional psychiatric disorders" and stated that fast activity was the predominant index of abnormality. It was greater among schizophrenics (17 per cent) and psychopathic states (21 per cent) than among depressives (6 per cent) and psychoneurotics (6 per cent). Finley and Campbell, in 1941 (16), were among the earliest to examine the EEGs of schizophrenics, comparing the records of 500 schizophrenics with those of 215 normals. They also found the presence of more fast activity in schizophrenics. The incidence among the normals was 3 to 8 per cent, among schizophrenics 10 to 35 per cent. It should be noted that the patients of both Newman and Finley were chronic patients residing in mental hospitals, and many were at the involutional age.

In 1956 Colony and Willis (9) carried out an electroencephalographic study of 1000 schizophrenic patients. These were compared with 474 control patients without discernible neurological disorder. The patients of both groups were naval personnel admitted to the Oakland California Naval Hospital, the range of age being 17 to 35 years. Of the controls 8.3 per cent showed EEG abnormality and of those in the schizophrenic group 5.0 per cent.

Particularly interesting was the fact that the nosological group of 18 patients with asocial, amoral, or aggressive personality disorders in the control group showed a comparatively higher incidence of EEG abnormality than either the control group as a whole or the schizophrenic group. This comparatively small group had an incidence of 27.7 per cent abnormal tracings. All had paroxysmal 4-to-6-per-second activity, generally in the fronto-temporal regions. It is obvious (from here on) that the findings of various examiners are totally different with regard to frequency of EEG abnormality among schizophrenics.

Among many who have found increased abnormality in the EEGS of schizophrenics are Mundy-Castle and his co-workers (57), Denis Hill (31), and Kennard (36). Koegler, Colbert, and Walter (44) stated correctly in 1961 that "up to now, attempts to correlate EEG abnormalities with psychiatric syndromes have resulted in a notable lack of success and a great deal of confusion due to the many conflicting reports." Both interpretation of the EEG and evaluation of psychopathology are responsible for the problem. They discussed problems of psychiatric evaluation, psychological testing, and neurological examination. Their conclusion was that "methods of studying the complex human psyche are still primitive." They suggested that the group of schizophrenics must be more meaningfully subdivided.

As a logical consequence of the above, well-qualified workers have made many attempts to analyze the factors within the schizophrenic syndrome which may relate to EEG patterning. Investigations centered upon the old diagnostic forms hebephrenic, simple, acute, and chronic yielded nothing. The periodicity of catatonia was studied by Bonkalo, Lovett-Doust, and Stokes in 1955 (7). They reported on a study of three cases showing periodic catatonia over a three-year period. "In all three patients it was found that, starting from a relatively normal baseline in the remission phase, fairly consistent physiological changes occurred with the onset of stupor or catatonic excitement. Both the EEG alpha incidence and alpha amplitude fell sharply and simultaneously with the disturbed phase. . . ." These authors reviewed the previous literature on the subject.

There has been no evidence that EEG pattern ever changes in relation to phases of clinical illness or recovery in schizophrenia. The periodic phases of acute agitation and of aggression or range have been found, in both the schizophrenic and the non-schizophrenic, to be associated with fast and irregular EEG activity. This appears in relation to the range phenomena rather than to the schizoid process. Denis Hill and his associates made this observation early in the last decade (30) and later followed the EEG pattern into the developing knowledge of temporal-lobe pathology and psychomotor seizures (29). Stafford-Clark and Taylor (77) carried this into a study of prisoners charged with murder and suggested that the EEG abnormality appeared in those whose crime appeared to be unmotivated. Of the entire group 32, or 50 per cent, had normal EEGs, but of the 14 severely disturbed who were judged "insane," only two showed normal records. Jarvie (33) discussed episodic rage, theta rhythm, and obsessions in his review of the literature. He commented upon the fact that earlier writers related obsessive states to organicity, thus adding another element to the analysis.

Since the EEG is known to be strongly related to visual stimuli and since some visual hallucinations occur in schizophrenia, there have been several studies of the effect of visual stimuli upon the EEG of psychotics. In 1955 Sem-Jacobsen and his associates (73) reported on intracerebral recordings from psychotic patients during hallucinations and agitation. Ninety psychotic patients were examined by depth electrodes placed in many cortical areas. Spontaneous episodic high-voltage waves were encountered in many from the frontal lobe and from the temporal lobes. Spike potentials appeared frequently among patients having no history of clinical epilepsy. A close relationship was observed between the recordings of paroxysmal activity and acute clinical symptoms.

There is a series of reports by Ulett and his associates on photic activation of the EEG as related to psychiatric disorders. In 1952 Ulett and Glaser (83) investigated the effects of experimental stress upon the photically activated EEG. They noted that occipital rhythms induced by intermittent photic stimulation are "blocked" by emotional tension. They offered a theory that during anxiety discharges from the diencephalic region interfere with cortical mechanisms of synchronization. Comparison of "normal" and schizophrenic individuals produced no notable difference in response. In 1953 Ulett (81) considered that "photic stimulation was a useful research tool in differentiation of psychiatric patterns." One finding in his paper was of considerable interest in relation to later work on sensory deprivation. "Rhythmic photic stimulation can, in susceptible subjects, induce subjective sensations, frequently of a dysphoric nature, and in psychiatric patients such sensations may take the form of previously experienced symptoms." Seizures were produced by photic stimulation in four cases with psychiatric disorders. In a later publication (84) response to photic stimulation was considered to be directly related to anxiety-proneness. Reviewing the matter in 1957, Ulett (82) found the use of photic stimulation valuable in many ways. It should be emphasized here that ten articles by Ulett are cited from 1953 to 1957, and in these a progressive serial study of methodology and the clinical and psychological correlation with EEG were made. Few others have so consistently and productively investigated the relations between the EEG and psychopathology. With the exception of Mundy-Castle (59) and Knott (43) in the field of investigation and Henry (27) in both investigation and bibliographical aid, most authors have touched somewhere upon this subject and then, for various reasons, moved rather rapidly to other matters.

EPILEPSY AND SCHIZOPHRENIA

It has long been known that schizophrenics tend to have epileptic seizures more often than normals. As cited above, Gibbs (20) in 1951 found similarities in EEG pattern between the two groups; and Smith, Ulett, and Johnson (76) noted what all electroencephalographers see occasionally—a focal spike potential appearing in an individual who is clinically schizophrenic and who has never been known to have had a seizure.

Denis Hill (29) gave an excellent review of the clinical interrelationships betwen epilepsy and schizophrenia. In his series 18 of the 80 schizophrenics had EEGs suggestive of epilepsy. These were found to be definitely related to epileptic clinical phenomena either in the patients themselves or in their relatives. But Lyketsos, Belinson, and Gibbs (51) in 1951 found no evidences of disorders of awake or sleeping EEG pattern in psychotic, non-epileptic patients, although fact activity was more prevalent among the schizophrenic than in other groups. In the same year Gibbs reported a large series of patients in whom temporal-lobe EEG foci and psychomotor seizures showed a strong positive correlation, psychiatric disorders being more than three times as common in this group as among individuals with normal EEGs.

Also in 1951, Bartlett (2) reported a relation of EEG abnormality to temporal-lobe dysfunction in psychotics. His initial inquiry had been into the nature or existence of epileptic psychosis, which had been observed many times prior to the present era of drug therapy. Like Gibbs and others, he concluded that there was a significant positive relationship between schizophrenia and temporal-lobe paroxysmal activity. His conclusion that "epilepsy in subjects liable to schizophrenia tends to manifest itself in the temporal lobe" made no attempt to separate cause and effect. It is somewhat contradictory to his original title, which was "Chronic Psychosis Following Epilepsy."

When Smith, Ulett, and Johnson (76) measured the convulsive thresholds of 30 schizophrenics as compared to 20 non-schizophrenics, using photopharmacological means, they found no differences in tendency to convulsion. These patients were a carefully selected group, all between the ages of 16 and 40, without abnormal cerebral dysrhythmia on EEG. Organic history was also negative. Again, young schizophrenics without sign of organic brain disorder did not produce abnormal EEGs beyond the normal average incidence.

An additional bit of evidence is contributed by the known fact that schizophrenic patients may develop seizures following frontal lobotomy. In the series of DeMille (13) more than twice as many catatonic patients (16 out of 33) developed epilepsy following lobotomy as would have been expected from the proportion in the sample. None had seizure of paroxysmal EEG patterns prior to the lobotomy.

TEMPORAL-LOBE PATTERNS

Our knowledge of psychomotor seizures and of the effects of temporal-lobe lesions on behavior is now fairly complete and consistent. With its growth another aspect of schizophrenic clinical syndromes has been discussed many times. In a Maudsley Lecture for 1955, Wilder Penfield (64) described the paroxysmal patterns of such disorders both from their physiological and psychological sides. Feelings of unreality and inability to comprehend immediate experience or to compare it with the past occur. The *déjà-vu* experience is a small part of this. His impression was that disturbances of behavior are more frequent among temporal-lobe epileptics than among others. This has, I believe, become even more evident in the years since his publication. The work of Hill and his associates in relation to aggression and paroxysmal rage is significant here (30, 77). Oldham (62) reported two interesting cases in which temporal-lobe lesions produced great changes when superimposed upon paranoid psychoses with violent outbursts. Calmness and apparent contentment initially supervened, but gradually disappeared. Rodin, Bagchi, and their associates (67) found that schizophrenia and certain forms of psychomotor seizures were positively related. These authors emphasized that many patients having both EEG and clinical evidence of paroxysmal psychomotor disturbances also show additional symptoms which may be considered as psychotic, while those who have never had grand mal seizures may be diagnosed as schizophrenic. In their series all patients showed lesions localized to the temporal lobes.

Weil (85) presented a unique group of 388 patients with "symptomatic epilepsy" in which seizures developed after "post-traumatic, atrophic, post-infectious vascular and/or expanding lesions." Of these there were 132 with clinical and EEG symptoms of temporal-lobe epilepsy. Twenty-eight of these experienced "ictal" emotions, which were largely fear or depression. A few were paranoid in nature. None were pleasurable. In some cases "a moment to moment correlation between the experience of ictal emotions and the occurrence of temporal lobe EEG abnormality could be established."

There have been a large number of articles relating to the effects of lobotomies of various kinds on clinical symptoms in schizophrenia, but there is no significant relationship between either the type of EEG abnormality or the amount of EEG change and clinical recovery. Occurrence of seizures after lobotomy also has no relation to recovery. This matter has been discussed by Greenblatt and Solomon (25), surveying nine years of lobotomy research. Krueger and Wayne (46) compared lobotomy with the less extensive topectomy and found that EEG changes as well as clinical changes are more extensive in the larger operation.

Green (24) examined behavior of children in relation to abnormal EEGs. Of ten children having disorders of behavior, there were spike foci in temporal or occipital areas in nine. None had ever had clinical seizures.

Effort to investigate indices other than the EEG in relation to schizophrenia should be mentioned briefly. Their number is vast and reviews are many. None have been conclusive. Histopathological changes in the brain of schizophrenics have been reported and denied. The matter was reviewed by Morton Weinstein in 1954 (86), and again by Winkelman and Brook in 1949 (**89**). Neither found convincing evidence of histological change. The techniques of study developed in this field since then have not uncovered any convincing findings that schizophrenia is organically originated. Recently more attention has been given to the metabolic status of the schizophrenic, particularly in studies relating to LSD and the adrenal cortex. Seymour Kety (**41**) has published an enlightening presentation of physiological concepts, neurochemistry, and the general field as related to the sociological and purely behavioral approaches.

Very recently there has been an inquiry into the vestibular and auditory dysfunction of schizophrenics. In 1959 Colbert, Koegler, and Markham (**8**) reviewed the literature of the matter, citing 50 previous articles. Their own tests showed that in the examination of vestibular and optokinetic functions in schizophrenic children, there was notable depression of function as compared to normal children or those with behavior disorders. Ludwig, Wood, and Downs (**50**) found no difference between schizophrenic and normal subjects in simple tone discriminations, but in tests involving tone decay and "delayed auditory feedback" the schizophrenics displayed significantly more abnormalities.

In 1958 Malamud and Overholzer (**53**) discussed multi-disciplinary research in schizophrenia. Here the literature on childhood schizophrenia began to be sorted and integrated. In this same year McKnight (**52**) examined "Historical Landmarks in Research in Schizophrenia in the United States." This article has a bibliography which divides research into clinical concepts, biological studies, genetic and epidemiological studies, interdisciplinary research, and investigations of somatic, psychotherapeutic, and social approaches to therapy.

CHILDHOOD SCHIZOPHRENIA

Developments in child psychiatry over the past 30 years have added more to the knowledge of childhood schizophrenia and its relation to the EEG. The development of the two disciplines intensified during the same decade. We are beginning to pick out significant points, but it is still true, as stated by Bergman and Green (**6**), that the significance of the EEG still stands on its clinical correlations alone.

In 1938 Jasper, Solomon, and Bradley (**34**) first reported that the EEGs of children with behavior disorders were relatively high in abnormal patterns. Many of the abnormal patterns were paroxysmal or "epileptoid." Again, seizures and paroxysmal activity appeared in relation to non-epileptic behavior. The finding of EEG abnormality in disorders of behavior is still true, and there have been many sorts of interpretation.

Recognition of a childhood condition which has a similar origin to that of adult schizophrenia was begun by Kanner (35) and by Lauretta Bender (5). In much more recent publications each has told in effect what had already been decided for the adult. Dr. Bender says that "schizophrenia is a psychobiological entity determined by an inherited predisposition, an early physiologic or organic crisis and a failure in an adequate defense mechanism." She feels that "in the early life of a child, schizophrenia tends to interfere with normal maturation in all behavioral levels." This she has demonstrated in regard to intellectual development. It can be traced in young children in relation to homeostatic equilibrium and to vaso-vegetative patterns. Sleeping-waking patterns are disturbed. Tone and mobility disturbances are also described in this same article with perceptual difficulties and distortion of body image. Later, during adolescence, these patterns convert into those of the neurotic, the psychopathic, or the psychotic types.

Over and over again in the discussion of abnormal EEGs in relation to childhood schizophrenia, we are told that the EEG pattern is abnormal for the age and that it is immature (34, 38). We then have to speculate as to whether the EEG is immature because of the psychological pattern or vice versa. Experience in relation to other types of behavior distortions in children which are known to have "organic" sources, such as psychomotor behavior or others relating to the temporal lobe, would indicate that the demonstrable lesion or distortion within the organic structures is primary. Behavior change may develop when known injury has occurred and has been reported as disappearing following operations or excisions of focal areas. The immaturity of the nervous system in other ways has been described recently in the infant by Fish (17, 18), who found that poor integration of early neurological development was related to a lowered early threshold for anxiety. Her discussion of the interrelationships involving lag in body image concepts is most interesting.

The author has recently compared the EEG patterns of young

children having disturbances of behavior with those described in the normal series of both Lindsley (**48**) in 1939 and Henry (**27**) in 1944. Having used their data as a base for many years, the author was amazed once again at the differences between the EEGs of their normal children and those seen in the children's wards in institutions and in the patterns of clinic subjects having lesser psychological disturbances.

Some of the following observations made by the author as an outgrowth of 20 years study can be proved statistically, others cannot (**36–40**).

1. Abnormal EEGs in children with behavior disorders are proportional to:
    a. The age at onset of the clinical pattern.
    b. The severity of the disturbance.
    c. The age at which the EEG is taken.
2. They are more frequent in autistic or schizophrenic children than in any other group.
3. They are sometimes, but not always, related to other signs of "organicity."
4. Those children having abnormal EEGs show a greater tendency toward fluctuations in awareness. They tend, under conditions of rest such as the recording of an EEG, to become drowsy very easily. Their sleep patterns tend toward paroxysmal elements to greater degree than do those of "normal" children.
5. None of the above tendencies is peculiar to autistic or schizophrenic children, but each occurs more frequently among this group.
6. Among the younger children, ages up to seven or eight, many with known organic brain injury show only behavioral changes, not gross motor or sensory defects. So many of these have autistic patterns that in one series we have reported three groups:
    a. Those children having clearly autistic tendencies without either retardation or known brain injury.
    b. Those children having known brain injury who have all the signs including abnormal EEG, and the symptoms of chronic brain syndrome.
    c. Those children having autistic patterns who show in-

dications of organic brain dysfunction in their psychological test results and clinical histories.

Pollack (**65**) analyzes and classifies childhood schizophrenia according to the observations made by others. His report is an excellent attempt to find the reasons for the inconsistencies. Neither childhood schizophrenia nor mental retardation can be accurately defined as a homogeneous entity. His final sentence expresses most clearly the fact that "the general disagreement and the lack of clarity in this field may be due largely to the paucity of systematic, controlled experimentation."

Hirschberg and Bryant (**32**) called attention in 1956 to similar observations which led them to conclude that in schizophrenic children different genotypical syndromes produce similar phenotypical patterns. Their conclusions thus suggested that interaction of the factors leads to the particular adaptive patterns in children. A year later Eisenberg (**14**) came to a similar conclusion, particularly in regard to prognostic evaluations.

According to our present knowledge, schizophrenia or autism appearing in childhood seems closely related to adult schizophrenia both in etiological factors and in clinical sequence relating to therapy and to behavioral consequences. It no longer seems possible that the increased incidence of EEG abnormality among children with such clinical patterns is entirely due to chance. Neither does it appear possible that the clinical pattern of childhood schizophrenia is directly and causally related to EEG abnormality in the relatively simple fashion in which epilepsy or other behavioral patterns may follow known focal and direct brain injury.

ABNORMAL EEG AND FLUCTUATIONS
IN CONSCIOUSNESS

The most interesting recent contributions have been those concerned with abnormalities or fluctuations in consciousness of which psychomotor seizures and temporal-lobe abnormalities are most important, as has been discussed above. As previously discussed, abnormalities in the EEGs of children may relate to paroxysmal behavior and to paroxysmal alterations of consciousness. In a series studied some years ago, we found that subjects with abnormal EEG rhythms, largely frontal dysrhythmia, showed a significant tendency to drowsiness in the EEG recording situation similar to that which occurs among children with delusions, hallucinations, and disturbances of thought.

The author is sure that paroxysmal wave patterns of the high-voltage positive spike type occur more frequently among this group of patients than among others. Here also, severity of clinical picture, duration of disturbance, and early onset have a positive correlation. There are a number of recent discussions of paroxysmal consciousness among adults (74). In what he described as "states of lowered vigilance," Roth (69) brought together a great number of clinical types, ranging from encephalitis to clinical exhaustion in normal subjects, in which lowered vigilance as shown by sleepiness and diminished awareness of surroundings was accompanied by "EEG rhythms corresponding to the period of transition from awakeness to sleep." He related these to disorders of the mesodiencephalic region and to "insufficiency" of subcortical activating mechanisms. Roth cited the hypnotic phases produced by Pavlov in dogs. If Pavlov had known the term, these might have been described by him as the result of "experimental neuroses."

There are, actually, some well-thought-out and controlled studies of this matter. Experimental insomnia has been related to changes in EEG. Increasing periods of insomnia result in increase in the rate of potential change in the brain (80). Gibbs, Lorimer, and Gibbs (19) in 1950 called attention to the "exceedingly fast activity" at 30–40 cycles per second, which never appeared in normal control subjects. It was definitely related to drowsiness in a group of their patients with various clinical patterns, and was considered as indicating "increased irritative factors."

SENSORY DEPRIVATION

An important matter in consideration of the EEG and schizophrenia is that of the effects of sensory deprivation. Sensory deprivation, the relative deficit of sensory input, results in impaired relationships to reality and may even produce hallucinations (47). There is a large literature on the subject, beginning with Hebb's original observation. Sensory deprivation has been compared to schizophrenia both in clinical manifestations and theoretically. Its results are called, by Rosenzweig, a "model psychosis" syndrome (68). Sensory deprivation has been used on psychiatric patients by Azima and Cramer

(1) and by Gibby, Adams, and Carrera (23). It is known that some subjects are more susceptible to change from such deprivation than others. Unfortunately, as far as the author knows, there has been no comparison of EEG patterns. Klein's discussion (42) of the adaptive properties of sensory function are of value here, as is Lindsley's (49).

PSYCHOLOGICAL ELEMENTS

There has been a great deal of experimental investigation of the individual psychological qualities as related to EEG pattern. This matter was extensively reviewed by Mundy-Castle in 1958 (59). He expounded on various theoretic circuits and psychological patterns which may underlie EEG types and personality structure. The process of conditioning the EEG is discussed. The psychopathology and personality patterns utilized do not seem, however, to be clearly defined. This author, together with many others, believes that the EEG will continue to be of increasing importance in relation to personality structure.

A number of types of investigation are undertaken as a result of our previous knowledge of EEG. The susceptibility of alpha activity to change as the result of visual stimuli has produced one group. A second has followed the discovery by Morell and his associates (55, 56) that the alpha rhythm can be conditioned when the unconditioned stimulus is light. Alpha rhythm and speed have been related to perception by Sugarman (78) in a group of 50 normal subjects. Positive correlation was found between alpha frequency and perception, the latter being directly related to intelligence.

In a study relating to psychological disturbances, Kooi and Hovey (45) examined EEG records during the administration of tests of higher integrative function to 21 patients who had previously shown paroxysmal EEG activity. Blocking of responses and other signs of confusion were found to be significantly related to the periods of paroxysmal cerebral activity. Frequency patterns have been found to relate to psychiatric disorders when the frequency profiles of schizophrenics are compared with those of a normal control group and those of a group of prison inmates (66). Fedio and associates (15) compared the reaction times of schizophrenics and normal subjects. They observed that the groups did not differ in speed of reaction when alpha activity was present, but that when alpha was blocked by an alerting response, the normal group improved in speed while schizophrenics failed to improve or even performed more slowly.

Matarazzo, Watson, and Ulett (**54**) have compared Rorschach findings to modes of perception induced by photic stimulation in normals and in individuals having high anxiety states. Responses of color and movement found in the control population were definitely related to the type of perceptive response to intermittent photic stimulation. In anxious patients and in anxiety-prone controls no such relationship appeared. These authors venture to suggest that since photic stimulation alters the EEG in varying degrees in various subjects, there may be some physiological relationship of the Rorschach and photic stimulation. It is a pity that they did not compare EEGs for these same subjects, for they should have found definite positive or negative correlations, either of which would be significant. Another objective study, dealing with mental imagery (**75**), is of related interest. Psychophysiological relationships are suggested between alpha EEG types and visual perceiving and imaging. Once again complex visual concepts were used.

Finally, it should be mentioned here that over all these twenty-five years of discussion of the EEG and psychopathology there has been a similar series of papers discussing the more complete defining of schizophrenia (**3**, **4**, **26**, **31**, **63**, **70**). Although schizophrenia remains a clinical entity, we can no longer say that this process is due to any single factor or to any group of factors. Genetic, sociological, familial, physiological, pharmacological, and structural processes have all been investigated. As with the EEG, the single relationship of any one factor is never more than partially contributory.

BIBLIOGRAPHY

1. Azima, H., and Cramer, F. J. Effects of partial perceptual isolation in mentally disturbed individuals. *Dis. nerv. Syst.* **17**: 117–122, 1956.
2. Bartlet, J. E. A. Chronic psychosis following epilepsy. *Amer. J. Psychiat.* **114**: 338–343, 1957.
3. Beck, A. R. Reliability of psychiatric diagnoses: 1. A critique of systematic studies. *Amer. J. Psychiat.* **119**: 210–216, 1962.
4. Beck, A. T., Ward, C. H., Mendelson, M., Mock, J. E., and Erbaugh, J. K. Reliability of psychiatric diagnoses: 2. A study of consistency of clinical judgments and ratings. *Amer. J. Psychiat.* **119**: 351–357, 1962.
5. Bender, L. Diagnostic and therapeutic aspects of childhood schizophrenia. Mental retardation. *Proc. First Internat. Conf.* pp. 453–468, July, 1959.
6. Bergman, P. S., and Green, M. A. The use of electroencephalography in differentiating psychogenic disorders and organic brain diseases. *Amer. J. Psychiat.* **113**: 27–31, 1956.
7. Bonkalo, A., Lovett-Doust, J. W., and Stokes, A. B. Physiological concomitants of the phasic disturbances seen in periodic catatonia. *Amer. J. Psychiat.* **112**: 114–122, 1955.

8. Colbert, E. G., Koegler, R. R., and Markham, C. H. Vestibular dysfunction in child-hood schizophrenia. *Arch. gen. Psychiat.* **1**: 600–617, 1959.
9. Colony, H. S., and Willis, S. E. Electroencephalographic studies of 1,000 schizophrenic patients. *Amer. J. Psychiat.* **113**: 163–169, 1956.
10. Davis, P. A. Evaluation of the electroencephalograms of schizophrenic patients. *Amer. J. Psychiat.* **96**: 851–860, 1940.
11. Davis, P. A. Electroencephalographic studies on three cases of frontal lobotomy. *Psychosom. Med.* **3**: 38–50, 1951.
12. Davis, P. A., and Davis, H. The electroencephalograms of psychotic patients. *Amer. J. Psychiat.* **95**: 1007–1025, 1939.
13. DeMille, R. An incidental observation of epilepsy in catatonic schizophrenics after prefrontal lobotomy. *J. nerv. ment. Dis.* **134**: 182–183, 1962.
14. Eisenberg, L. The course of childhood schizophrenia. *Arch. Neurol. Psychiat.* **78**: 69–83, 1957.
15. Fedio, P., Mirsky, A. F., Smith, W. J., and Parry, D. Reaction time and EEG activation in normal and schizophrenic subjects. *Electroenceph. clin. Neurophysiol.* **13**: 923–926, 1961.
16. Finley, K. H., and Campbell, C. M. Electroencephalography in schizophrenia. *Amer. J. Psychiat.* **98**: 374–381, 1941.
17. Fish, B. Involvement of the central nervous system in infants with schizophrenia. *Arch. Neurol.* **2**: 115–121, 1960.
18. Fish, B. The study of motor development in infancy and its relationship to psycho-logical functioning. *Amer. J. Psychiat.* **117**: 1113–1118, 1961.
19. Gibbs, E. L., Lorimer, F. M., and Gibbs, F. A. Clinical correlates of exceedingly fast activity in the electroencephalogram. *Dis. nerv. Syst.* **11**: 323–326, 1950.
20. Gibbs, F. A. Ictal and non-ictal psychiatric disorders in temporal lobe epilepsy. *J. nerv. ment. Dis.* **113**: 522–528, 1951.
21. Gibbs, F. A., and Davis, H. Changes in the human electroencephalogram associated with loss of consciousness. *Amer. J. Physiol.* **113**: 49–50, 1935.
22. Gibbs, F. A., Gibbs, E. L., and Lennox, W. G. The likeness of the cortical dysrhythmias of schizophrenia and psychomotor epilepsy. *Amer. J. Psychiat.* **95**: 255–269, 1938.
23. Gibby, R. G., Adams, H. B., and Carrera, R. N. Therapeutic changes in psychiatric patients following partial sensory deprivation. *Arch. gen. Psychiat.* **3**: 33–42, 1960.
24. Green, J. B. Association of behavior disorder with an electroencephalographic focus in children without seizures. *Neurology.* **11**: 337–344, 1961.
25. Greenblatt, M., and Solomon, H. C. Survey of nine years of lobotomy investigations. *Amer. J. Psychiat.* **109**: 262–265, 1952.
26. Gregory, I. Genetic factors in schizophrenia. *Amer. J. Psychiat.* **116**: 961–972, 1960.
27. Henry, C. E. Electroencephalograms of normal children. *Monogr. Soc. Res. Child Develop.* **9**: No. 3, 1944.
28. Henry, C. E., and Knott, J. R. Electroencephalography. *Progr. Neurol. Psychiat.* **14**: 270–297, 1959.
29. Hill, D. The relationship between epilepsy and schizophrenia: EEG studies. *Folia Psychiat. Neurol. et Neurochir. Neerl.* pp. 1–19, 1948.
30. Hill, D. EEG in episodic psychotic and psychopathic behavior. A classification of data. *Electroenceph. clin. Neurophysiol.* **4**: 419–442, 1952.
31. Hill, D., Theobald, J., Waddell, M., and Loe, P. S. A central homeostatic mechanism in schizophrenia. *J. ment. Sci.* **97**: 111–131, 1951.
32. Hirschberg, J. C., and Bryant, K. N. Problems in the differential diagnosis of child-hood schizophrenia. *Res. Publ. Ass. Res. Nerv. Ment. Dis.* **34**: 454–461, 1954.
33. Jarvie, H. F. Episodic rage, theta rhythm, and obsessions. *J. ment. Sci.* **99**: 252–256, 1953.
34. Jasper, H. H., Solomon, P., and Bradley, C. Electroencephalographic analyses of be-havior problem children. *Amer. J. Psychiat.* **95**: 641–658, 1938.
35. Kanner, L. The thirty-third Maudsley lecture: Trends in child psychiatry. *J. ment. Sci.* **105**: 581–593, 1959.
36. Kennard, M. A. The electroencephalogram and disorders of behavior. A review. *J. nerv. ment. Dis.* **124**: 103–124, 1956.
37. Kennard, M. A. Behavior problems and the brain injured child. *Northwest. Med.* **58**: 1535–1541, 1959.
38. Kennard, M. A. The characteristics of thought disturbance as related to electro-encephalographic findings in children and adolescents. *Amer. J. Psychiat.* **115**: 911–921, 1959.
39. Kennard, M. A. Value of equivocal signs in neurologic diagnosis. *Neurology.* **10**: 753–764, 1960.

40. Kennard, M. A., Schwartzman, A. E., and Miller, T. P. Sleep, consciousness, and the alpha electroencephalographic rhythm. *Arch. Neurol. Psychiat.* **79**: 328–335, 1958.
41. Kety, S. S. A biologist examines the mind and behavior. *Science.* **132**: 1861–1867, 1960.
42. Klein, G. S. Adaptive properties of sensory functioning: Some postulates and hypotheses. *Bull. Menninger Clin.* **13**: 16–23, 1949.
43. Knott, J. R. Brain and behavior. Symposium, 1959. 1. EEG and behavior. *Amer. J. Orthopsychiat.* **30**: 292–297, 1960.
44. Koegler, R. R., Colbert, E. G., and Walter, R. D. Problems in the correlation of psychopathology with electroencephalographic abnormalities. *Amer. J. Psychiat.* **117**: 822–824, 1961.
45. Kooi, K. A., and Hovey, H. B. Alterations in mental function and paroxysmal cerebral activity. *Arch. Neurol. Psychiat.* **78**: 264–271, 1957.
46. Krueger, E. G., and Wayne, H. L. Clinical and electroencephalographic effects of prefrontal lobotomy and topectomy in chronic psychoses. *Arch. Neurol. Psychiat.* **67**: 661–671, 1952.
47. Leiderman, H., Mendelson, J. H., Wexler, D., and Solomon, P. Sensory deprivation. *Arch. intern. Med.* **101**: 389–396, 1958.
48. Lindsley, D. B. A longitudinal study of the occipital alpha rhythm in normal children: Frequency and amplitude standards. *J. genet. Psychol.* **55**: 197–213, 1939.
49. Lindsley, D. B. Basic perceptual processes and the EEG. *Psychiat. Res. Rep. Amer. Psychiat. Ass.* **6**: 161–170, 1956.
50. Ludwig, A. M., Wood, B. S., and Downs, M. P. Auditory studies in schizophrenia. *Amer. J. Psychiat.* **119**: 122–127, 1962.
51. Lyketsos, G., Belinson, L., and Gibbs, F. A. Electroencephalograms of non-epileptic psychotic patients awake and asleep. *Arch. Neurol. Psychiat.* **69**: 707–712, 1953.
52. McKnight, W. K. Historical landmarks in research on schizophrenia in the United States. *Amer. J. Psychiat.* **114**: 873–881, 1958.
53. Malamud, W., and Overholser, W. Multidisciplinary research in schizophrenia. *Amer. J. Psychiat.* **114**: 865–872, 1958.
54. Matarazzo, R. G., Watson, R. I., and Ulett, G. A. Relationship of Rorschach scoring categories to modes of perception induced by intermittent photic stimulation—a methodological study of perception. *J. clin. Psychol.* **8**: 368–374, 1952.
55. Morrell, F., and Jasper, H. H. Electrographic studies of the formation of temporary connections in the brain. *Electroenceph. clin. Neurophysiol.* **8**: 201–215, 1956.
56. Morrell, F., and Ross, M. H. Central inhibition in cortical conditioned reflexes. *Arch. Neurol. Psychiat.* **70**: 611–616, 1953.
57. Mundy-Castle, A. C. The electroencephalogram in relation to temperment. *Acta psychol.* **11**: 397–411, 1955.
58. Mundy-Castle, A. C. The electroencephalogram and mental activity. *Electroenceph. clin. Neurophysiol.* **9**: 643–655, 1957.
59. Mundy-Castle, A. C. An appraisal of electroencephalography in relation to psychology. *J. Nat. Inst. Personnel Res. Monograph.* Suppl. **2**: 43, May, 1958.
60. Newman, H. W. Electroencephalography. *Amer. J. med. Sci.* **196**: 882–887, 1938.
61. Newman, H. W., and Lawrence, R. The electroencephalogram in functional psychiatric disorders. *Stanford med. Bull.* **10**: 76–77, 1952.
62. Oldham, A. J. The effects of temporal lobe lesions on behavior in paranoid states. *J. ment. Sci.* **99**: 580–587, 1953.
63. Ovshinsky, S. R. A concept of schizophrenia. *J. nerv. ment. Dis.* **125**: 578–586, 1957.
64. Penfield, W. The twenty-ninth Maudsley lecture: The role of the temporal cortex in certain psychical phenomena. *J. ment. Sci.* **101**: 451–465, 1955.
65. Pollack, M. Brain damage, mental retardation and childhood schizophrenia. *Amer. J. Psychiat.* **115**: 422–428, 1958.
66. Rabinovitch, M. S., Kennard, M. A., and Fister, W. P. Personality correlates of electroencephalographic patterns: Rorschach findings. *Canad. J. Psychol.* **9**: 29–41, 1955.
67. Rodin, E. A., DeJong, R. N., Waggoner, R. W., and Bagchi, B. K. Relationship between certain forms of psychomotor epilepsy and "schizophrenia." *Arch. Neurol. Psychiat.* **77**: 449–463, 1957.
68. Rosenzweig, N. Sensory deprivation and schizophrenia: Some clinical and theoretical similarities. *Amer. J. Psychiat.* **116**: 326–329, 1959.
69. Roth, B. The clinical and theoretical importance of EEG rhythms corresponding to states of lowered vigilance. *Electroenceph. clin. Neurophysiol.* **13**: 395–399, 1961.
70. Rusinov, V. S., and Rabinovitch, M. Y. Electroencephalographic researchers in the laboratories and clinics of the Soviet Union. *Electroenceph. clin. Neurophysiol.* Suppl. **8**: May, 1958.

71. Saul, L. J., Davis, H., and Davis, P. A. Psychologic correlations with the electro-encephalogram. *Psychosom. Med.* **11**: 361–376, 1949.
72. Saunders, M. G. Electroencephalography and psychiatry. *Canad. Psychiat. Ass. J.* **6**: 3–8, 1961.
73. Sem-Jacobsen, C. W., Petersen, M. C., Lazarte, J. A., Dodge, H. W., and Holman, C. B. Electroencephalographic rhythms from the depths of the frontal lobe in 60 psychotic patients. *Electroenceph. clin. Neurophysiol.* **7**: 193–210, 1955.
74. Sherwood, S. L. Consciousness, adaptive behavior and schizophrenia. In: *Schizophrenia: Somatic Aspects.* Pergamon Press, London, pp. 131–146, 1957.
75. Short, P. L. The objective study of mental imagery. *Brit. J. Psychol.* **44**: 38–51, 1953.
76. Smith, K., Ulett, G. A., and Johnson, L. C. The convulsive threshold in schizophrenia. *Arch. Neurol. Psychiat.* **77**: 528–532, 1957.
77. Stafford-Clark, D., and Taylor, F. H. Clinical and electroencephalographic studies of prisoners charged with murder. *J. Neurol. Neurosurg. Psychiat.* **12**: 325–330, 1949.
78. Sugarman, L. Alpha rhythm, perception and intelligence. *J. Nat. Inst. Personnel Res.* **8**: 170–179, 1961.
79. Thiesen, J. W. Effects of certain forms of emotion on the normal electroencephalogram. *Arch. Psychol.* **40**: No. 285, 1943.
80. Tyler, D. B., Goodman, J., and Rothman, T. The effect of experimental insomnia on the rate of potential changes in the brain. *Amer. J. Physiol.* **149**: 185–193, 1947.
81. Ulett, G. A. Photically-activated electroencephalogram: Research tool in psychiatry; preliminary observations. *Psychosom. Med.* **15**: 66–83, 1953.
82. Ulett, G. A. Experience with photic stimulation in psychiatric research. *Amer. J. Psychiat.* **114**: 127–133, 1957.
83. Ulett, G. A., and Gleser, G. The effect of experimental stress upon the photically activated EEG. *Science.* **115**: 678–682, 1952.
84. Ulett, G. A., Gleser, G., Winokur, G., and Lawler, A. The EEG and reaction to photic stimulation as an index of anxiety-proneness. *Electroenceph. clin. Neurophysiol.* **5**: 23–32, 1953.
85. Weil, A. A. Ictal emotions occurring in temporal lobe dysfunction. *Arch. Neurol.* **1**: 87–97, 1959.
86. Weinstein, M. R. Histopathological changes in the brain in schizophrenia. A critical review. *Arch. Neurol. Psychiat.* **71**: 539–553, 1954.
87. Williams, A. C., Jr. Some psychological correlates of the electroencephalogram. *Arch. Psychol.* **34**: No. 240, 1939.
88. Williams, D. The significance of an abnormal electroencephalogram. *J. Neurol. Psychiat.* **4**: 257–268, 1941.
89. Winkelman, N. W., and Book, M. H. Observations on the histopathology of schizo phrenia. *Amer. J. Psychiat.* **105**: 889–896, 1949.

THE ELECTROENCEPHALOGRAM IN OLD AGE [1]

Walter D. Obrist, Ph.D., and Ewald W. Busse, M.D.

In 1941 Pauline Davis (**10**) reported the presence of a slow alpha rhythm and delta waves in the EEGs of elderly psychiatric patients. She suggested that the senescent EEG undergoes a shift toward the slow end of the frequency spectrum relative to young adult standards. Berger (**4**) had previously noted similar changes in patients with senile dementia, but regarded them as purely pathological, denying the existence of an age trend. Subsequent research has confirmed Davis' hypothesis that the EEG becomes slower in old age, while at the same time supporting the view of Berger that intellectual impairment is an important correlate of such changes.

The general question of whether aging can proceed independently of pathological processes has received some attention in the geriatric literature (**39**). In the case of EEG, many of the so-called age changes occur in subjects who manifest varying combinations of mental and physical deterioration. During senescence individual differences in EEG are pronounced, perhaps more so than at any other time in life. Some people over 80 years of age have tracings indistinguishable from young adults, whereas others only 60 show marked deviations. The basic problem of geriatric electroencephalography is the extent to which these individual differences are related to variations in mental and physical function.

Methodological considerations are particularly relevant to EEG research in aging. Wide variations exist in the composition of the different groups studied, ranging from healthy community volunteers to chronically ill institutionalized patients. Selective factors operate to determine the nature of a given sample, so that generalizations to the elderly population as a whole are rarely possible. For this reason it is desirable to survey a variety of investigations, with careful attention to the sampling techniques employed.

[1] Portions of this work were supported by PHS Grants M-900 and HD-00668, National Institutes of Health.

Of equal importance are the methods used for describing and evaluating EEG changes in senescence. Gross characterizations of normal or abnormal, although frequently made, are practically meaningless at this age level. Such concepts presume a knowledge of statistical normality and clinico-pathologic correlates not yet obtained. A more adequate understanding requires a detailed description of the EEG, including quantitative measurements.

It is the purpose of the present paper to describe the major EEG characteristics of senescence and to indicate, when possible, the nature and extent of their correlation with declining mental and physical function. Four types of EEG change have been consistently observed in old age: (1) a slow alpha rhythm, (2) increased fast activity, (3) diffuse slowing, and (4) focal disturbances. Each of these topics is discussed in detail below.

1. Alpha Rhythm

Alpha rhythm may be defined as a sequence of 8 to 13 c/sec waves from the posterior region, present during relaxation and eye closure, and attenuated by visual stimulation. Because of the tendency for such rhythms to become slower in old age, investigators have often used a more liberal frequency classification, including waves of 7 c/sec or less. Whether one calls a 7 c/sec rhythm "slow alpha" or "theta activity" is problematical. In the present discussion, these rhythms will be referred to as slow alpha when morphologically and functionally they appear to be similar to the dominant activity of young adults.

Alpha slowing is perhaps the most common finding in senescence, where it occurs as a function of both age and health status. In comparison with a young adult average of 10.2 to 10.5 c/sec (**5, 30**), the alpha rate of mentally normal old subjects is significantly lower. Mengoli (**41**) found alpha frequencies of 8 c/sec or less in a quarter of healthy subjects over 60 years of age. Among residents of an old age home, Obrist (**48**) obtained a mean alpha frequency of 9.1 c/sec in the seventh and eighth decades, and 8.6 c/sec beyond age 80. Mundy-Castle *et al.* (**46**) reported a mean of 9.4 c/sec for normal control subjects with an average age of 75 years. Similar findings have been obtained in general hospital patients by Friedlander (**13**) and Harvald (**20**), both of whom noted an increasing incidence of frequencies around 8 c/sec with advancing age.

Table I presents the mean and standard deviation of alpha frequency for a group of elderly community volunteers recently studied by the authors (**9**). A comparison of the two age groups below and above 75 years reveals a significant downward shift in frequency of more than a half cycle. Of particular interest is the finding that males have a reliably lower mean frequency than females, a phenomenon observed previously (**45**).

Table I. EEG Findings in 256 Elderly Community Subjects: Age and Sex Differences

	60-74 years		75-94 years	
	male	female	male	female
Number of cases	89	96	37	34
Alpha freq. (c/sec) Mean* † S. D.	9.4 0.7	9.7 0.8	8.9 0.9	9.1 0.6
Percentage of cases Fast activity† Diffuse slowing*	6 6	22 8	3 27	15 18

* Age differences are significant for alpha frequency and diffuse slowing at the .01 level.
† Sex differences are significant for alpha frequency and fast activity at the .02 level.

Associated with a lower mean alpha frequency is a decrease in the incidence of tracings with rates above 10 c/sec. Only 16 per cent of the elderly subjects described in Table I had alpha frequencies greater than 10 c/sec, the median for young adults. Rhythms in the 11 to 12 c/sec range were relatively rare, being less than 2 per cent. Thus the entire distribution shifts to the slow side, suggesting either a selective drop-out of subjects with higher rates, or a general slowing down that affects most individuals. The latter interpretation is supported by a longitudinal study (**56**) in which two-thirds of a group of mentally normal old people underwent progressive reductions in alpha frequency over a 10-year period. Drop-outs due to death occurred more often among subjects with slower rhythms. Although well within the young adult range, an alpha frequency of 9 c/sec in an elderly person may actually represent a considerable reduction from some earlier level.

Figure 1 illustrates one of the more precipitous declines observed by Obrist and co-workers in their longitudinal study. A fairly regular 9.4 c/sec rhythm between the ages of 79 and 82 decreases to an irregular 8.0 c/sec rhythm, interrupted by occasional 6 to 7 c/sec theta waves. This mixture of alpha and theta activity occurs commonly in subjects where the alpha rhythm slows to around 8 c/sec. The appearance of such irregular patterns may be a precursor to the development of more severe diffuse slowing.

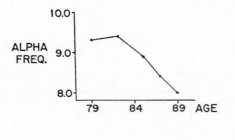

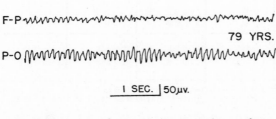

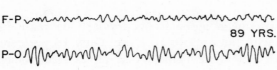

Figure 1. Alpha frequency plotted as a function of age for a mentally "normal" old man over a ten-year period. The top tracing was recorded at age 79, the bottom tracing at age 89. The latter EEG was associated with mild signs of intellectual impairment. F-P = Fronto-Parietal; P-O = Parie-to-Occipital. Taken from a study by Obrist et al. **(56).**

Intellectual impairment is associated with a slow alpha frequency in neuropsychiatric patients (**70**). Such a relationship, however, is not found in relatively healthy old people where mental function is well preserved and alpha frequency remains moderately high (**45, 49**). Thus, Obrist et al. (**52**) obtained no relationship between alpha rate and intelligence test performance in community volunteers, but did find significant correlations of +.20 to +.60 in institutionalized subjects where both variables underwent appreciable decline. Patients with clinical evidence of arteriosclerosis yielded higher correlations than subjects with negative physical findings. These authors concluded that pathological factors are responsible for the relationship between EEG and intellectual function during senescence. It is interesting to note that the subject in Figure 1 showed a 36 per cent decline in intelligence test performance that paralleled his EEG changes.

Memory function may also be related to alpha frequency in old age. Hoagland (**21**) obtained a correlation of +.87 between memory test scores and dominant occipital frequency in elderly psychiatric patients. The present authors, however, have been unable to replicate this finding in mentally normal old people. Again, the occurrence of a relationship probably depends upon the degree of pathology existing in the particular sample studied.

The association of alpha slowing and intellectual deficit is quite apparent in elderly patients with chronic brain syndrome (**64**). Such cases are more likely to have slow alpha rhythms than patients with functional disorders (**32, 54**). Two groups of aged psychiatric patients studied by Frey and Sjögren (**12**) are compared in Figure 2. As indicated by the graph, an alpha frequency of 7 c/sec is six times more prevalent in cases with organic dementia than in those without.

Although the etiology of alpha slowing in old age is obscure, there is some suggestion that vascular disease is a contributing factor (**50**). When age-matched groups of arteriosclerotic and normal subjects are compared, the former are found to have significantly lower alpha frequencies, regardless of whether the arteriosclerosis is clinically manifest in the heart or brain (**51**). Even subjects with asymptomatic arteriosclerosis, detectable only by extensive laboratory and physical examinations, have reliably lower frequencies than healthy controls (**49**). The fact that such cases have reduced cerebral blood flow and increased vascular resistance (**69**) suggests that a declining alpha rate may be an early sign of cerebral vascular insufficiency. Cardiovascular disease, however, is certainly not the only factor responsible for senescent alterations in alpha frequency, since subjects with completely negative findings show minor, but significant, EEG changes.

Characteristics of the alpha rhythm other than frequency also undergo changes with age. Mengoli (**41**) noted a general reduction in voltage among elderly control subjects, a finding confirmed by Mundy-Castle *et al*. (**46**). Both studies reported that a decrease in the proportion of time alpha activity is present, a result, however, that has not been consistently obtained (**45, 48**). Definite reductions in percent-time alpha occur in mentally deteriorated patients where the rhythms have been replaced by slower theta and delta waves (**10, 55**). Recently Gaches (**14**) observed an increased spatial distribution of alpha activity in elderly people, principally a greater extension into the frontal and temporal areas, which he related to the occurrence of cardiovascular disease. This interesting aspect of the senescent EEG, largely neglected, deserves further study.

An intriguing recent development in aging research is the more dynamic use of EEG in studies of sensory stimulation and reaction time. Wilson (**88**) found that mentally normal old people show less desynchronization of the alpha rhythm in response to a visual stimulus than do young adults. Habituation curves based on summated voltage revealed a tendency for the older person to adapt sooner and more completely with repeated stimulation. Reduced alpha blocking has also been noted among elderly institutionalized cases (**1**) and in aged psychiatric patients (**81**). The findings of Wells (**86**) suggest that cerebral pathology, including vascular disease, may result in lowered EEG reactivity.

There is some evidence that response speed in the elderly person is related to EEG frequency. Surwillo (**73**, **74**) obtained positive correlations between simple reaction time and the average duration of waves occurring between stimulus and response, many of which were in the alpha range. Thus, alpha slowing in old age may bear a functional relationship to increased reaction time. More research of this type is desirable as a means of elucidating relationships between CNS variables and senescent behavior.

2. Fast Activity

Waves with a frequency above the alpha range are considered fast activity. In the waking adult, such activity usually takes the form of an 18 to 30 c/sec beta rhythm, averaging less than 25 microvolts, and maximal over the precentral region (**24**). Both the magnitude and incidence of these rhythms increases during middle life. Gibbs and Gibbs (**17**) noted a twofold rise in the incidence of "F_1" ratings between 20 and 60 years of age among normal control subjects. Greenblatt (**19**) made a similar observation on middle-aged psychiatric patients.

Fast activity clearly persists into old age, where it is found in a relatively high proportion of cases (**17**, **38**, **40**, **44**, **48**). The exact incidence, however, varies from study to study, depending upon the criteria used. It might be conservatively estimated that 50 per cent of all elderly people show at least traces of low-voltage beta rhythm in one or more leads (see Figure 3). In some samples, as many as a quarter of the cases have fast rhythms that dominate the anterior tracings.

Table I presents the combined incidence of the Gibbses' F_1 and F_2 ratings in the elderly community group studied by the present authors. It is quite apparent that fast records occur more often among females than males, a finding which is statistically significant. Sex differences have previously been reported by Mundy-Castle (**44**) for young adults. The present authors, however, have been unable to confirm his observation of racial differences in fast activity among old people. Negroes, who comprised 78 of the 256 cases in Table I, did not differ significantly from white subjects on any EEG variable.

Fast activity is not a constant feature of the senescent EEG, but varies with age and mental status. Busse *et al.* (**7**) found that elderly community subjects with fast activity had lower mean ages than those with other EEG characteristics. Silverman and co-workers (**65**) reported a decreasing incidence of fast rhythms with increasing age and intellectual impairment. They found no instances of the Gibbses' F_1 or F_2 tracings in community volunteers beyond age 80. Consistent with this finding is the observation that only one male and one female out of 34 cases in Table I had fast tracings after 80 years of age. A decline in the amount of fast activity at advanced ages has also been noted in subjects studied longitudinally (**56**).

A relative absence of fast rhythms in deteriorated senile patients has been reported by a number of investigators (**2, 41, 46, 47, 55**), where it appears to be inversely related to the occurrence of diffuse slowing. Deteriorated and non-deteriorated elderly patients studied by Frey and Sjögren (**12**) are compared in Figure 2. As can be seen, beta activity occurred only one-third as often in the group with dementia. Because fast activity is most prevalent among intellectually well-preserved subjects during early senescence, its presence in an elderly person's EEG can probably be regarded as a favorable sign.

3. Diffuse Slowing

Diffuse slowing consists of theta (4–7 c/sec) and delta (1–3 c/sec) waves that have a diffuse as opposed to focal distribution, involving the anterior as well as posterior regions of both hemispheres. In its milder form diffuse slowing is contiguous in frequency with a slow alpha rhythm, from which it may be difficult to distinguish. Only tracings with a considerable amount of activity below 7 c/sec will be regarded as diffusely slow in the present discussion.

In contrast to other age-related EEG characteristics, diffuse slow waves are rarely found among community volunteers during early senescence. As shown in Table I, only 6 to 8 per cent of the authors' subjects under age 75 revealed slow activity in sufficient quantity to be rated as "S_1" by the Gibbses' classification, an incidence comparable to that of healthy young adults (17). With advancing age, however, there is a significant increase in diffuse slow activity, which occurs in more than one out of five cases over 75 years, according to Table I. The apparent sex difference for the older group is not statistically reliable. It should be noted that the severity of the slowing in community subjects never reaches the degree observed among mental hospital patients. None of the tracings in the present series were rated "S_2" according to the Gibbses' criteria. These results are essentially the same as those obtained by earlier studies on community groups (7, 65).

Diffuse slow activity, more than any other EEG variable, is related to senile intellectual deterioration. As in the case of alpha frequency, the magnitude of the correlation between EEG and mental function varies with the sample studied. Community subjects who have mild slowing and minimal intellectual impairment yield no relationship (7). On the other hand, institutionalized subjects who deviate more along these dimensions show significant correlations. Biserial coefficients of $+.20$ to $+.50$ have been reported between the presence or absence of diffuse slow activity and intelligence test performance, both for residents of an old age home and hospitalized psychiatric patients (52). This is consistent with previous findings of significantly lower intelligence test scores in cases with diffusely slow, as opposed to normal, EEGs (2, 66, 76).

Studies employing intelligence tests are necessarily limited to cases with mild deterioration because of the cooperation required by the examination. Using a psychiatric rating scale, McAdam and Robinson (34, 36) were able to assess a greater range of intellectual deficit. They obtained a rank-order correlation of $+.79$ between ratings of senile dementia and a quantitative index of theta and delta activity in hospitalized patients, thus confirming the earlier work of McAdam and McClatchey (33). This finding is particularly important because it indicates that the degree of EEG slowing is related to the severity of intellectual impairment; i.e., the slower and more abundant the waves, the greater the deterioration. Similar relationships have been reported by Mundy-Castle et al. (46)

and Weiner and Schuster (**84**), who also rated the severity of dementia.

If EEG slowing is quantitatively related to intellectual deterioration, it is not surprising that diffuse slow activity has been used to differentiate functional from organic mental disorders in old age. The early studies of Hoch and Kubis (**22**) and Liberson and Seguin (**28**) suggested that diffuse slowing is more prevalent in confused senile and arteriosclerotic patients than in cases with schizophrenic, affective, or involutional psychosis. This distinction has been emphasized by Luce and Rothschild (**32**) and Obrist and Henry (**54**), who studied aged psychiatric patients. In the latter investigation, 79 per cent of the cases with diffuse slow activity were found to have chronic brain syndrome, while 88 per cent of those with normal EEGs had functional disorders, consisting primarily of depressions and paranoid reactions. Figure 2 illustrates the kind of differentiation that can be made between elderly patients with and without organic dementia (**12**). Almost four times as

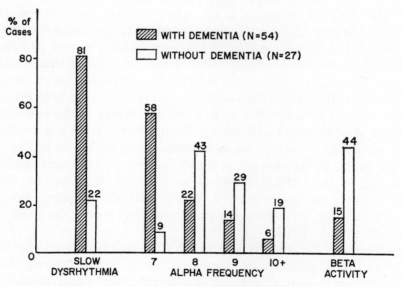

Figure 2. A comparison of EEG characteristics in two psychotic groups of patients over 60 years of age studied by Frey and Sjögren (**12**). Patients with dementia showed severe intellectual deterioration, while those without manifested little or none. The two groups are approximately equal in age.

many of the demented patients have slow dysrhythmias of the diffuse type.

Not only is diffuse slowing related to psychiatric diagnosis, but also to prognosis and life expectancy. Obrist and Henry (54) found that the majority of elderly patients with diffuse slow activity either remained hospitalized or died within a year after their EEG. Patients with normal or focal tracings, on the other hand, tended to be discharged or transferred to convalescent homes. Both McAdam and Robinson (35, 36) and Pampiglione and Post (59) have made similar observations.

The value of EEG in geriatric psychiatry has been the subject of some controversy. Turton (77) and Turton and Warren (78) take issue with investigators who suggest that the EEG is useful in assessing the degree of dementia in patients where coexisting functional disorders obscure the picture. They argue that the EEG offers definitive diagnostic information only when the presence of organic dementia is already clinically obvious. This conclusion begs the question, however, because there are no adequate criteria for evaluating the EEG in equivocal cases of dementia, other than the uncertain signs of dementia itself. Thus Turton and Warren (78) obtained rather poor agreement between EEG and mental status in a sample heavily weighted with long-term schizophrenics who were difficult to assess psychologically. When cases with questionable dementia were excluded, the relationship improved, even though only gross characterizations of EEG normality were made. Presumably the correlation would have been still higher if the amount of diffuse slow activity had been specifically rated. It should be noted that only diffuse slowing bears a positive relationship to intellectual impairment. Focal slowing is poorly correlated (see next section), and excess fast activity tends to be inversely related. The lumping together of diffusely slow, focal, and fast tracings into one broad category of abnormal almost certainly lowers the predictive efficiency of the EEG.

Admittedly the correlation between EEG and behavior is far from perfect, being particularly puzzling when a normal tracing is obtained from a patient with obviously advanced brain disease, or vice versa. The authors agree with Turton and co-workers that the only reliable EEG sign of senile intellectual deterioration is moderately severe diffuse slowing. The presence or absence of such a tracing may nevertheless be of considerable help in a few cases where profound depression or delusions make accurate psychologic assessment impossible. This alone would seem to justify the cautious optimism of several investigators regarding the usefulness of EEG in geriatric psychiatry (**36, 59**).

Some clue to the possible etiology of diffuse slow activity in senescence is offered by experiments on cerebral blood flow and metabolism. It is well established that cerebral ischemia and anoxia produce EEG slowing (**16**). Lassen and associates (**26**) observed that deteriorated senile patients with abnormally slow EEGs have a low cerebral oxygen consumption. Obrist *et al.* (**57**) reported a correlation of −.78 between the amount of occipital slow activity and cerebral oxygen uptake in elderly patients with chronic brain syndrome and diffusely slow EEGs. Significant correlations were also obtained between brain wave frequency and cerebral blood flow and vascular resistance. These findings suggest that diminished cerebral blood flow and metabolism in elderly people give rise to diffuse slowing. They shed little light, however, on whether circulatory or metabolic variables are primary.

There is some evidence that cerebral vascular insufficiency contributes to diffuse slowing in aged psychiatric patients. Obrist *et al.* (**53**) observed that patients with low blood pressure had three times as many diffusely slow tracings as individuals with high blood pressure. In fact, when low blood pressure occurred in combination with clinically detectable vascular disease, over 70 per cent of the EEGs were diffusely slow (**50**). This interaction of blood pressure and vascular disease suggests that the observed EEG changes may represent the accumulative effects of chronic cerebral ischemia. It might be speculated that an adequate regulation of blood pressure, particularly in cases with vascular disease, is crucial for the maintenance of EEG normality in old age.

Little is known about the anatomic correlates of senescent EEG changes. Studies on presenile dementia have shown that cerebral atrophy is usually associated with diffuse slowing (**27, 29**), although normal EEGs are occasionally found (**75**). The only systematic investigation on aged psychiatric patients was undertaken by Sheridan *et al.* (**64**), who reported EEG and postmortem findings in 14 cases. Nine mentally deteriorated patients with diffuse slow activity revealed evidence of senile or arteriosclerotic brain disease, or both. Unfortunately, there were not enough cases to attempt an EEG differentiation of the two types of pathology. Of special interest is the fact that three patients showed focal slowing that was not explainable by localized pathologic changes, and three cases had normal EEGs in the face of moderately severe postmortem findings. This suggests that physiologic factors such as hemodynamic or metabolic variables may influence the EEG independently of structural CNS changes. A fuller understanding of the pathologic mechanisms underlying EEG alterations in the senium would seem to require a combined anatomic-physiologic approach.

4. Focal Disturbances

The term focal disturbances is employed here to designate localized EEG patterns that clinical electroencephalographers generally regard as abnormal. These consist of focal theta or delta waves, marked amplitude asymmetries, and localized sharp waves or spikes. The foci may be unilateral or bilateral, the latter being distinguished from diffuse disturbances by their restriction to a limited brain region.

Busse and co-workers (8) were the first to report a high incidence of focal slow activity in elderly people. They found that 30 to 40 per cent of community volunteers over age 60 had slow wave foci, predominantly from the left anterior temporal area. Silverman et al. (65) observed that three-quarters of the focal disturbances were lateralized to the left hemisphere, while 80 per cent appeared maximally over the anterior portion of the temporal lobe. Amplitude asymmetries and random spiking were also noted, usually in association with the slow waves. These findings were later replicated on a different community sample by Busse et al. (7). An even higher incidence of focal slowing (50 per cent) was reported by Mundy-Castle (45) for residents of an old age home. Again, three-quarters were left-sided, with maximal involvement of the anterior temporal area. In all of these studies, some of the severest foci occurred among mentally and neurologically normal subjects who were making adequate social adjustments.

A high incidence of temporal-lobe disturbances has also been noted in elderly hospital samples (12, 20). Barnes et al. (2) found temporal foci in 30 per cent of aged psychiatric patients, four-fifths of whom were left-sided. In comparison with community subjects, the slow waves tended to have a wider distribution, extending into the posterior and mid-temporal areas. Among patients with chronic brain syndrome, the foci often took the form of a localized accentuation of diffuse slow activity. Obrist and Henry (**54**) obtained similar findings, but emphasized the frequent involvement of the frontal as well as temporal areas in mentally deteriorated patients, an observation made earlier by Schwab (**63**). It would appear that focal slowing, when restricted to the anterior temporal region, is compatible with good social adjustment. However, when it involves adjacent areas or becomes part of a diffuse disturbance, chronic brain syndrome is more probable.

Not all studies have observed such a high incidence of focal slow activity among old people, a discrepancy that might be attributed to differences in recording technique. Using mid-temporal electrodes with an ear reference, Obrist (**48**) and Sheridan *et al.* (**64**) failed to obtain foci in more than a small percentage of their elderly subjects. Silverman *et al.* (**65**) stressed the importance of electrode placement, particularly the proximity of leads to the anterior tip of the temporal lobe. They applied electrodes only one to

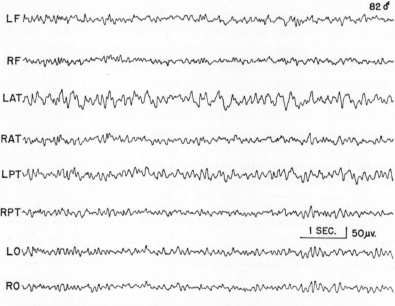

Figure 3. Illustration of a temporal-lobe focus in an 82-year-old community volunteer who is mentally and neurologically normal.   L = Left;   R = Right;   F = Frontal;   AT = Anterior Temporal; PT = Posterior Temporal; O = Occipital. All leads are referred to the vertex.

two cm above the zygomatic arch, one-third of the distance between
the auditory meatus and external canthus of the eye. A central
vertex reference was employed. It should be noted that a temporal
electrode in this location is at least four cm away from the nearest
placement of the International System, a fact that could lead to dis-
crepant results (**67**).

Figure 3 is an example of a moderately severe temporal focus in
an 82-year-old man. A mixture of theta and delta waves is seen over
the left anterior temporal area, with minor spread to the left frontal
and posterior temporal leads. Foci as severe as this occur in about
10 per cent of community volunteers. Although fairly continuous
in this particular sample, such slowing is typically episodic, being
interspersed by sections of normal tracing. The subject remains
active and mentally alert after four years of retirement. Neurological
and physical findings are negative, except for a moderate hearing
loss and EKG signs of an old anterior infarct. His IQ is 135, there
being little or no intellectual impairment indicated by his pattern
of test scores.

In a recent study by the authors (**9**), focal disturbances were
found in 36 per cent of community volunteers over age 60. Five-
sixths of these cases (30 per cent of the sample) revealed focal
slow activity over the temporal lobe, the remainder showing either
amplitude asymmetries, spikes or sharp waves, predominantly of
temporal origin. Only 2 out of 256 cases had a slow wave focus
outside of the temporal area (one frontal and one occipital). Table
II presents the laterality and distribution of slow activity involving

Table II. Localization of Temporal Slow Activity in Elderly Community
Subjects (Waking EEG)

	Per cent of 78 Foci*
Unilateral	
Left	40
Right	5
Bilateral	
Left > Right	40
Right > Left	4
Symmetrical	11
Anterior temporal	75
Ant. & post. temporal	22
Posterior temporal	3

* Temporal slowing occurred in 78 out of 256 cases (30%).

the temporal lobe. As shown, 40 per cent of the foci were confined to the left hemisphere, while another 40 per cent were bilateral with a left-sided emphasis. The slow waves were localized to the anterior temporal area in 75 per cent of the subjects, and to the posterior temporal area in only 3 per cent. They appeared equally from the anterior and posterior leads in the remaining cases.

Several other interesting observations were made by the authors on the same series of community subjects. The prevalence of foci did not increase with age; i.e., the proportion of cases remained roughly constant from 60 years on. Temporal slowing did occur, however, more often among females than males (36 and 25 per cent, respectively). Contrary to a previous report by Silverman et al. (65), the incidence of temporal foci did not vary inversely with socioeconomic level. In the earlier study, lower-class subjects were recruited from a medical clinic, while upper-class subjects were solicited through social organizations. It seems likely that the previous findings were due to differences in health, rather than to variations in social class. The authors have also recorded from 250 young and middle-aged control subjects. Although temporal-lobe disturbances rarely appear before the age of 40, they become increasingly prevalent in the fifth and sixth decades.

In contrast to diffuse slow wave abnormalities that bear a significant relation to intellectual impairment, focal disturbances over the temporal lobe tend to be clinically silent. No definitive correlations have been obtained with routine psychological or psychiatric assessments, even in severe cases with high amplitude delta waves (7, 45, 52, 66, 76). Although the literature suggests a relationship between temporal-lobe damage and memory impairment (43, 60, 82), our own unpublished attempts to correlate senescent EEG foci with learning and memory function have been largely unsuccessful. Temporal foci do not appear to be related to cerebral dominance, aphasia, or seizures (9, 12, 65). A relationship to senile cataract has been observed by Strauss et al. (71), but this is probably fortuitous. As noted earlier, temporal slowing is associated with intellectual deterioration only when the focus extends widely into adjacent areas, suggesting a mass-action effect. The possibility of a highly specific psychological correlate remains an intriguing prospect for future research.

Focal disturbances are not a constant feature of the senescent EEG, but vary with the level of consciousness or arousal. Figure

4 compares the waking, drowsy, and sleep states of 77 elderly community subjects studied by the authors. Whereas the number of cases with focal slow activity is approximately equal during wakefulness and drowsiness, amplitude asymmetries and sharp waves (including spikes) tend to increase during the drowsy state. On the other hand, light sleep (early spindle stage) is accompanied by a decrease in all types of focal disturbance. The foci are overwhelmingly temporal, there being only three instances of non-temporal localization. In the case of asymmetry, the higher amplitude appears on the left side in three-quarters of the tracings. The asymmetries usually consist of an accentuation of alpha-like activity over the temporal area, often in association with slow and sharp waves from the same region.

Little is known about the exact origin of temporal foci in elderly people. Following Silverman and Groff (68), it might be speculated that the disappearance of slow waves during sleep is indicative of a relatively deep lying lesion, possibly in the hippocampal region. Strauss *et al.* (72) pointed out that temporal foci frequently accompany pathology in other areas of the brain, thus giving rise to false localization. In patients with cerebral vascular accidents,

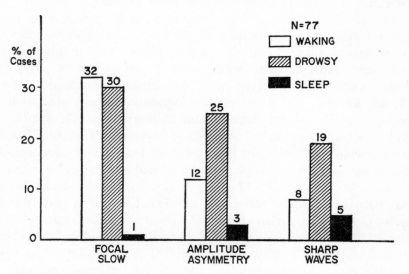

Figure 4. Incidence of different focal abnormalities in elderly community subjects at three levels of arousal; awake, drowsy, and asleep. All foci except three asymmetries involve the temporal area.

Frantzen and Lennox-Buchthal (11) localized all foci to the temporal lobe, regardless of the site of the lesion. Hughes (23) performed a statistical analysis of EEG foci on a heterogeneous collection of cases and found that more than 50 per cent were localized to the temporal lobe, with a definite predilection for the left hemisphere. Temporal slowing, in particular, occurred twice as often on the left side as on the right. He suggested that a greater susceptibility to vascular pathology may account for the more frequent involvement of the left hemisphere and temporal lobe.

The possibility that temporal foci have a vascular etiology is suggested by the relatively high incidence of such patterns in patients with clinical evidence of cerebral vascular disease (11, 12, 20). Bruens *et al.* (6) studied a group of aged clinic patients with moderately severe temporal foci and found that 89 per cent had neurologic findings suggestive of a vascular disorder. Hyperventilation, compression of the carotid artery, or inhalation of low oxygen mixtures exacerbated the slowing, while breathing CO_2 tended to reduce it. This was considered support for the hypothesis that "chronic" cerebral circulatory insufficiency is responsible for temporal-lobe slowing in old age. The applicability of these findings to the average old person is open to question, however, due to the highly select nature of the sample. Although approximately one-third of elderly community volunteers have temporal foci, very few of them reveal neurologic impairment. Further investigation of "normal" aged subjects is definitely indicated.

Activation techniques offer a possible means of assessing the role of cerebral ischemia in senescent EEG changes. With few exceptions, their use has been limited to patients with specific neurologic complaints. Several studies have suggested an increased sensitivity of the older person's EEG to procedures that alter cerebral hemodynamics. Approximately 25 per cent of elderly control subjects give focal slow wave responses to unilateral carotid compression (31, 37, 85). Although hyperventilation produces relatively little generalized buildup in old age (3, 48, 87), the authors have noted an exacerbation of temporal slowing in one out of five community cases with foci. Inhalation of low oxygen mixtures elicits less slow activity in healthy aged subjects (62) than in patients with cerebral vascular disease, where the response is often generalized (15, 42). Inhalation of CO_2 has been found to reduce focal slowing in cases with cerebral infarction (61, 83). The provocation or modification of foci by these techniques provides inferential evidence of underlying vascular insufficiency. It is hoped that more direct evidence of localized cerebral ischemia can be obtained from radioisotopic determinations of regional blood flow (25) for possible correlation with EEG (18).

The occurrence of temporal foci in a fair proportion of the elderly population presents certain difficulties in the interpretation of clinical tracings. Van der Drift and Magnus (79, 80) have discussed the problem of differentiating space-occupying lesions from cerebral vascular disorders in senescence. The fact that many old people have clinically silent foci argues for considerable caution in attributing diagnostic significance to such abnormalities (58). The prognostic value of temporal slowing at this age is probably no greater than its diagnostic value. A majority of foci observed by the authors over a three-to-four-year period have remained stable without the development of clinical symptomatology. Much more knowledge is needed about this type of EEG finding before meaningful interpretations can be made.

BIBLIOGRAPHY

1. Andermann, K., and Stoller, A. EEG patterns in hospitalized and non-hospitalized aged. *Electroenceph. clin. Neurophysiol.* **13**: 319, 1961.
2. Barnes, R. H., Busse, E. W., and Friedman, E. L. The psychological functioning of aged individuals with normal and abnormal electroencephalograms. II. A study of hospitalized individuals. *J. nerv. ment. Dis.* **124**: 585–593, 1956.
3. Barnes, T. C., and Amoroso, M. D. The effect of age of the human brain on the electroencephalogram during hyperventilation. *Anat. Rec.* **99**: 622, 1947.
4. Berger, H. Über das Elektrenkephalogramm des Menschen. Fünfte Mitteilung. *Arch. Psychiat. Nervenkr.* **98**: 231–254, 1933.
5. Brazier, M. A. B., and Finesinger, J. E. Characteristics of the normal electroencephalogram. I. A study of the occipital cortical potentials in 500 normal adults. *J. clin. Invest.* **23**: 303–311, 1944.
6. Bruens, J. H., Gastaut, H., and Giove, G. Electroencephalographic study of the signs of chronic vascular insufficiency of the Sylvian region in aged people. *Electroenceph. clin. Neurophysiol.* **12**: 283–295, 1960.
7. Busse, E. W., Barnes, R. H., Friedman, E. L., and Kelty, E. J. Psychological functioning of aged individuals with normal and abnormal electroencephalograms. I. A study of non-hospitalized community volunteers. *J. nerv. ment. Dis.* **124**: 135–141, 1956.
8. Busse, E. W., Barnes, R. H., Silverman, A. J., Shy, G. M., Thaler, M., and Frost, L. L. Studies of the process of aging: Factors that influence the psyche of elderly persons. *Amer. J. Psychiat.* **110**: 897–903, 1954.
9. Busse, E. W., and Obrist, W. D. Significance of focal electroencephalographic changes in the elderly. *Postgrad. Med.* **34**: 179–182, 1963.
10. Davis, P. A. The electroencephalogram in old age. *Dis. nerv. Syst.* **2**: 77, 1941.
11. Frantzen, E., and Lennox-Buchthal, M. Correlation of clinical electroencephalographic and arteriographic findings in patients with cerebral vascular accident. *Acta psychiat. scand.* **36**: Suppl. 150, 133–134, 1961.
12. Frey, T. S., and Sjögren, H. The electroencephalogram in elderly persons suffering from neuropsychiatric disorders. *Acta psychiat. scand.* **34**: 438–450, 1959.
13. Friedlander, W. J. Electroencephalographic alpha rate in adults as a function of age. *Geriatrics.* **13**: 29–31, 1958.

14. Gaches, J. Étude statistique sur les traces "alpha largement développé" en fonction de l'age. *Presse med.* **68**: 1620–1622, 1960.
15. Gastaut, H., Bostem, F., Fernandez-Guardiola, A., Naquet, R., and Gibson, W. Hypoxic activation of the EEG by nitrogen inhalation. III. Preliminary results in patients suffering from cerebrovascular disease. In H. Gastaut and J. S. Meyer (Editors), *Cerebral Anoxia and the Electroencephalogram.* Charles C. Thomas, Springfield, pp. 365–382, 1961.
16. Gastaut, H., and Meyer, J. S. (Editors). *Cerebral Anoxia and the Electroencephalogram.* Charles C. Thomas, Springfield, 617 pp., 1961.
17. Gibbs, F. A., and Gibbs, E. L. *Atlas of Electroencephalography.* Vol. I. *Methodology and Controls.* Addison-Wesley Press, Cambridge, Mass., 324 pp., 1950.
18. Gleichmann, U., Ingvar, D. H., Lassen, N. A., Lübbers, D. W., Siesjö, B. K., and Thews, G. Regional cerebral cortical metabolic rate of oxygen and carbon dioxide, related to the EEG in the anesthetized dog. *Acta physiol. scand.* **55**: 82–94, 1962.
19. Greenblatt, M. Age and electroencephalographic abnormality in neuropsychiatric patients: A study of 1593 cases. *Amer. J. Psychiat.* **101**: 82–90, 1944.
20. Harvald, B. EEG in old age. *Acta psychiat. scand.* **33**: 193–196, 1958.
21. Hoagland, H. Studies of brain metabolism and electrical activity in relation to adreno-cortical physiology. In G. Pincus (Editor), *Recent Progress in Hormone Research.* Academic Press, New York, **10**: 29–63, 1954.
22. Hoch, P. H., and Kubis, J. Electroencephalographic studies in organic psychoses. *Amer. J. Psychiat.* **98**: 404–408, 1941.
23. Hughes, J. R. A statistical analysis on the location of EEG abnormalities. *Electroenceph. clin. Neurophysiol.* **12**: 905–909, 1960.
24. Jasper, H. H., and Andrews, H. L. Electroencephalography. III. Normal differentiation of occipital and precentral regions in man. *Arch. Neurol. Psychiat. (Chic.).* **39**: 96–115, 1938.
25. Lassen, N. A., Höedt-Rasmussen, K., Sörensen, S. C., Skinhöj, E., Cronquist, S., Bodforss, B., and Ingvar, D. H. Regional cerebral blood flow in man determined by krypton[85]. *Neurology.* **13**: 719–727, 1963.
26. Lassen, N. A., Munck, O., and Tottey, E. R. Mental function and cerebral oxygen consumption in organic dementia. *Arch. Neurol. Psychiat. (Chic.).* **77**: 126–133, 1957.
27. Letemendia, F., and Pampiglione, G. Clinical and electroencephalographic observations in Alzheimer's disease. *J. Neurol. Neurosurg. Psychiat.* **21**: 167–172, 1958.
28. Liberson, W. T., and Seguin, C. A. Brain waves and clinical features in arteriosclerotic and senile mental patients. *Psychosom. Med.* **7**: 30–35, 1945.
29. Liddell, D. W. Investigations of EEG findings in presenile dementia. *J. Neurol. Neurosurg. Psychiat.* **21**: 173–176, 1958.
30. Lindsley, D. B. Electrical potentials of the brain in children and adults. *J. genet. Psychol.* **19**: 285–306, 1938.
31. Loeb, C. Effects of alternate carotid compression in aged and apparently normal subjects. In H. Gastaut and J. S. Meyer (Editors), *Cerebral Anoxia and the Electroencephalogram.* Charles C. Thomas, Springfield, pp. 415–427, 1961.
32. Luce, R. A., Jr., and Rothschild, D. The correlation of electroencephalographic and clinical observations in psychiatric patients over 65. *J. Geront.* **8**: 167–172, 1953.
33. McAdam, W., and McClatchey, W. T. The electroencephalogram in aged patients of a mental hospital. *J. ment. Sci.* **98**: 711–715, 1952.
34. McAdam, W., and Robinson, R. A. Senile intellectual deterioration and the electroencephalogram: A quantitative correlation. *J. ment. Sci.* **102**: 819–825, 1956.
35. McAdam, W., and Robinson, R. A. Prognosis in senile deterioration. *J. ment. Sci.* **103**: 821–823, 1957.
36. McAdam, W., and Robinson, R. A. Diagnostic and prognostic value of the electroencephalogram in geriatric psychiatry. In H. T. Blumenthal (Editor), *Medical and Clinical Aspects of Aging.* Columbia Univ. Press, New York, pp. 557–564, 1962.
37. McBeath, J., Winston, R., and Friedlander, W. J. Evaluation of controlled digital artery compression in cerebral vascular insufficiency. *Neurology.* **11**: 143–150, 1961.
38. Maggs, R., and Turton, E. C. Some EEG findings in old age and their relationship to affective disorder. *J. ment. Sci.* **102**: 812–818, 1956.
39. Magladery, J. W. Neurophysiology of aging. In J. E. Birren (Editor), *Handbook of Aging and the Individual.* Univ. Chicago Press, Chicago, pp. 173–186, 1959.
40. Markovich, S. E. Electroencephalographic patterns in elderly patients: A longitudinal study. In H. T. Blumenthal (Editor), *Medical and Clinical Aspects of Aging.* Columbia Univ. Press, New York, pp. 547–556, 1962.
41. Mengoli, G. L'elettroencefalogramma nei vecchi. *Riv. Neurol.* **22**: 166–193, 1952.
42. Meyer, J. S., and Waltz, A. G. Arterial oxygen saturation and alveolar carbon dioxide

during electroencephalography. Comparison of hyperventilation and induced hypoxia in subjects with cerebral vascular disease. In H. Gastaut and J. S. Meyer (Editors), *Cerebral Anoxia and the Electroencephalogram*. Charles C. Thomas, Springfield, pp. 329–342, 1961.

43. Meyer, V. Cognitive changes following temporal lobectomy for relief of temporal lobe epilepsy. *A.M.A. Arch. Neurol. Psychiat.* **81**: 299–309, 1959.
44. Mundy-Castle, A. C. Theta and beta rhythm in the electroencephalograms of normal adults. *Electroenceph. clin. Neurophysiol.* **3**: 477–486, 1951.
45. Mundy-Castle, A. C. Central excitability in the aged. In H. T. Blumenthal (Editor), *Medical and Clinical Aspects of Aging*. Columbia Univ. Press, New York, pp. 575–595, 1962.
46. Mundy-Castle, A. C., Hurst, L. A., Beerstecher, D. M., and Prinsloo, T. The electroencephalogram in the senile psychoses. *Electroenceph. clin. Neurophysiol.* **6**: 245–252, 1954.
47. Noël, M. G. L'EEG dans l'artériosclérose cérébrale. *Rev. neurol.* **87**: 198–199, 1952.
48. Obrist, W. D. The electroencephalogram of normal aged adults. *Electroenceph. clin. Neurophysiol.* **6**: 235–244, 1954.
49. Obrist, W. D. The electroencephalogram of healthy aged males. In PHS Publ. No. 986, *Human Aging: A Biological and Behavioral Study*. U. S. Govt. Print. Off., Washington, pp. 79–93, 1963.
50. Obrist, W. D. Cerebral ischemia and the senescent electroencephalogram. In E. Simonson and T. H. McGavack (Editors), *Cerebral Ischemia*. Charles C. Thomas, Springfield, pp. 71–98, 1964.
51. Obrist, W. D., and Bissell, L. F. The electroencephalogram of aged patients with cardiac and cerebral vascular disease. *J. Geront.* **10**: 315–330, 1955.
52. Obrist, W. D., Busse, E. W., Eisdorfer, C., and Kleemeier, R. W. Relation of the electroencephalogram to intellectual function in senescence. *J. Geront.* **17**: 197–206, 1962.
53. Obrist, W. D., Busse, E. W., and Henry, C. E. Relation of electroencephalogram to blood pressure in elderly persons. *Neurology.* **11**: 151–158, 1961.
54. Obrist, W. D., and Henry, C. E. Electroencephalographic findings in aged psychiatric patients. *J. nerv. ment. Dis.* **126**: 254–267, 1958.
55. Obrist, W. D., and Henry, C. E. Electroncephalographic frequency analysis of aged psychiatric patients. *Electroenceph. clin. Neurophysiol.* **10**: 621–632, 1958.
56. Obrist, W. D., Henry, C. E., and Justiss, W. A. Longitudinal study of EEG in old age. *Excerpta med., Int. Congr. Series* No. 37, 180–181, 1961.
57. Obrist, W. D., Sokoloff, L., Lassen, N. A., Lane, M. H., Butler, R. N., and Feinberg, I. Relation of EEG to cerebral blood flow and metabolism in old age. *Electroenceph. clin. Neurophysiol.* **15**: 610–619, 1963.
58. O'Leary, J. L. The electroencephalogram in geriatric practice. *Geriatrics.* **12**: 413–420, 1957.
59. Pampiglione, G., and Post, F. The value of electroencephalographic examinations in psychiatric disorders of old age. *Geriatrics.* **13**: 725–732, 1958.
60. Penfield, W., and Milner, B. Memory deficit produced by bilateral lesions in the hippocampal zone. *A.M.A. Arch. Neurol. Psychiat.* **79**: 475–497, 1958.
61. Potes, J., and Wells, C. E. The electroencephalogram during administration of 100% oxygen and of 5% carbon dioxide in patients with cerebral infarction. *Neurology.* **11**: 738–741, 1961.
62. Rossen, R., Simonson, E., and Baker, J. Electroencephalograms during hypoxia in healthy men. *Arch. Neurol.* **5**: 648–654, 1961.
63. Schwab, R. S. *Electroencephalography in Clinical Practice*. W. B. Saunders, Philadelphia, pp. 143–148, 1951.
64. Sheridan, F. P., Yeager, C. L., Oliver, W. A., and Simon, A. Electroencephalography as a diagnostic and prognostic aid in studying the senescent individual: A preliminary report. *J. Geront.* **10**: 53–59, 1955.
65. Silverman, A. J., Busse, E. W., and Barnes, R. H. Studies in the processes of aging: Electroencephalographic findings in 400 elderly subjects. *Electroenceph. clin. Neurophysiol.* **7**: 67–74, 1955.
66. Silverman, A. J., Busse, E. W., Barnes, R. H., Frost, L. L., and Thaler, M. B. Studies on the processes of aging. 4. Physiologic influences on psychic functioning in elderly people. *Geriatrics.* **8**: 370–376, 1953.
67. Silverman, D. The anterior temporal electrode and the ten-twenty system. *Electroenceph. clin. Neurophysiol.* **12**: 735–737, 1960.
68. Silverman, D., and Groff, R. A. Brain tumor depth determination by electrographic recordings during sleep. *A.M.A. Arch. Neurol. Psychiat.* **78**: 15–28, 1957.

69. Sokoloff, L. Cerebral circulatory and metabolic changes associated with aging. *Res. Publ. Ass. Res. Nerv. Ment. Dis.* **41**, in press.
70. Stoller, A. Slowing of the alpha rhythm of the electroencephalogram and its association with mental deterioration and epilepsy. *J. ment. Sci.* **95**: 972–984, 1949.
71. Strauss, H., Linn, L., and Ostow, M. Electroencephalographic and neuropsychiatric observations in patients with senile cataract. *Mschr. Psychiat. Neurol.* **130**: 321–327, 1955.
72. Strauss, H., Ostow, M., Greenstein, L., and Lewyn, S. Temporal slowing as a source of error in electroencephalographic localization. *J. Mt. Sinai Hosp.* **22**: 306–315, 1955.
73. Surwillo, W. W. Frequency of the "alpha" rhythm, reaction time and age. *Nature (Lond.).* **191**: 823–824, 1961.
74. Surwillo, W. W. The relation of simple response time to brain-wave frequency and the effects of age. *Electroenceph. clin. Neurophysiol.* **15**: 105–114, 1963.
75. Swain, J. M. Electroencephalographic abnormalities in presenile atrophy. *Neurology.* **9**: 722–727, 1959.
76. Thaler, M. Relationships among Wechsler, Weigl, Rorschach, EEG findings, and abstract-concrete behavior in a group of normal aged subjects. *J. Geront.* **11**: 404–409, 1956.
77. Turton, E. C. The EEG as a diagnostic and prognostic aid in the differentiation of organic disorders in patients over 60. *J. ment. Sci.* **104**: 461–465, 1958.
78. Turton, E. C., and Warren, P. K. G. Dementia: A clinical and EEG study of 274 patients over the age of 60. *J. ment. Sci.* **106**: 1493–1500, 1960.
79. Van der Drift, J. H. A., and Magnus, O. Space occupying lesions in older patients. *Psychiat. Neurol. Neurochir. (Amst.).* **64**: 192–201, 1961.
80. Van der Drift, J. H. A., and Magnus, O. The EEG with space occupying intracranial lesions in old patients. *Electroenceph. clin. Neurophysiol.* **14**: 664–673, 1962.
81. Verdeaux, G., Verdeaux, J., and Turmel, J. Étude statistique de la fréquence et de la réactivité des électroencéphalogrammes chez les subjets agés. *Canad. Psychiat. Ass. J.* **6**: 28–36, 1961.
82. Walker, A. E. Recent memory impairment in unilateral temporal lesions. *A.M.A. Arch. Neurol. Psychiat.* **78**: 543–552, 1957.
83. Waltz, J. M., Von Weiss, J. F., and Stevens, J. The effect of CO_2 inhalation on the electroencephalogram of patients with cerebral infarction. *Electroenceph. clin. Neurophysiol.* **9**: 527–530, 1957.
84. Weiner, H., and Schuster, D. B. The electroencephalogram in dementia: Some preliminary observations and correlations. *Electroenceph. clin. Neurophysiol.* **8**: 479–488, 1956.
85. Weiss, S., and Froelich, W. Tilt table electroencephalography in insufficiency syndromes. *Neurology.* **8**: 686–693, 1958.
86. Wells, C. E. Alpha wave responsiveness to light in man. In G. H. Glaser (Editor), *EEG and Behavior.* Basic Books, New York, pp. 27–59, 1963.
87. Whittier, J. R., and Dhrymiotis, A. D. Age differences in the human electroencephalographic response to hyperventilation. *J. Geront.* **17**: 461–462, 1962.
88. Wilson, S. Electrocortical reactivity in young and aged adults. Unpublished doctoral dissertation, George Peabody College, Nashville, Tenn., 1962.

RELATIONSHIPS BETWEEN THE EEG AND OTHER PHYSIOLOGICAL MEASURES IN MAN

J. A. Stern, Ph.D.

If we can assume the EEG to be a measure of the activity of the brain, and if we further wish to assume that the brain is the "master organ" exerting a dominant influence on the other physiological systems within the organism, we would then expect to see reasonable and predictive relationships between EEG measures and measures of other physiological systems. One of the factors which, of course, immediately will confound the picture is the other side of the coin, namely, the effect of other physiological systems on central nervous system functioning. The question of which system turns out to be the "master organ" will not be answered by this review. Our goal will be to sketch some of the interrelations between physiological measures.

This review is limited to studies pertaining to man and to a lesser extent the specific interests of the reviewer. Rather than attempting to organize the review about specific measures, we have organized it around more general physiological states such as cortical and autonomic disturbances, sleep, sleep deprivation, states of alertness, and response to stimulation. It is not an exhaustive review; rather, representative studies for the various areas specified have been included.

EEG ABNORMALITY AS REFLECTED IN OTHER MEASURES

Jung (17) studied 10 normal subjects and 10 subjects with petit mal epilepsy using the following physiological measures: EEG,[1]

[1] Glossary of abbreviations used in text

BP	Blood pressure	EEG	Electroencephalograph
ED	Electrodermal	EKG	Electrocardiograph
EDR	Electrodermal response (PGR)	EMG	Electromyograph
EDRe	Electrodermal resistance	HR	Heart rate

EKG, EDR, plethysmograph, and respiration. Under conditions of rest subjects were stimulated with "arousing" stimuli such as shouts, pistol shots, and pin pricks. Petit mal discharges could be effectively blocked by intense sensory stimulation, the most effective ones being loud noise and pain. When such blocking was effective, it was always followed by sympathetic discharge as recorded in the EDR and plethysmograph. If the stimuli were ineffective in blocking the spike-and-wave phenomena, they also did not elicit such peripheral autonomic discharge. Jung apparently did not observe any changes in his other physiological measures which accompanied EEG signs of petit mal activity. Johnson *et al.* (16) studying EEG, HR, EDR, and skin temperature in 19 subjects with bursts of abnormal EEG activity also were unable to find any physiological correlates with bursts of EEG abnormality regardless of whether such bursts were spontaneous in origin or induced by photic stimulation. The only deviation from this finding was obtained if the abnormal activity persisted for more than 10 seconds. If this occurred, they observed a slight (2 beats/min) increase in heart rate and more rapid and deeper respiration. In seven patients who demonstrated "clinical discharges" it was found that an EDR was seen if a motor response accompanied EEG abnormality or if the patient was subjectively aware of the discharge. This occurred close to the onset of the motor response. Otherwise, no uniform pattern of responding was observed in the other physiological measures in these patients. Five patients with petit mal discharges were also studied during such discharges. Some types of autonomic alterations after the onset of the discharge were seen in all patients, the more typical pattern of response involving an increase in HR, a decrease in skin temperature, and erratic respiratory patterns. A decrease in skin resistance occurred in all patients, not during, however, but upon termination of, the abnormal EEG activity. Johnson *et al.* wondered whether the autonomic alterations which occurred during or after the EEG changes were directly attributable to the discharge or might more properly be a function of the subject's awareness that something unusual was occurring to him. In any case, with the possible exception of petit mal attacks, no consistent pattern of autonomic changes could be demonstrated to accompany specific types of seizure discharges as measured in the EEG.

Van Buren (35) and Van Buren and Ajmone-Marsan (36) studied autonomic concomitants (EDR, EKG, BP, respiration, skin temperature, plethysmograph) accompanying EEG components of ictal automatism and temporal-lobe epilepsy. Some of the seizures observed were spontaneous; others were induced by Metrazol administration, hyperventilation, and depth stimulation. In the second of these studies the authors report that "autonomic recording gave evidence of a remarkably stereotyped response consisting predominantly of hypertension, tachycardia, fall of skin resistance, esophageal peristalsis, inhibition of gastric motility and inhibition of respiration. Variations in this pattern lay predominantly in the failure of a given change to appear or in the sequence of the changes. In nearly all instances, however, failure of the patient to respond was preceded by some alteration in autonomic functioning (36). In the earlier study Van Buren stated that, "Indeed the various autonomic functions showed a remarkable lack of interdependence in the seizure state" (35). These studies thus also demonstrate that autonomic alterations do accompany ictal automatisms. However, the specific nature of these autonomic responses cannot be stated, though there tended to be some patterning of autonomic features during an attack. The earliest responses were a decrease in skin resistance and swallowing, followed by respiratory changes: expiratory apnea, the most common of these (these changes might appear early, though they were noted at other times as well), and tachycardia with or without blood pressure rise, followed by aura or unconsciousness, although these latter phenomena also occurred concurrently with the tachycardia in many instances.

Obrist, Busse, and Henry (27) in a study of elderly patients demonstrated some relationships between EEG and blood pressure. These authors studied 233 psychiatric patients and 261 mentally normal controls, all over 60 years of age. They demonstrated that in their group of psychiatrically disturbed patients elevated blood pressures were associated with a higher incidence of normal EEGs while reduced blood pressure was related to the observance of diffuse slow wave abnormalities. These authors suggest that with relatively low blood pressure and cerebral arteriosclerosis there is impairment in cerebral blood flow resulting in the EEG abnormality observed. Interestingly, the control subjects did not demonstrate this relationship nor was there as high an incidence of diffuse slow activity in the EEGs of these subjects. Obrist, Busse, and Kleemeier (personal communication, Kleemeier) further demonstrated that in an aged population arteriosclerotic disturbances were associated with changes in EEG alpha frequency. They found a decrease in the dominant frequency (alpha activity) related to cerebrovascular accidents. A relationship between decreases in alpha frequency and "impending death" was also related to impairment in intellectual functioning of the aged subject.

EEG AND PHYSIOLOGICAL CHANGES ASSOCIATED WITH GENERAL PHYSIOLOGICAL STATES

Sleep and Sleep Deprivation

We are all familiar with the concept that more or less specific EEG patterns are associated with different levels of sleep. Let us first concur with Ackner and Pampiglioni (1) that "the variability of the EEG in normal subjects, from alertness to sleep, is wide with much individual diversity." However, the general patterns observed are that a wide-awake, alertly attending subject's EEG is characterized by a desynchronized EEG (low-voltage fast activity). With reduction of alertness, or reduction of sensory input, alpha activity (in alpha producers) appears in the EEG. As the subject becomes drowsy, bursts of alpha activity decrease in frequency of appearance and are observed against a background of low amplitude and low frequency (4–7 cps) activity. Under conditions of light sleep one can observe the generalized background of low frequency activity with sleep spindles (12–15 cps) occasionally or periodically appearing in the central and anterior lead placements. As sleep deepens the incidence of slow activity increases and the number of sleep spindles decrease. In deep sleep we observe more rhythmic slow wave activity which in many subjects appears more synchronously from various electrode locations.

Ackner and Pampiglioni investigated the relationship between EEG and peripheral vasomotor (finger plethysmograph) changes as subjects went from wakefulness to sleep. In the relaxed subject they observed that when the EEG demonstrated a considerable number of alpha bursts they could often observe an increase in the number of spontaneous fluctuations in pulse-volume amplitude. As the subject became more relaxed and lapsed into drowsiness, fluctuations in pulse-volume amplitude tended to become more periodic. During this period diminution in pulse-volume amplitude was associated with a return of alpha activity. Under conditions of light sleep, if a burst of alpha activity appeared, it was often followed by peripheral vasoconstriction. Sleep spindles had no observable effect on ongoing peripheral vasomotor activity. As sleep deepened the appearance of spontaneous K complexes in the EEG were often associated with vasoconstriction. In general, they found then that EEG indicators of decreasing alertness (or increasing drowsiness leading to sleep) were associated with peripheral vasodilatation and an increase in pulse-volume variability. However, these changes were not observed in all records. The authors attributed the non-appearance of the vasomotor phenomena to such factors as tension in the subject and speed with which he fell asleep.

Krump (19) in a study of 50 patients found that during drowsiness and sleep there was a relationship between frequency and amplitude of the EEG and tonus of the peripheral autonomic nervous system. During periods of transition from wakefulness to sleep he reported marked fluctuations in heart rate, respiratory arhythmias, and greater blood pressure variation than during the waking state. K complexes as well as spontaneous bursts of alpha activity were often observed to be accompanied by acceleration in heart rate and respiration.

A number of recent studies have dealt with the relationship between eye movements and dreaming. The findings in general indicate that rapid conjugate vertical or horizontal eye movements are occasionally seen during light sleep (Stages A & B), and that these periods range from 3 to 50 minutes in length and tend to occur periodically between 70 to 100 minutes apart. When subjects are awakened during periods of eye movement, approximately 80 per cent report dreams, while subjects awakened at other times report dreams as occurring between 5 and 10 per cent of the time. Dreaming is apparently a necessary evil, since subjects who are monitored for dreaming and awakened during the dream period demonstrate an increase in dreaming on subsequent nights as evaluated by incidence of eye movement as well as subjective report.

A study of Goodenough (13) in which he evaluated eye movement and EEG in a group of subjects who reported that they did not dream as compared to a group of dreamers demonstrated no difference in the incidence of eye movement between the two groups. Non-dreamers were less likely than dreamers to recall their dreams; but all subjects, including those who said they had never dreamt before, reported at least one dream during the study. The factor discriminating non-dreamers from dreamers was a higher incidence of eye movement during the A phase (any presence of alpha spindles), suggesting that non-dreamers perhaps do their dreaming during a period where it can be confused with daydreaming. Perhaps non-dreamers have less need to guard against the welling up of unconscious urges and need less active censoring of their "dream-life."

The following discussion presents data on the relationship between different physiological measures during sleep, which were collected by two medical students, Mr. Richardson and Mr. Yamshon (deceased) during a summer fellowship in the Bliss laboratory. The measures used were peripheral skin temperature (back of hand), heart rate, electrodermal activity (measured from electrodes attached to the index and ring finger of the left hand), electro-encephalographic activity (bipolar recording occipital to parietal area on left side), observations of the subject's motor activity obtained by a device which measured bed movement, EMG recording from the bicep muscle of the left leg, as well as direct observation of the subject. The output of the EEG was fed through a frequency analyser, and the results presented are the dominant frequency observed during a 10-second recording at the beginning of each hour. The EDRe measure was obtained at this same period of time, skin temperature was also recorded, and heart rate was based on a count of R waves over a 20-second period starting with the onset of the 10-second period of EEG analysis. All subjects were young men between the ages of 17 and 26 who were working in the laboratory. We thus are dealing with a highly select sample. The following are four randomly selected records out of a series of nine in which all systems could be recorded most of the night.

Subject M. P. demonstrated consistency in EEG and EDRe measures. At 5:45 when the subject awakened there was a return of alpha activity accompanied by a sudden drop in skin resistance as well as a sudden rise in heart rate. The subject then returned to a state of light sleep in which resistance again increased. When he finally woke up at 7:45, we saw a sudden drop in skin resistance and a return of alpha activity. Skin temperature, heart rate, and EDRe bear a close relationship to each other. All three show steady decreases till the early morning hour (5–6 A.M.). The only measure which does not reflect this short period of wakefulness is the skin-temperature measure.

Subject D. A., who fell asleep while electrodes were being attached, showed a different pattern (if indeed it can be called a pattern at all). His skin temperature showed a relatively steady drop from 36.4° at the beginning of recording to 32.8° at time of awakening. His heart-rate pattern is quite erratic, with periods of

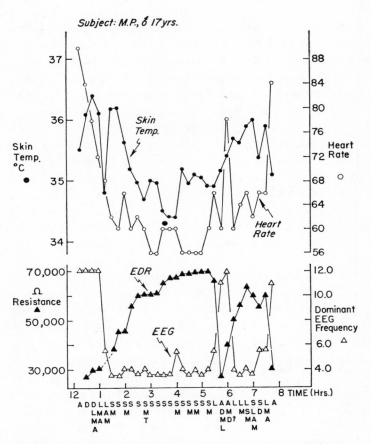

Figure 1. Physiological recording during sleep. *Subject MP.* Legend: A—awake; L—light sleep; S—medium or deep sleep; D—"dream" activity; M—movement; T—talking. Dominant EEG frequency refers to 10-second sample evaluated at the beginning of each 15-minute period. EDR and skin temperature were measured at beginning of each period, while heart rate is based on a 20-second sample at the beginning of each period.

HR increase showing little relationship to any other measure. EDRe and EEG frequency showed a reciprocal relationship. EDRe was high where EEG dominant frequency was low, and vice versa.

Subject T. M. again showed an over-all pattern of skin-temperature drop from beginning to end. HR shows no consistent nocturnal pattern, except for increases in HR occurring at about the same time that we observe increases in dominant frequency of EEG. EDRe shows a consistent trend to increase during the night with a sudden drop upon awakening. The EEG at two points in time showed increases in dominant frequency occurring during light sleep with "dream" activity in the later two periods, while the increase observed at 4 A.M. could not be related to any observable event.

A. N. again showed a tendency toward a decrease in skin temperature during the night. HR after a rapid drop early in the night remained depressed, except for a period at 4 A.M. when he awakened.

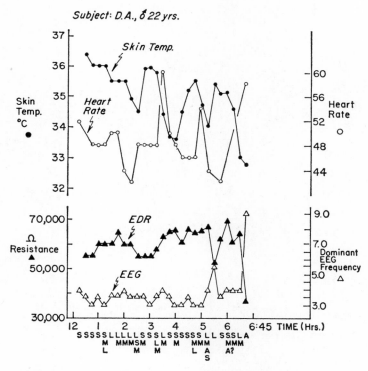

Figure 2. Physiological recording during sleep. *Subject DA.*

It is of interest to note how rapidly his HR returned to the baseline level after this period of wakefulness. Unlike the other three subjects, EDR showed a steady drop during sleep interrupted by a period of wakefulness at 4 A.M.

Summarizing the results for our nine subjects, we find six showed a fairly consistent drop in skin temperature throughout the night, one showed a persistent rise, and two a U-shaped curve. Heart rate decreased rapidly and then showed considerable vacillation in most subjects, generally increasing during periods of wakefulness and in one subject during "dreaming." Skin resistance in all but one subject showed a steady increase throughout the night with a rapid drop at time of awakening. When the subject awakened, there was a sudden drop in skin resistance with a relatively rapid return to the pre-awakening level, similar to changes in heart rate. The EEG changes analyzed, i.e. dominant frequency measured from occipito-

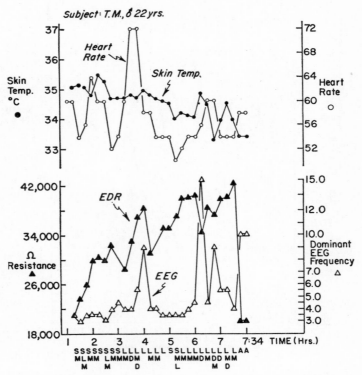

Figure 3. Physiological recording during sleep. *Subject TM.*

parietal leads relate nicely to our criterion measures of sleep (bed movement, leg-muscle action potentials recorded from left biceps, and direct observation of the subject). The deeper the level of sleep, the lower the dominant frequency. Return to sleep after awakening was most rapidly and consistently reflected in the EEG.

Studies have been conducted in which EEG and other physiological measures were recorded during periods of enforced wakefulness. Bjerner (6) reported diurnal fluctuations in dominant alpha frequency. Four of his five subjects showed their lowest alpha frequency between 4 and 6 A.M. These shifts in alpha frequency were poorly related, if at all, to the heart-rate changes. The one factor which related to the decrease in alpha frequency was percentage of errors

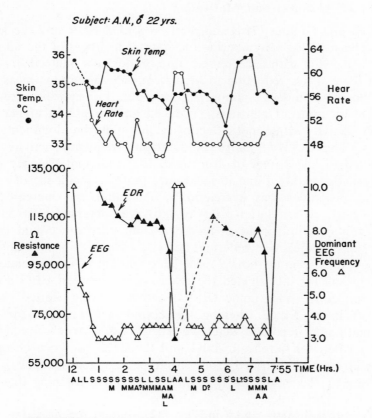

Figure 4. Physiological recording during sleep. *Subject AN.*

in motor task. At the lowest alpha frequency four out of five subjects showed the highest percentage of errors.

William *et al.* (37) studied the EEG and finger-pulse volume as predictors of reaction time during sleep. These authors found vasodilatation to be related to impaired performance, and periods of vasoconstriction related to times when responses were found to be brisk. They reported that reaction time was fast in the presence of high amplitude alpha on the EEG, while with alpha depression in which alpha is replaced by theta activity, both fast and slow responses occurred. These results demonstrated that periods of vasodilatation and the replacement of alpha activity by theta may be accompanied by impaired performance and may be interpreted as indicants of the subject drifting off to sleep.

Studies of Alertness and Motivation

Burch and Greiner (7) concurrently recorded EDR and the EEG while pharmacologically altering the state of alertness of the subject. They found that with a decreased state of alertness induced by Pentothal there was a reduction in high frequency activity as measured by a decrease in EEG minor period count. Epinephrine, used to increase the state of alertness, produced an increase in higher frequency activity while not affecting activity at the dominant frequency. The lack of change in dominant frequency activity was attributed to low dosage of drug used. Electrodermal changes were concurrently recorded and it was found that the incidence of "nonspecific" responses was decreased by Pentothal and increased by epinephrine. A correlation (rho) of 0.61 was obtained between the EEG minor period count as recorded from parieto-occipital leads, and "non-specific" electrodermal activity. These two measures of alertness thus seem to show a reasonable amount of correspondence.

Bartoshuk (4) investigated the relationships between EEG amplitude and electromyographic (EMG) activity during alerted conditions as in motivated listening. He found that only on the first presentation of recorded detective stories could a relationship be obtained between forehead EMG and the EEG (desynchronization of alpha activity recorded from fronto-parietal leads). The EMG was found to be more closely related to attentive listening than the EEG.

Lansing, Schwartz, and Lindsley (22) studied reaction time and EEG activation under "alerted" conditions in which a warning signal was given prior to presentation of stimulus and the "non-alerted" conditions. They found no consistent relationship between reaction time and alpha desynchronization. Under non-alerted conditions there was no reduction in reaction time when alpha activity was absent as compared to when it was present. They did, however, find that under alerted conditions the relationship between alpha blocking (percentage of alpha blocking) and the length of the foreperiod was similar in shape to the plot of reaction time against length of foreperiod. The unexpected results found during non-alerted conditions are attributed to the hypothesis that alpha desynchronization can occur in response to local cortical conditions as well as to input from the ARAS. It is only in response to desynchronization produced through the latter channel that one would expect to see relationships between reaction time and alpha desynchronization. Unfortunately, there are no techniques currently available to differentiate between alpha desynchronization produced by ARAS and that produced by local events.

Yoshii (38) studied time estimation as related to EEG in normal and fatigued subjects. He found that in fatigued subjects there was an increase in slow wave activity associated with distortion of time judgment, with real time longer than judged time ($r = .74$). Subjects who were less fatigued showed an increase in fast activity in the EEG but the correlation between EEG and time estimation was not statistically significant.

Larson (23) manipulated the state of alertness by instruction and studied eye-blink response, EEG, heart rate, and respiration. The magnitude of the (startle) eye-blink response and non-specific EEG responses (alpha desynchronization) were both related to the degree of significance of the stimulus. The more significant the stimulus material was to the subject, the more marked his reaction. Under conditions of high significance he further found that there was an increase in the incidence of non-specific EEG responses to irrelevant stimuli, with no changes reported for the eye-blink response. For both cardiac and respiratory rates the pattern of response to stimulation as a function of significance of the stimuli was different from that observed for EEG and eye blink.

Sternbach (33) evaluated EEG, BP, EDRe, EKG, temperature from various body sites, finger-pulse volume, and stomach motility in response to being startled by sudden intense stimulus (a pistol shot), in a group of subjects who reacted rapidly and a group who showed a delayed reaction time to electric shock.

In response to the pistol shot he observed no differences in the speed with which alpha activity was either desynchronized or the speed with which it returned. The correlation between these two measures also was surprisingly low ($r = .268$). He did, however, observe differences between the two groups on some of his other measures. The slow reactors were found to develop significantly greater increases in systolic blood pressure, pulse pressure, heart rate, and decreases in EDRe and finger-pulse volume.

Response to Stimulation as Reflected in the EEG and Other Physiological Measures

In response to stimulation one can observe responses which are not specific to the stimulus presented. These responses are called orienting responses (OR), and they are non-specific in that a wide variety of stimuli will produce the same response. With stimulation one can observe alpha desynchronization in the EEG of an awake subject, return of alpha in the drowsy subject, and K complexes in the sleeping subject. These are all examples of OR. Some examples of ORs in other physiological measures are decreases in skin resistance (at relatively specific latencies), vasoconstriction, decreases in finger-pulse volume, increases or decreases in HR and blood pressure (dependent upon resting level), alterations in breathing rate, and decreases in peripheral skin temperature.

ORs further have the attribute of being subject to habituation or extinction. That is, if the same stimulus is presented a number of times the OR will diminish in amplitude and will finally disappear. Two types of ORs can be described, the generalized OR and a localized OR. The latter differs from the former in that it is specific to the "analyzer" being stimulated. It also shows habituation but at a slower rate than the generalized OR. For example, in response to visual stimulation alpha desynchronization will adapt out more slowly in the visual than the auditory area. Most of the research involving the OR is to be found in the Russian literature, though there are allusions to it in the American literature of the 1930's and 1940's dealing with the conditioning of alpha activity.

Charan and Goldstein (8) studied the relationship between EEG ORs and ED ORs to tone. These authors divided their subjects into two groups, one with much, the other with little, alpha activity, and further divided the groups by sex. For male subjects they found significantly more ED ORs in their low, when compared to their high, alpha group, while for female subjects the difference was not significant. No significant difference in EEG ORs was observed between the high and low alpha groups. In comparing EEG ORs with ED ORs they observed that the former were more resistant to extinction than the latter.

Roger, Voronin, and Sokolov (28) evaluated ORs in the EEG, HR, respiration, EDR, and EMG. In response to a proprioceptive stimulus (passive arm movement) both occipital and rolandic alpha desynchronization could be habituated in 8 out of 10 subjects in approximately 15 to 20 trials. The ED OR extinguished after 10 to 15 applications of the stimulus and EMG ORs were not consistently obtained.

Mundy-Castle and McKiever (26) related ED OR to tone stimulation to EEG measures. Unfortunately their EEGs were not obtained concurrently with the ED measures. They did, however, find a significant correlation ($r = .40$) between alpha frequency and speed of adaptation of ED ORs to tone in a group of stable subjects who demonstrated few spontaneous fluctuations in the ED system under conditions of rest. None of the other EEG measures were found to be significantly related to ED OR adaptation. These authors were unable to substantiate the findings of Darrow, Pathman, and Kronenberg (12) with respect to relationships between ED conductance and alpha frequency and amplitude.

Sokolov (29) studied habituation of ORs in response to dark stimulation. He found that the first exposure of darkness produced a reduction in amplitude of the EEG OR (desynchronization) in all subjects, while for the other measures (EDR, eye movement, respiration, EMG) some subjects responded in one system but none responded in all of the other systems. One of the interesting points made in this as well as other papers by Sokolov *et al.* was that during habituation of ORs slow waves appeared in the occipital and motor areas and "paradoxical disinhibition" of the generalized OR was observed. This was manifested by the return of ED ORs, as well as respiratory changes and return of alpha activity, in response to stimulation. Sokolov has developed an interesting theoretical model to account for these effects (29), but space limitation prevents its development here. Another interesting finding is that the source of alpha rhythm activity in the rolandic and occipital areas must differ since one can produce differential adaptation in the EEG (alpha desynchronization) in these regions.

Atayev (2), as described by Rusinov and Rabinovitch (2),

studied the OR in the EEG and pupillary response. The author
found that in a conditioning experiment (sound CS, light UCS)
alpha depression followed by pupillary constriction was observed
as a conditioned response.

That EEG alpha desynchronization is not the most sensitive measure under all experimental conditions is reflected in a study by
Kats (18). Utilizing 81 subjects he studied EEG, finger pressure,
EMG (flexor muscle of arm), and the EDR. The stimuli used were
acoustic, tactual, and visual. Kats reports that with the first application of the indifferent stimulus (CS) alpha depression and an ED
OR were observed. The depression of alpha activity was found to
habituate more rapidly than the ED OR. Similarly, with conditioning
(CS was verbal stimulus PRESS) EEG desynchronization disappeared after 3–4 combinations while ED OR reappeared and persisted after the motor response was well established. This author
also observed a conditioned response localized in the motor regions
of both hemispheres (slow waves 3–4 cps, 50–60 μV or higher in
amplitude). These slow waves appeared after a short latency from
onset of CS and persisted until the verbal signal was given, terminating before the motor response was performed.

We have only scratched the surface of the empirical findings in
this area and feel this is an exciting area toward which research
in this country might well develop. The major difficulty with evaluating the Russian as well as American literature is the lack of quantification: terms such as many, most, some, etc., stud the reports
reviewed.

The findings that do appear consistently are that one can observe
ORs in a wide variety of physiological response systems, and that
speed of habituation of ORs is a function of both the stimulus as
well as response specificity inherent in the subject.

DISCUSSION

Our review of the general literature attempting to relate EEG
variables to measures in other physiological response systems has, in
general, failed to come up with consistent results. There appear to
be no consistent correlations between measures of electroencephalographic disturbance and measures of autonomic activity, between
EEG alterations indicative of sleep or sleep deprivation and other
physiological measures, between EEG correlates of alertness and

autonomic measures, or between EEG orienting or conditioned responses and similar measures in other physiological systems. Although many interesting relationships emerge, none are of a great enough magnitude to be very predictive. It should be remembered that correlations of .50 look quite respectable and formidable (and were seldom seen in the literature reviewed) but account for only 25 per cent of the variance.

Should we be perturbed by these inconsistencies and disturbingly low correlations? Are they a function of faulty measuring techniques or is there something basically wrong with our expecting perfect, or even high, correlations between various measures of physiological activity? We feel that the latter rather than the former seems to be the case. If we look at the relationship between activity in physiological systems in response to stimulation, we again find lack of covariation between such measures to be more obvious and more frequent than covariation (**3, 5, 33**). We tend to find less evidence than expected to support the assumed "stimulus induced specificity," i.e., that along with a given type of stimulus or physiological state of the organism we get highly invariant responses in physiological systems. Thus, drinking a given quantity of wood alcohol should be expected to kill everyone who drinks it—it doesn't; administering a given amount of anesthetic should anesthetize everyone—it doesn't, etc. One can, however, predict with a better chance of success that if a given quantity of wood alcohol does not kill the drinker, an equivalent dose ingested a week later also will not kill him, or that under similar conditions if a given dose of anesthetic does not anesthetize a patient on day one, it also will not anesthetize him on day 21. The point we wish to make is that rather than looking for stimulus specificity, we should be looking for consistency of action in physiological systems within the individual. Lacey (**20, 21**) has presented an impressive amount of evidence that normal subjects exhibit organized and idiosyncratic patterns of somatic responses to stressors which are reliable over time.

Most of the research reviewed has been constructed with the hope of finding stimulus specificity or at least signs of covariation in different physiological systems. What little evidence we have seems to indicate that a more fruitful line of endeavor would be to look for response specificity and response consistency to a wide variety of stressful or alerting agents.

What kind of response specificity can be observed in the EEG, if by response specificity we mean that regardless of the type of stimulation we will see fairly specific changes in the system measured? Certainly alpha desynchronization, and under certain conditions alpha enhancement and the appearance of K complexes, would be good examples of response specificity. Regardless of the type of stimulus used, a person who produces a reasonable amount of alpha activity will, when stimulated with noise, light, odors, cutaneous stimulation, ideational stimulation, etc., show alpha desynchronization as well as signs of disturbance in other physiological systems. He may thus show breathing disturbances, bradycardia, tachycardia, peripheral vasoconstriction, vasodilation of the forehead, electrodermal, electromyographic responses, gastric motility changes, etc.

All of these signs of response of physiological systems can be broadly defined as generalized orienting responses. One of the consistent features of such orienting responses is that under most conditions one observes habituation of such responses. Thus, if a tone of a given frequency and intensity is presented on a varied time schedule to a subject, he will, after a given number of trials, fail to show the alpha desynchronization that was regularly observable during the early phase of stimulus presentation. He will also demonstrate habituation of orienting responses in other physiological response systems.

Limiting ourselves to a single stimulus, we can get quite consistent results if we use a crude enough measuring tool. A large proportion of subjects will, in response to a sudden noise, show alpha desynchronization, a decrease in skin resistance, a decrease in skin temperature, an increase in heart rate, peripheral vasoconstriction, etc. (10, 31, 32). However, if we attempt to correlate the "intensity" or the OR in two physiological systems as measured, for example, by length of alpha desynchronization period, amount of skin resistance change, amount of time for skin resistance to return to basal level, amount of vasodilation, etc., we find that our correlations again become rather small.

On the one hand with intense enough stimulation we can demonstrate consistency in responding of different physiological systems while on the other hand we find differential speed of habituation of the OR in the different systems. This may be all we should expect at our present level of sophistication. If one hypothesis, the evidence for which we have briefly presented elsewhere (32), is valid, then we should be able to make some statement about the likelihood that a given physiological system will respond to a stimulus as well as predicting the intensity of the response and the speed with which ORs to a series of stimuli will adapt. To be more specific, we would predict that a person who under condition of "rest" shows many periods of alpha activity interspersed between periods of low-voltage fast (LVF) activity would demonstrate many ORs (alpha desynchronization) to an aperiodically or periodically presented stimulus such as a light, a tone, etc., while a person with either little or consistent alpha activity would show quite rapid adaptation of the OR. The same relationship is predicted to hold for other physiological systems. Systems with high levels of spontaneous fluctuations (or high degree of variability) in the absence of external stimulation will show slower adaptation of ORs than systems characterized by a high degree of stability. Similarly, labile systems are more easily conditioned in both the laboratory as well as by "life stresses." What remains unpredictable is the relationship between lability and stability in physiological systems either within or across individuals. It is expected that constellations of labile and stabile systems will emerge, but to date we have come across no investigations specifically conducted to answer this question. We suspect that the predispositions toward lability of specific systems are in part genetically determined and in part determined by early (infantile) life experiences, but again these suspicions await experimental investigation.

We should like to conclude with a statement of faith: consistent relationships between physiological response systems will be demonstrated if we switch our research design from studies looking for stimulus-induced specificity across subject to specificity of response to a variety of stimuli within subjects.

BIBLIOGRAPHY

1. Ackner, B., and Pampiglioni, G. Some relationships between peripheral vasomotor and EEG changes. *J. Neurol. Neurosurg. Psychiat.* **20**: 58–64, 1957.
2. Atayev, M. Methods of the simultaneous recording of pupil reaction and EEG during the elaboration of pupillary conditioned reflexes in man. In: V. S. Rusinov and M. Y. Rabinovitch (Editors), *Electroenceph. clin. Neurophysiol.* Suppl. **8**: 1958.
3. Ax, A. F. The physiological differentiation between fear and anger in humans. *Psychosom. Med.* **15**: 433–442, 1953.
4. Bartoshuk, A. K. EMG gradients and EEG amplitude during motivated listening. *Canad. J. Psychol.* **10**: 156–164, 1956.
5. Berger, L. Interrelationships of autonomic and personality variables. Ph. D. dissertation, University of Pittsburgh, 1959.
6. Bjerner, B. Alpha depression and lowered pulse rate during delayed actions in a serial reaction test: A study in sleep deprivation. *Acta physiol. scand.* **19**: Suppl. 65, 1949.

7. Burch, N. R., and Greiner, T. H. A bioelectric scale of human alertness: Concurrent recordings of the EEG and GSR. *Psychiat. Res. Rep. Amer. Psychiat. Ass.* **12**: 183–193, 1960.
8. Charan, K. K., and Goldstein, R. Relation between EEG pattern and ease of eliciting electrodermal responses. *J. Speech Hearing Dis.* **22**: 651–661, 1957.
9. Chertok, L., and Kramarz, P. Hypnosis, sleep and electroencephalography. *J. nerv. ment. Dis.* **128**: 227–238, 1959.
10. Corah, N. L., and Stern, J. A. Stability and adaptation of some measures of electrodermal activity in children. *J. exp. Psychol.* **65**: 80–85, 1963.
11. Darrow, C. W. The relation of cerebral to autonomic activity in the conditioned emotional reactions of children. *Ann. N. Y. Acad. Sci.* **56**: 289–306, 1953.
12. Darrow, C. W., Pathman, J., and Kronenberg, G. Level of autonomic activity and electroencephalogram. *J. exp. Psychol.* **36**: 355–365, 1946.
13. Goodenough, D. R., Shapiro, A., Holden, M., and Steinschriber, L. A comparison of "dreamers" and "non-dreamers": Eye movements, electroencephalograms, and the recall of dreams. *J. abnorm. soc. Psychol.* **59**: 295–302, 1959.
14. Holubar, J. Elektroencefalograficke projevy kozniho galvanickeho reflexu u cloveka (Electroencephalographic manifestations of the cutaneous reflex in man). *Cesk. Fysiol.* **7**: 179–180, 1958.
15. Holubar, J. EEG manifestations of the unconditioned and conditioned skin galvanic reflex. *Electroenceph. clin. Neurophysiol.* **11**: 177–178, 1959.
16. Johnson, L. C., Davidoff, R. A., and Mann, S. H. Brain activity, seizure discharges and behavior. Unpublished manuscript.
17. Jung, R. Correlations of bioelectric and autonomic phenomena with alterations of consciousness and arousal in man. In: E. D. Adrian, F. Bremer, and H. H. Jasper (Editors), *Brain Mechanisms and Consciousness: A Symposium.* C. C. Thomas, Springfield, Ill., pp. 310–344, 1954.
18. Kats, K. EEG study of reflex activity in man. *Zh. Vyssh. Nerv. Deiat. Pavlov.* **8**: 466–470, 1958.
19. Krump, J. E. Polygraphic investigations in states of diminished awareness. *Electroenceph. clin. Neurophysiol.* **12**: 257, 1960.
20. Lacey, J. I. Individual differences in somatic response patterns. *J. comp. physiol. Psychol.* **43**: 338–350, 1950.
21. Lacey, J. I., and Lacey, B. C. Verification and extension of the principle of autonomic response-stereotypy. *Amer. J. Psychol.* **71**: 50–73, 1958.
22. Lansing, R. W., Schwartz, E., and Lindsley, D. B. Reaction time and EEG activation under alerted and non-alerted conditions. *J. exp. Psychol.* **58**: 1–7, 1959.
23. Larsson, L. E. Correlation between the psychological significance of stimuli and the magnitudes of the startle blink and evoked EEG potentials in man. *Acta physiol. scand.* **48**: 276–294, 1960.
24. Malmo, R. B., and Surwillo, W. W. Sleep deprivation: Changes in performance and physiological indicants of activation. *Psychol. Monogr.* **74**: No. 15, 1960.
25. Mnukhina, R. S. EEG evaluations of trace conditioned reflex in man. In: V. S. Rusinov and M. Y. Rabinovitch (Editors), *Electroenceph. clin. Neurophysiol.* Suppl. **8**: 1958.
26. Mundy-Castle, A. C., and McKiever, B. L. The psychophysiological significance of the galvanic skin response. *J. exp. Psychol.* **46**: 15–24, 1953.
27. Obrist, W. D., Busse, E. W., and Henry, C. E. Relation of electroencephalogram to blood pressure in elderly persons. *Neurology.* **11**: 151–158, 1961.
28. Roger, A., Voronin, L. G., and Sokolov, E. N. Elektroentsefalograficheskoi issledovanie vremennoi sviazi pri ugashenii orientirovochnogo refleksa u cheloveka (Electroencephalographic investigations of temporary bonds during extinction of orientation reflex). *Zh. Vyssh. Nerv. Deiat. Pavlov.* **8**: 3–16, 1958.
29. Sokolov, E. N. Neuronal models and the orienting reflex. In: M.A.B. Brazier (Editor), *Conference on the Central Nervous System and Behavior.* Josiah Macy Found., New York, 1959.
30. Stern, J. A. Spontaneous fluctuations in physiological response systems. Paper presented at Third Physiological Psychology Symposium, Pensacola, March, 1962.
31. Stern, J. A., Stewart, M. A., and Winokur, G. An investigation of some relationships between various measures of galvanic skin response. *J. psychosom. Res.* **5**: 215–223, 1961.
32. Stern, J. A., Winokur, G., Stewart, M., and Leonard, C. GSR conditioning: Some further correlates. Manuscript, 1963.
33. Sternbach, R. A. Correlates of differences in time to recover from startle. *Psychosom. Med.* **22**: 143–148, 1960.

34. Sternbach, R. A. Some relationships among various "dimensions" of autonomic activity. *Psychosom. Med.* **22**: 430–434, 1960.
35. Van Buren, J. M. Some autonomic concomitants of ictal automatisms; a study of temporal lobe attacks. *Brain.* **81**: 505–528, 1958.
36. Van Buren, J. M., and Ajmone-Marsan, C. A correlation of autonomic and EEG components in temporal lobe epilepsy. *Arch. Neurol.* **3**: 683–703, 1960.
37. Williams, H. L., Granda, A. M., Jones, R. C., Lubin, A., and Armington, J. C. EEG frequency and finger pulse volume as predictors of reaction time during sleep loss. *Electroenceph. clin. Neurophysiol.* **14**: 64–70, 1962.
38. Yoshii, N. Methodological principles of electroencephalographic investigation on conditioned behavior. *Folia Psychiat. Neurol. Jap.* **9**: 341–365, 1956.

QUANTITATIVE EEG AND HUMAN PSYCHOPHARMACOLOGY [1]

Changes on Acute and Chronic Administration of Chlorpromazine, Imipramine, and Placebo (Saline)

Max Fink, M.D.

Changes in electroencephalographic patterns have been demonstrated with many of the newer psychotropic agents on both chronic and acute administration and have been related to the principal psychopharmacological activity of these compounds (**7**). These observations were viewed as consistent with the suggestion by Wikler (**14**) that compounds that apparently increased EEG abundance[2] were associated with sedation, behavioral tranquilization, and decreased excitement, while drugs that decreased EEG abundance were associated with behavioral excitement, alertness, illusory sensations, and hallucinations. These data provided the basis for the selection of compounds in a recently completed psychotropic drug evaluation program.

Chlorpromazine was selected as a psychotropic agent that increased electrographic abundance and provoked slowing and imipramine as one that decreased abundance with or without frequency change (**5**). This report details our electrographic observations on acute and chronic administration of chlorpromazine, imipramine, and saline placebo in psychiatric subjects. Two techniques of quanti-

[1] This study was done at the laboratories of the Department of Experimental Psychiatry, Hillside Hospital, New York, and is the third in a series.

The assistance of Dr. Karl Andermann and of Mrs. Hannah Mosquera in the visual analyses and Dr. Dean Clyde of the Biometric Laboratory of the University of Miami in the statistical computations are gratefully acknowledged.

This study was aided, in part, by grant MY-2715, National Institute of Mental Health, National Institutes of Health, U.S.P.H.S.

[2] For this report the recommended terminology of the International Federation for Electroencephalography will be followed (**2**). In this terminology, *abundance* is the term recommended for total activity; and increase or attenuation in abundance are similar to the earlier terms *synchronization* and *desynchronization*.

tative analysis of the EEG records were used—hand measurement and electronic resonator-integrator frequency determinations.

MATERIAL AND METHODS

1. Electronic Frequency Analysis

a. **Chronic oral administration.** In a voluntary psychiatric hospital, consecutive patients referred for psychotropic drug therapy randomly received one of three medications in liquid form. Chlorpromazine was combined with procyclidine in initial dosages of 300 mg chlorpromazine and 3.75 mg procyclidine daily, increased weekly to a final dosage of 1200 mg chlorpromazine and 15 mg procyclidine. A second group received imipramine, begun at 75 mg daily and increased weekly to a final dosage of 300 mg during the fourth week. A third group received the saline vehicle as a placebo in daily volumes equivalent to the liquid medication.

EEG records were taken prior to medication and during the fifth week at a time of maximum drug dosage. The electrode placement and recording techniques followed that of Strauss *et al.* (**12**).

EEG frequency spectra were determined by a wave analyzer of the Grey Walter type (**13**) responsive to 24 frequencies from 3 to 33 cycles per second with a 10-second epoch. For each record, six 10-second samples of activity of the left fronto-occipital leads were averaged for each frequency. The mean millimeters of pen deflection for each of the 24 frequencies for 60 seconds became the raw data used to describe each record, and these data were used in a variety of statistical procedures. In these analyses, frequencies were combined according to conventional "frequency bands" of delta, 3–4.5 cps; theta, 5–7 cps; alpha, 8–12 cps; beta-[1], 13.5–20 cps; and beta-[2], 22–33 cps.

In this study 144 subjects were assigned to the three treatments with 49 subjects receiving chlorpromazine, 52 imipramine, and 43 placebo. Of these subjects, 93 were classified as schizophrenia, 49 as depressive psychosis, and 13 as personality disorder.

b. **Acute intravenous administration.** Prior to the start of drug therapy, 64 patients selected at random from the referrals received intravenous injections of one of three solutions. Sixteen patients received 10 cc of physiological saline at a rate of 1 ml/minute; 23

patients received chlorpromazine, 0.10–0.30 mg/kg diluted in 1 ml
solution and injected at 0.1 ml/minute; and 25 patients received
imipramine, 0.25–2.0 mg/kg in 10 ml solution at 1 ml/minute. Each
patient was told that the injection would have effects recorded by
the instruments but relatively little effect that he could experience.

Records were examined immediately after the end of injection and
60 seconds of activity of the left-frontal leads were measured in a
fashion identical to that above.

2. Visual Analyses

a. Chronic oral administration. In concurrent visual analyses, the
records of 20 of the subjects in each chronic drug treatment group
were selected at random. Epochs of 105 seconds were measured for
the percent-time alpha (8–12 cps) and slow activity (3–7 cps),

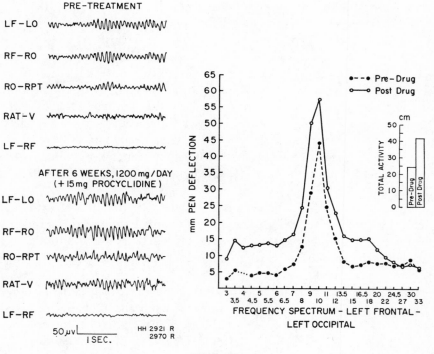

Figure 1

using a map measure. Only waves of maximum to half-maximum amplitude were measured. Samples were obtained from the same lead combinations and from samples used for electronic analysis. Because of the small amount of theta and delta activity and the tediousness of the measurements, all frequencies slower than 7 cps were combined in one measure. The "central alpha frequency" was defined as the mean frequency of identifiable waves of 8–12 cps.

b. Acute intravenous administration. In the visual analyses after acute drug injection, the EEG tracings of epochs lasting 105 seconds were measured prior to injection, after needle insertion, at the end of injection, and after 30 minutes. Measurements were similar to those described for the visual analyses on chronic administration.

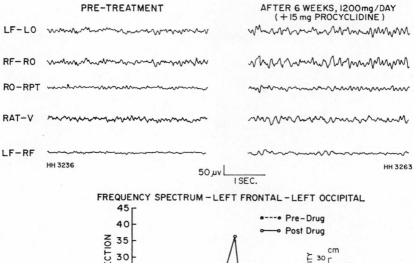

EFFECT OF CHRONIC ORAL CHLORPROMAZINE
INITIAL LOW PER-CENT TIME ALPHA
(17 YRS., MALE, J.G.)

Figure 2

RESULTS

1. Electronic Frequency Analyses

a. Chronic oral drug administration. In the electronic frequency analyses no consistent changes were observed in the placebo treated subjects other than an increase in theta abundance. With chlorpro-

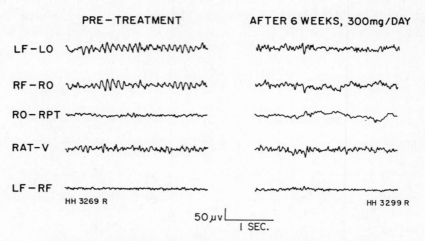

EFFECT OF CHRONIC ORAL IMIPRAMINE
INITIAL HIGH PER-CENT TIME ALPHA
(59 YRS., MALE , I.C.)

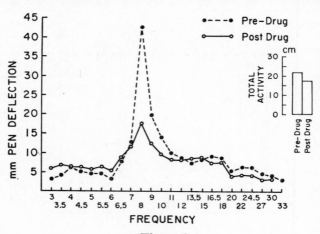

FREQUENCY SPECTRUM — LEFT FRONTAL — LEFT OCCIPITAL

Figure 3

mazine there was an increase in percent-time delta and theta and a shift of the mean alpha frequency toward a lower rate. With imipramine, there was a decrease in percent-time alpha, an increase in fast activity, and some increase in the slow frequencies. These changes are demonstrated in the EEG samples and analyzer spectra (Figs. 1, 2).

In statistical analyses of the data for each of the five frequency bands, drug-induced changes are reflected in the significant F ratios of the means for all bands except beta-[1] in the covariance analyses

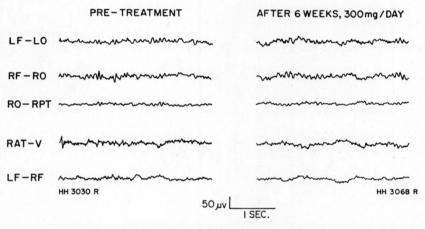

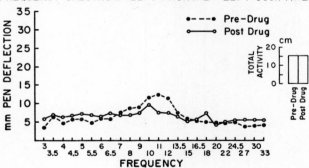

Figure 4

Table I. Mean mm Pen Deflection for Frequency Bands on Chronic Drug Administration

(Final Analysis of Covariance)

Frequency Band	3.0–4.5 cps (Delta)		5.0–7.0 cps (Theta)		8.0–12.0 cps (Alpha)		13.5–20 cps (Beta-1)		22.0–23.0 cps (Beta-2)	
	Before	During	Before	During	Before	During	Before	During	Before	During
Placebo	29.95	29.68	49.93	53.17	136.6	136.9	50.29	51.37	30.93	30.46
Imipramine	28.50	31.56	47.71	53.35	128.5	108.6	52.27	51.02	33.00	37.54
Chlorpromazine-procyclidine	33.83	42.19	53.49	66.00	128.1	129.9	55.36	53.85	32.74	32.21
F ratio for regression coefficients	0.52		0.22		7.29**		2.41		1.76	
F ratio for means		8.41****		4.79***		4.78*		0.44		6.83****
t test of adjusted means:										
Placebo-imipramine	1.41		0.59		3.03***		0.87		3.20***	
Placebo-chlorpromazine	4.01****		2.88***		1.09		0.76		0.16	
Imipramine-chlorpromazine	2.72***		2.39*		2.01*		0.14		3.16***	

$* \ p < .05$
$*** \ p < .01$
$**** \ p < .001$

(Table I). Significant *t* tests are observed for delta and theta bands with chlorpromazine and placebo, and for alpha and beta-[2] bands with imipramine and placebo. Significant *t*-test values are also found between chlorpromazine and imipramine, indicating that these compounds can be distinguished from each other, with the greatest difference in beta-[2] and with lesser differences in delta and alpha activities.

To determine changes in mean alpha frequency, the mean mm pen deflection for each frequency in the alpha band (8–12 cps) was calculated for each treatment group (Table II). The changes in the placebo group are small and not statistically significant. With imipramine, the abundance of each frequency shows a significant decrease, but in proportion to each individual frequency, or to total alpha activity, there is no greater change in one frequency than in any other. With chlorpromazine, however, there is a decrease in abundance of frequencies 10, 11, and 12 cps, and an increase in 8 cps. Relative to each frequency and to total alpha activity, there is an increase in slower alpha frequencies and a decrease in the faster alpha frequencies, with a decrease in mean alpha frequency.

b. Acute intravenous drug administration. After saline injection the changes in abundance in each frequency band measured as mean

Table II. Mean mm Pen Deflection for Each Frequency of the Alpha Band

(Chronic Drug Administration)

	8 cps	9 cps	10 cps	11 cps	12 cps
Placebo					
Pre-Treatment	20.67	35.49	38.11	23.65	17.01
On-Treatment	20.78	35.55	38.12	22.99	17.21
Difference#	+ 0.11	+ 0.06	+ 0.01	− 0.66	+ 0.20
Imipramine					
Pre-Treatment	21.35	29.63	32.73	25.44	19.42
On-Treatment	18.22	25.72	25.80	20.92	17.40
Difference#	− 3.13*	3.91*	− 6.93****	− 4.52***	− 2.02
Chlorpromazine-procyclidine					
Pre-Treatment	21.85	34.97	38.04	24.37	19.15
On-Treatment	24.88	35.01	33.11	20.45	17.03
Difference#	+ 3.03***	+ 0.04	− 4.93***	− 3.92***	− 2.12***

* $p < .05$ # Significance for differences by *t* test for correlated means
*** $p < .01$ indicated by *.
**** $p < .001$

Table III. Mean mm Pen Deflection for Frequency Bands on Acute Drug Administration

	N	Delta		Theta		Alpha		Beta-1		Beta-2	
		Before	During	Before	During	Before	During	Before	During	Before	During
Placebo	15	27.1	26.7	46.1	49.8	137.5	147.3	56.5	54.8	31.4	27.7
Imipramine	25	29.2	29.6	49.1	46.6	136.6	80.8	52.3	40.8	31.8	31.8
Chlorpromazine	23	30.5	35.8	46.9	64.9	127.9	141.5	57.1	62.6	33.1	35.7
t test of means:											
Placebo-imipramine		0.35		0.22		9.65****		1.97		1.51	
Placebo-chlorpromazine		2.99***		2.53*		0.80		3.32***		3.36***	
Imipramine-chlorpromazine		1.98		4.43****		5.55****		4.10****		1.30	

* $p < .05$
*** $p < .01$
**** $p < .001$

millimeters pen deflection were insignificant (Table III). With each drug, significant changes were observed. Following imipramine, the abundance of the alpha frequency band was reduced. Little change occurred in the slow or the fast frequencies. In contrast, after intravenous chlorpromazine, there was an increase in the amount of slow and of all fast frequencies. Significant differences were observed between chlorpromazine and imipramine in the amounts of theta, alpha, and beta-[1] abundance. On acute administration, chlorpromazine increased these activities in comparison to imipramine.

Comparing the group data for the intravenous and the oral routes of administration demonstrated two differences. With imipramine, chronic oral administration was associated with an increase in beta-[2] activity, which was not seen on acute administration. On acute intravenous chlorpromazine administration, an increase in beta-[2] activity was demonstrated, which was not noted on chronic oral administration.

c. **Comparison of acute and chronic drug effects.** Changes in frequency spectra by oral and intravenous routes were also measured in the same subjects in 23 receiving chlorpromazine and in 10 receiving imipramine. Rank order correlations of the change on acute and chronic administration of chlorpromazine ranged from $+.54$ to $+.85$ for each of the frequency bands ($p < .01$). Similar analyses for imipramine showed a greater variation of the correlations, with those for alpha, beta-[1] and beta-[2] being $+.66$ to $+.70$ ($p < .05$). Correlations for delta ($+.30$) and theta ($+.05$) were not significant (Table IV).

Table IV. Acute-Chronic Administration Correlations

	N	Delta	Theta	Alpha	Beta-[1]	Beta-[2]
Chlorpromazine	23	$+.54$***	$+.68$***	$+.80$***	$+.83$***	$+.85$***
Imipramine	10	$+.30$	$+.05$	$+.66$*	$+.70$*	$+.66$*

* $p < .05$
*** $p < .01$

d. **Relation to resting percent-time alpha.** The availability of quantitative measures permitted the determination of a variety of other relationships. Examination of the covariance data derived from electronic analysis demonstrated that the degree of change with each drug depended on the initial amount of alpha abundance, while changes with placebo were related little to initial level (Table I). This is seen in the significant F ratio for the regression coefficients for alpha activity ($Frc = 7.29$; $p < .01$[3]). Examination of a scattergram plot of the pretreatment and posttreatment measures of alpha activity demonstrated that subjects with small amounts of alpha activity on the pretreatment recording showed an increase in alpha, while those with large amounts showed a decrease with drug treat-

Table V. Changes on Chronic Drug Administration by Visual Analysis

	Percent-Time Slow Activity (3–7 cps)			Percent-Time Alpha Activity (8–12 cps)			Mean Alpha Frequency		
	< 3.1 %	± 3 %	< 3.1 %	< 5.1 %	± 5 %	< 5.1 %	< 0.3 cps	± 0.2 cps	< 0.3 cps
Placebo	0	16	4	1	17	2	3	15	2
Imipramine	0	13	7	13	6	1	3	12	5
Chlorpromazine-procyclidine	1	4	15	6	6	8	14	6	0
chi square–Placebo-imipramine	0.6			13.3***			0.2		
chi square–Placebo-chlorpromazine	10.1***			3.3			9.3***		
chi square–Imipramine-chlorpromazine	4.9*			3.6			9.0**		

* $p < .05$
** $p < .02$
*** $p < .01$

ment. (Regression coefficients for alpha were +0.92 for placebo, +0.69 for imipramine, and +0.57 for chlorpromazine).

2. Hand Analyses and Electronic-Derived Data

On chronic oral administration an increase in slow wave and alpha activities and a decrease in mean alpha frequency were observed with chlorpromazine, while an increase in slow activity, decrease in alpha abundance, and absence of central frequency change were observed with visual measurement in the case of imipramine (Table V). The electronic analyzer data, however, permitted better

[3] A significant Frc generally precludes interpretation of the Fm. The changes in mean alpha activity with imipramine in relation to placebo were found significantly decreased by non-parametric U-test and sign-test methods.

estimates of total activity change, and with imipramine indicated changes in the higher beta frequencies that were not seen in the visual analyses.

These changes were also observed after the intravenous injection of the two compounds. When the changes on acute administration of chlorpromazine were compared directly with the effect of chronic chlorpromazine administration in 20 subjects, the correlation in alpha percent-time was $+.72$ ($p < .01$). The correlation for alpha frequency was $+.77$ ($p < .01$), and for theta and delta percent-time $+.56$ ($p < .01$).

The relationship between changes in alpha activity to pretreatment alpha activity was examined, and in subjects with low initial percent-time alpha an increase in this value was measured on both acute and chronic chlorpromazine administration. In subjects with high initial values, however, the changes were small and in a random fashion.

In subjects whose mean alpha frequency was 12 cps or higher, there was a decrease of more than 10 per cent in this value with chlorpromazine. In subjects with initially lower mean alpha frequencies, the change was less than 10 per cent by either route of administration.

DISCUSSION

Electrographic changes have been demonstrated after the acute intravenous and chronic oral administration of chlorpromazine and imipramine, using both visual and electronic techniques of analysis. Despite individual differences in initial records and individual and instrumental variability, significant electrographic effects of these compounds were readily demonstrable, and the changes were consistent with our expectations at the onset of the study.

The electronically derived frequency analyses provided data that reflected accurately the changes derived on visual inspection and by hand measurement (1). In addition, these data were obtained more readily, at less expense in staff time, and in quantitative form allowing considerable statistical exploration and study. The differences between the compounds were clearly demonstrated. Relationships to pretreatment levels of activity were observed, as were correlations between the acute and chronic routes of administration. Although the observations are not novel, frequency analysis places them on a quantitative basis, providing a significant step in raising the arts of electroencephalography and psychopharmacology to quantitative sciences.

Electronic analysis. Various objections have been voiced against the use of electronic analyses, including instability of the instrumentation (8) and the lack of a conceptual framework with which to interpret the analyzer-derived data.

For the instruments of this study, examination of the mean pen deflection for each frequency band of the placebo-treated subjects (Table I) and of each frequency in the alpha band (Table II) shows a remarkably stable mean for each band except theta, with the latter increase possibly reflecting the behavioral relaxation of subjects on retesting.

The absence of a satisfactory conceptual framework to assess electronically derived data is a more serious objection to such studies. Despite extensive investigations there is still no theoretic basis for identifying significant aspects of the electroencephalogram. In a recent review of the methods of automatic EEG analysis, Burch (3) indicated that "as long as neurophysiological coding remains unknown and mathematical criteria appropriate to the EEG have not been established, information can be extracted from the EEG wave only on a 'best guess' basis. . . ." Such "best guess" measures include frequency change, amplitude, time series, wave form, and more recently, the specialized techniques of evoked potentials and cross-correlation. Unfortunately, the absence of an adequate theoretical framework for understanding electrographic activity leaves no choice but to continue such pragmatic data collections as may eventually provide reasonable conceptualizations. The limitations of the electronic analyzer system do not appear to be any greater than the limitations of the EEG recording systems following the International Federation specifications. It is our impression that such studies should be extended with concurrent explorations of other techniques of measuring brain electrical activity. FM tape recording and amplifier systems, evoked potential patterns derived from averaging techniques, and configurational pattern analyses warrant study and may provide the basis for more adequate theories for understanding scalp-recorded and electronic-resonator-derived data. Also, the analyses of the electronically derived data presented here are only initial statistical approaches. Other methods of using electronically derived frequency data are to be found in the reports of Gleser (**9**), Kennard *et al.* (**10**), Corbin and Bickford (**4**), and Lettich and Margerison (**11**).

Applications of analyses. Electronic analysis provides quantitative measures of aspects of the electroencephalogram generally studied. Such analyses of drug-induced EEG change provide a criterion for the determination of pharmacological dose-response curves. Such measures may also be a criterion of minimal effective drug dosage in clinical studies of the comparative efficacy of psychotropic compounds. A classification of psychopharmaceuticals and standards for the identification of new active agents (**7**) is provided by a catalogue of the variety of electrographic patterns associated with known active compounds.

Over the past decade more than 500 reports of the effects of new compounds on the human electroencephalogram have been published (**7**). These reports are primarily qualitative, often assessed in terms of "abnormal," "normal," or "without significant difference," and present ambiguous and conflicting views of drug effects. Besides the overwhelming problems of identification of populations, drug dosage, route and duration of drug administration, the lack of EEG quantification has made comparisons among studies even more difficult. Electronic analyzer techniques for EEG provide a way of describing and quantifying a physiological change of significance to drug therapy.

SUMMARY

EEG tracings of 144 psychiatric patients were recorded before, and six weeks after, the start of oral placebo, chlorpromazine, or imipramine. Changes before and after intravenous administration also were recorded in 64 patients. Abundance and shift in mean frequencies were measured both by an electronic wave-analyzer and a visual analysis method.

Both on acute intravenous and chronic oral administration, imipramine reduced alpha abundance and moderately increased slow activity. Chlorpromazine increased alpha abundance in subjects having a low alpha index, but reduced alpha abundance in subjects having a high alpha index. It also reduced the mean alpha frequency and increased the amount of slow wave activity.

The EEG effects of these psychotropic drugs by the chronic oral route correlated with those by the acute intravenous route.

EEG patterns derived by visual methods were similar to the electronic wave-analyzer measurements.

Similar analyses are suggested for the description of physiological effects as criteria in the classification of psychoactive compounds, the establishment of pharmacologic dose response curves, and in the screening of new psychotropic agents.

BIBLIOGRAPHY

1. Andermann, K., and Fink, M. EEG changes on acute and chronic administration of chlorpromazine and imipramine. *Electroenceph. clin. Neurophysiol.* **15**: 133, 1963.
2. Brazier, M. A. Preliminary proposal for an EEG terminology by the Terminology Committee of the International Federation for Electroencephalography and Clinical Neurophysiology. *Electroenceph. clin. Neurophysiol.* **13**: 646–650, 1961.
3. Burch, N. R. Automatic analysis of the electroencephalogram: A review and classification of systems. *Electroenceph. clin. Neurophysiol.* **11**: 827–834, 1959.
4. Corbin, H. P. F., and Bickford, R. G. Studies of the electroencephalogram of normal children: Comparison of visual and automatic frequency analyses. *Electroenceph. clin. Neurophysiol.* **7**: 15–28, 1955.
5. Fink, M. Quantitative electroencephalography and human psychopharmacology: I. Frequency spectra and drug action. *Med. Exp.* **5**: 364–369, 1961.
6. Fink, M. Quantitative EEG in human psychopharmacology: II. Drug patterns. In: G. H. Glaser (Editor), *EEG and Behavior.* Basic Books, New York, pp. 177–197, 1963.
7. Fink, M. A selected bibliography of electroencephalography in human psychopharmacology. *Electroenceph. clin. Neurophysiol.* Supp. **23**: 68 pp., 1964.
8. Gibbs, F. A., and Grass, A. M. Frequency analysis of electroencephalograms. *Science.* **105**: 132–134, 1947.
9. Gleser, G. C. A method of statistical treatment for electronically analyzed EEG data. *Electroenceph. clin. Neurophysiol.* **6**: 329–333, 1954.
10. Kennard, M. A., Rabinovitch, M. S., and Fister, W. P. The use of frequency analysis on the EEGs of patients with psychological disorders. *Electroenceph. clin. Neurophysiol.* **7**: 29–38, 1955.
11. Lettich, E., and Margerison, J. H. Presentation of data from low frequency analysis to illustrate serial changes in the electroencephalogram. *Electroenceph. clin. Neurophysiol.* **13**: 606–611, 1961.
12. Strauss, H., Ostow, M., and Greenstein, L. *Diagnostic Electroencephalography.* Grune and Stratton, New York, 1952.
13. Ulett, G. A., and Loeffel, R. G. A new resonator-integrator unit for the automatic brain wave analyzer. *Electroenceph. clin. Neurophysiol.* **5**: 113–115, 1953.
14. Wikler, A. Clinical and electroencephalographic studies on the effects of mescaline, n-allylnormorphine and morphine in man. *J. nerv. ment. Dis.* **120**: 157–175, 1954.

THE EFFECT OF PSYCHOTROPIC DRUGS ON THE EEG OF THE CHRONIC PSYCHOTIC PATIENT

George A. Ulett, M.D., Anton F. Heusler, M.D., and
Thomas J. Word, A.B.

PSYCHOTROPIC DRUGS

During the past several years hundreds of studies (4) have been completed in which it was the investigators' aim to describe the electroencephalographic changes which occur following the administration of psychotropic agents. Frequently the investigators' interest was primarily to determine whether a particular drug produced paroxysmal activity in the electroencephalogram. Such studies are a natural sequel to the clinical reports of drug-induced convulsions. It is now well established that convulsive seizures do occur in some patients following the administration of certain tranquilizers and a number of electroencephalographic studies have demonstrated that these agents produce paroxysmal discharges in non-epileptic subjects.

However, as the results presented here indicate, much further work must be accomplished before the effect of tranquilizing drugs on the EEG can be fully evaluated. Such factors as individual differences in subjects, clinical response to drugs, the nature of the predrug EEG, dosage level, and a host of other variables influence the results of any study in this area.

The present study is of a single group of 21 chronic psychotic female patients upon whom EEGs were taken at weekly intervals, over a period of 15 months, during which time they were given eight different psychotropic agents in similar dosages. This long-term study carried out in a clinical setting was in certain respects unique, affording as it did an opportunity to study intensively the effect of tranquilizing drugs in a group of patients who served as their own controls. The difficulties encountered, however, in analyzing this large

241

body of EEG data from a clinical viewpoint have served to reinforce our own belief that the important questions regarding EEG and drugs will be answered only by the use of quantitative analysis.

METHODS AND MATERIALS

The 21 patients used in this study were chronically psychotic females between the ages of 25 and 77 years; the mean age of the group was 51. Fourteen patients were diagnosed as schizophrenic reaction types, six were classified as mental defectives, and one was diagnosed as manic-depressive.

Electroencephalograms were taken before initiation of medication, during the last week of medication, and for a minimum of one week post drug withdrawal. In those cases in which the drug effects persisted for a longer period, recording was continued at weekly intervals until drug effects were no longer evident in the record.

Records were obtained with a Grass Eight-Channel Electroencephalograph. Eight scalp leads were employed with ear ground. The

Table I. Pertinent Clinical Data on 21 Patients Studied Electroencephalographically

Name	Age	Diagnosis	Treatment Record	Basic EEG
BLA-BOR	53	Schizophrenia (Unclassified)		N
ETT-EBE	60	Schizophrenia (Hebephrenic)		N
SHI-EIC	25	Mental Deficiency		N
ETH-HIC	54	Schizophrenia (Hebephrenic)	50–1ST–'40–'41	N
JOS-RES	47	Schizophrenia (Catatonic)	130–Metra. '39	N
RUT-TYL	37	Schizophrenia (Hebephrenic)	93–EST–'47–'57	N
ELS-WIT	44	Schizophrenia (Catatonic)		N
MAR-BER	62	Schizophrenia (Paranoid)	10–EST–'47	LVF
			24–EST	
GLO-SHI	32	Schizophrenia (Catatonic)	94–EST–'51–'54	LVF
MAR-TOU	37	Mental Deficiency	15–EST–'45	LVF
			16–EST–'53	
MAR-BAC	45	Schizophrenia (Catatonic)	60–EST–'43–'54	MFS
KAT-FOR	77	Schizophrenia (Unclassified)		MFS
MAR-KNO	55	Schizophrenia (Hebephrenic)		MFS
DOR-ROS	56	Mental Deficiency		MFS
FLO-WAR	52	Schizophrenia (Paranoid)	1–EST–'53	MFS
MAR-WEL	61	Mental Deficiency		MFS
JOS-DEF	75	Manic-Depressive		Parox.
MAB-KIL	54	Mental Deficiency		Parox.
BAR-McC	28	Mental Deficiency	84–EST–'49–'51	Parox.
CLA-RAS	60	Schizophrenia (Unclassified)		Parox.
CLA-STE	63	Schizophrenia (Unclassified)		Parox.

lead combinations were: fronto-parietal, parieto-temporal, parieto-occipital, and temporal-occipital. Recordings were made from these areas bilaterally. On the basis of their initial resting records the 21 patients were categorized as follows: Normal—seven, Low Voltage Fast (LVF)—three, Mixed Fast and Slow (MF&S)—six, and Paroxysmal—five. Relevant clinical data, including the type of resting EEG for each patient, are given in Table I.

Subsequent interpretations of the electroencephalograms obtained during the serial administration of drugs were made relative to pre-drug records. Changes in the EEG were noted by comparing the total predrug record to the total experimental record. Concordance of judgment of two electroencephalographers was required for inclusion of a record in the series. Changes in the EEG, with the exception of dysrhythmic activity, were described using a simple quantitative rating scale. Dysrhythmic activity was defined as either classical paroxysmal patterns or high-voltage delta activity. To prevent contamination of the data by slow wave patterns due to sleep or drowsiness, the technicians were instructed to be particularly alert to, and to note, slow activity related to drowsiness. Records in which sleep-induced slow activity was present were excluded from the analysis. The final classification of the EEGs was on the basis of: (1) an increase or decrease in frequency, (2) an increase or decrease in amplitude, (3) an increase or decrease in the presence of alpha activity, and (4) the presence of dysrhythmic activity. The

Table II. Drug Dosage Schedule and Recovery Time

Drug	Daily Dosage in mgs			Recovery Period in weeks
	1 wk	2 wk	3 wk	
Thioridazine[1]	200	400	800	3
Oxanamide[2]	800	1600	3200	2
Hydroxyzine[3]	400	600	800	6
Tetrabenazine[4]	75	125	200	10
Chlorpromazine[5]	200	400	800	9
Phenobarbital	200	200	400	5
Fluphenazine[6]	5	10	20	6
Chlorprothixene[7]	150	150	200	3
Thioridazine	200	400	800	3

[1] Thioridazine—"Mellaril," Sandoz
[2] Oxanamide—"Quiactin," Merrell
[3] Hydroxyzine—"Vistaril," Pfizer
[4] Tetrabenazine—"Nitoman," Roche
[5] Chlorpromazine—"Thorazine," Smith, Kline & French
[6] Fluphenazine—"Prolixin," Squibb
[7] Chlorprothixene—"Taractan," Roche

drugs administered in this study were given on a variable time schedule since no new drug was given until the electroencephalographic changes produced by the preceding drug were no longer seen in the record. The drugs administered, the dosage schedule, the period of administration, and the recovery period between drugs can be seen in Table II.

RESULTS

In attempting to report in summary form conclusions based on a sample of 756 EEG records interpreted from a clinical viewpoint, we are obviously faced with a severe problem in data reduction. In the following presentation general statements will be made concerning drug effects on the EEG. However, these summary descriptions are intended to present only an overview of the relationship between drugs and the EEG, providing, as it were, a basis for the more detailed analysis to follow.

A number of factors must be considered in the interpretation of the results. For example, individual variation in response to drugs was not unusual. Figure 1 illustrates records from a patient in whom dysrhythmias commonly occurred. Also, as can be seen, the EEG response of this patient was not constant from drug to drug.

Other patients, in contrast, did show a consistent EEG response to the drugs studied. Figure 2 illustrates records from a patient who showed increased EEG amplitude to all drugs. Our results also strongly indicate that the changes seen in the EEG following drug administration must be viewed in relation to the predrug EEG.

In some of the summary graphs we have found it necessary to exclude the five patients whose predrug records were classified as paroxysmal. The complete series of records was not available for this group, and it was also extremely difficult, because of the disturbed character of their resting records, to describe adequately changes in terms of the usual EEG parameters. Such conclusions as we could form on this group will be presented separately.

Alpha activity during drug administration. Alpha activity was rated on a five-point scale, which represented a continuous range from no alpha to alpha present in more than 50 per cent of the record, with some weight also being given to the amplitude of the alpha waves. This scale proved to be the least adequate measure employed.

On the basis of this rating, a judgment was made as to whether in any given EEG record there had been an increase or decrease in alpha activity, as compared to the resting EEG. The numbers in Figure 3 indicate those patients who showed an increase or a decrease in alpha activity on each of the drugs. It can be seen that

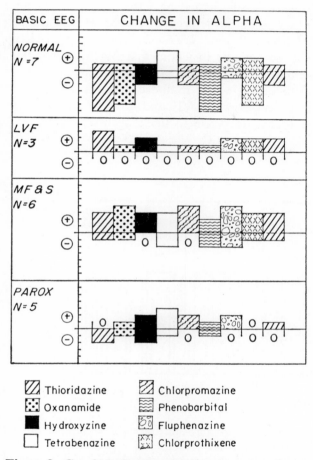

Figure 3. Graph indicating the number of patients of each basic EEG category who show either increase or decrease of alpha activity with the administration of eight different psychotropic drugs.

there is some relationship between the predrug EEG and the changes in alpha seen during drug administration. The decrease in alpha in the normal group is influenced in part, however, by the dominant alpha rhythm in the predrug records of these patients.

Our rating scale did not weigh increases and decreases in alpha equally in this group. On the other hand, since the patients in the LVF group were without alpha in their predrug records, alpha could only increase in response to medication or show no change.

This was to a lesser degree also true of the MF&S group. The mean rating for alpha in the predrug records for the three groups was N—2.1, MF&S—1.3, and LVF—0. Our results indicate that, in general, in those patients in whom a stable alpha rhythm is a characteristic of the predrug record, a slight decline in alpha may occur in response to drugs, while in those patients whose predrug EEG shows little or no alpha (LVF and MF&S) an increase in alpha is the more typical response to these agents.

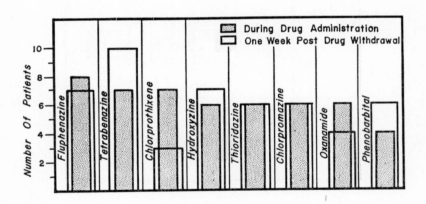

Figure 4. Bar graphs illustrating the number of patients showing an increase in alpha activity during the period of maximum drug dosage and one week following drug withdrawal. In this graph the 16 patients with normal, LVF, and mixed fast and slow records are treated as a single group.

Alpha activity following drug withdrawal. As Figure 4 shows, alpha activity was essentially similar to the on-drug period during the first week following drug withdrawal. Only following chlorprothixene and oxanamide withdrawal did the patients show a significant return to baseline levels. With three drugs, tetrabenazine, hydroxyzine, and phenobarbital, a greater number of patients showed alpha enhancement during the first week postdrug than during the period of drug administration.

Amplitude of the EEG during drug administration. All of the drugs studied increased the amplitude of the EEG (Fig. 5). With chlorprothixene, 15 of the 16 patients showed an increase in EEG amplitude. A decrease in amplitude was usually seen in a few patients with all drugs, but increased EEG amplitude was the more general finding.

Amplitude of the EEG following drug withdrawal. As Figure 5 shows, most patients continue to show increased amplitude one week postdrug. Recovery from the drug-induced increase in amplitude is

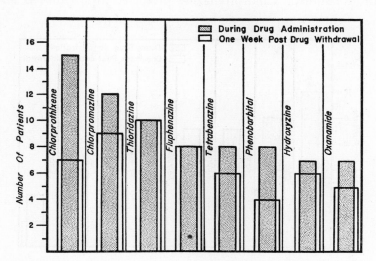

Figure 5. Bar graphs illustrating the number of patients showing an increase in EEG amplitude during the period of maximum drug dosage and one week following drug withdrawal. In this graph the 16 patients with normal, LVF, and mixed fast and slow records are treated as a single group.

most rapid with chlorprothixene and phenobarbital. With the other drugs studied, the amplitude changes persist for a longer period.

Frequency changes during drug administration. As demonstrated in Figure 6, with the exception of phenobarbital and oxanamide, slowing of the EEG was characteristic of the drugs investigated. The incidence of slowing ranged from a high of 12 patients showing a decrease in basic frequency on chlorprothixene, to only 4 exhibiting a decrease on oxanamide.

Frequency changes following drug withdrawal. Of the parameters studied, the most rapid return to baseline levels was seen in the case of the frequency decline produced by these drugs. With the exception of fluphenazine and phenobarbital a significant return to baseline is seen following one week off drug (Fig. 6).

Dysrhythmias during drug administration. As Figure 7 shows, while classical paroxysmal patterns were only rarely seen, severe slow dysrhythmias were a prominent finding in the case of two of the drugs studied. Chlorpromazine produced dysrhythmias in 12

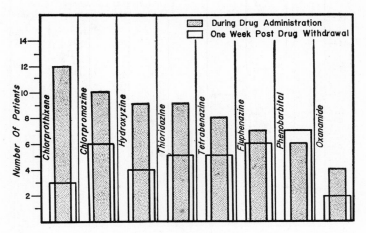

Figure 6. Bar graphs illustrating the number of patients showing slowing in the EEG during the period of maximum drug dosage and one week following drug withdrawal. In this graph the 16 patients with normal, LVF, and mixed fast and slow records are treated as a single group.

patients and hydroxyzine so affected 10 patients. Tetrabenazine and fluphenazine each produced abnormal EEG activity in six patients, chlorprothixene and oxanamide in four patients, thioridazine in two patients, and phenobarbital in one patient.

Dysrhythmias following drug withdrawal. Figure 7 shows that a significant number of patients continued to show dysrhythmic activity one week post drug withdrawal. All of the patients so affected by tetrabenazine continued to show dysrhythmias and only one patient had returned to baseline on fluphenazine. Thioridazine is notable in that while two patients showed abnormal patterns during the administration of this drug, four patients exhibited dysrhythmias one week following its withdrawal. In the case of all of the drugs studied, some patients still displayed abnormal EEG rhythms one week off drug.

Duration of drug effects on the EEG. As the preceding analysis indicates, both the nature and duration of drug-induced EEG change is highly variable, relative both to the specific drug given and to the

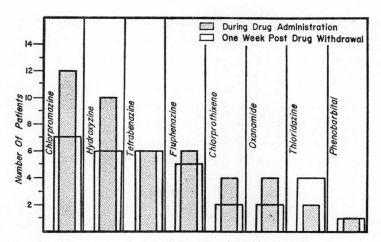

Figure 7. Bar graphs showing the number of patients showing the appearance of marked EEG dysrhythmias during the period of maximum drug dosage and one week following drug withdrawal. In this graph, the 16 patients with normal, LVF, and mixed fast and slow records are treated as a single group.

patient. The patients were followed until the drug-induced changes were no longer clinically evident in the EEG.

For the sample as a whole, as Table II shows, the recovery period was between three and six weeks for all of the drugs studied with the exception of chlorpromazine and tetrabenazine. Nine and ten weeks, respectively, had to elapse before the EEG changes produced by these drugs were no longer evident. Again, some of the patients showed a more rapid return to the predrug level from these and the other compounds studied.

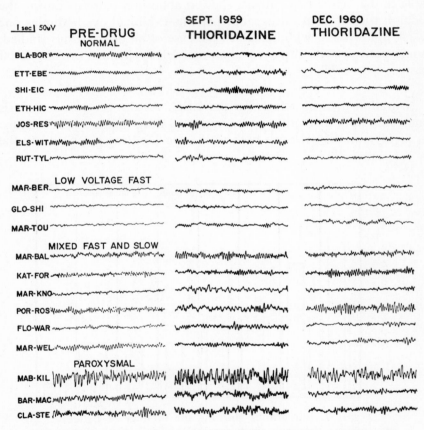

Figure 8. Sample strips from the EEGs of 19 patients with different types of predrug resting patterns. This figure illustrates the essentially similar individual responses of these patients when given the same three-week dosage schedule of thioridazine on two occasions 15 months apart.

Replication of EEG response. In order to see whether the serial administration of these drugs had produced any lasting effect on the CNS, we repeated, as the last in the series, the drug that was administered initially. This drug, thioridazine, gave essentially the same EEG changes on both occasions (Fig. 8), indicating to us that the EEG changes here described were non-cumulative and replicable.

Drug effects on the paroxysmal EEG. As previously mentioned, 5 of our 21 patients had predrug EEGs which were classified as paroxysmal. These patients were subjected to the same regimen of drug administration as the experimental group, but constant record sampling was not available on these patients, and two failed to complete the series. From the data available, however, it was apparent that with the exception of one patient on phenobarbital, all of the drugs given failed to ameliorate the existing paroxysmal dysrhythmia. Although in most cases these drugs produced a worsening of the existing paroxysmal activity which persisted after drug withdrawal, it is of interest that no seizures were observed in these patients. On the experimental ward of 86 patients (**10**), however, from which the entire EEG group was drawn, 12 patients convulsed during the administration of high dosages of hydroxyzine. Three of these 12 patients were in the EEG series. The predrug EEG of two of these patients had been classified as normal and one as MF&S. One patient convulsed on tetrabenazine, one on chlorpromazine, and one on chlorprothixene.

Individual patterns of EEG response in relation to drugs. The data relating to decreased frequency and dysrhythmias brought about by drug administration were placed in a simple matrix so that patterns of EEG response of individual patients could be detected. Two of the 16 patients showed a decrease in frequency during the period of drug administration for all eight drugs. Three other patients were consistent in responding with slowing to six of the eight drugs. The frequency response to the drugs was quite random in the remaining 11 patients. The two patients who had shown slowing to all eight of the drugs manifested severe slow wave dysrhythmic activity to six of the eight drugs. Two patients did not exhibit dysrhythmias to any drug. Ten of the 16 patients showed dysrhythmias to two or more of the drugs tested.

Patterns of EEG response in relation to the predrug records. We have emphasized the great variability that exists in our data. One source of this variability, which is frequently unrecognized in EEG drug studies, is the relationship between the predrug EEG and the drug record. Grouping the patients according to similarity of resting EEG allows certain generalizations to be made with greater confidence despite the variation in the EEG which occurs during drug therapy. For example, the six patients classified as MF&S represented 38 per cent of our sample, yet they accounted for 59 per cent of the dysrhythmic records seen.

Figures 9 and 10 illustrate samples of the EEG for each patient during drug administration and one week following drug withdrawal

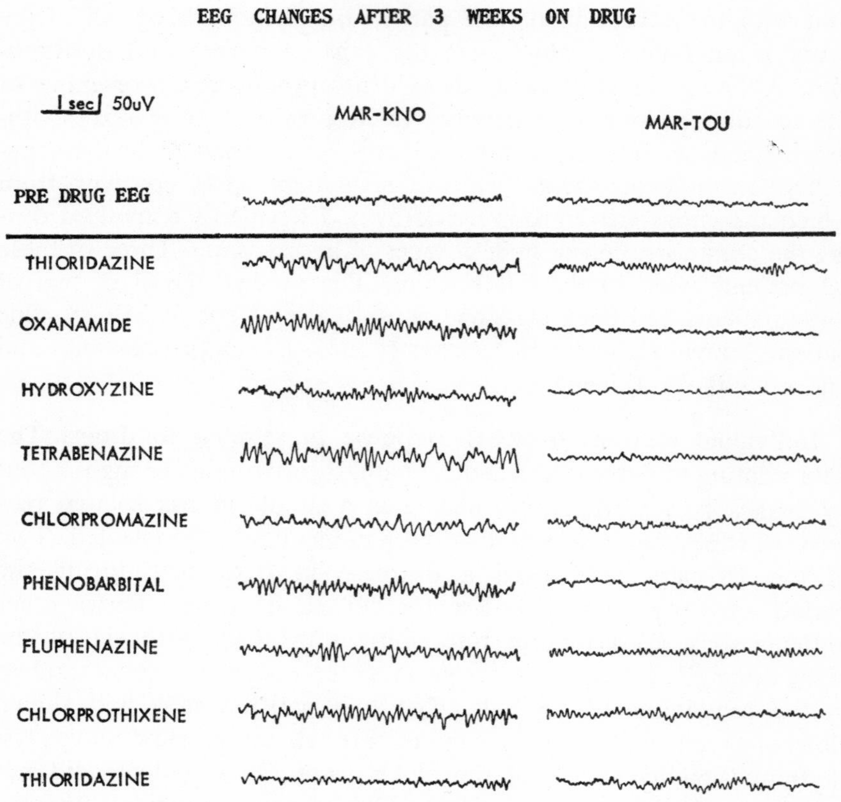

Figure 11. Sample strips from the EEGs of two patients with similar low-voltage resting patterns. These two patients showed markedly different responses during the administration of the eight drugs studied.

for each of the drugs studied. A representative sample of each patient's predrug EEG is also shown for comparison.

Figures 11 through 14 show the wide individual variations that may occur in response to drugs.

DISCUSSION

All of the drugs employed in this study affected the EEG. In general, more alpha was seen, the amplitude was increased, and the frequency was decreased by these agents. The parameter of greatest interest would appear to be change in frequency, with the produc-

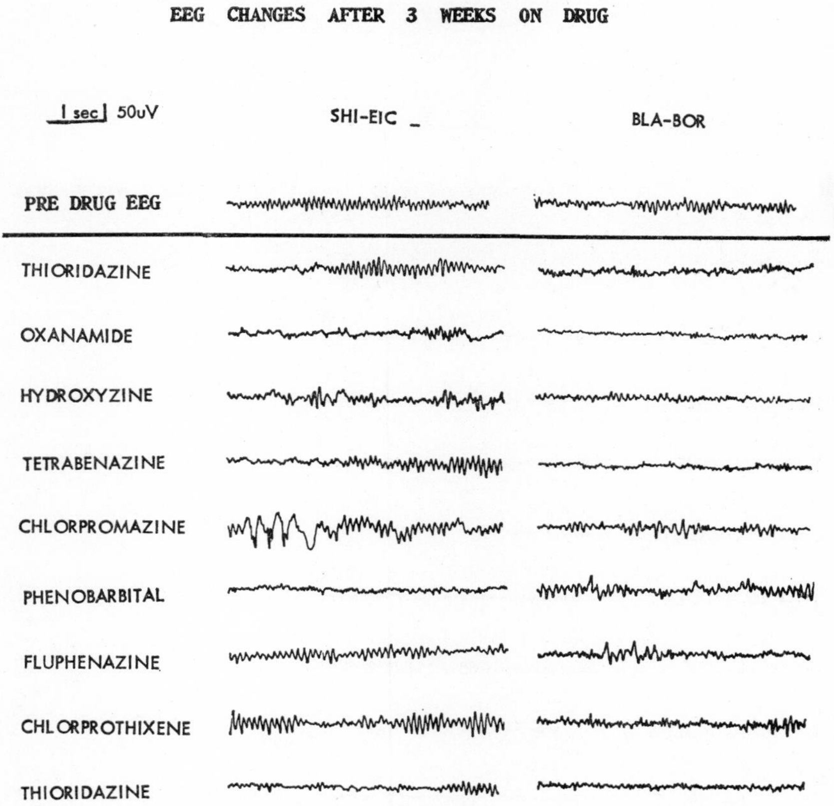

EEG CHANGES AFTER 3 WEEKS ON DRUG

Figure 12. Sample strips from the EEGs of two patients with similar normal resting EEG patterns. Different response patterns are seen to the eight drugs administered.

tion of severe dysrhythmias the next most striking finding. EEGs taken during tranquilization tend to be lower in frequency, and when high-dosage levels are employed dysrhythmias are commonly seen. Slowing as a characteristic of the phenothiazines has been reported by Bennet and Kooi (2). Swain and Litteral found that 45 per cent of a group of patients on chlorpromazine showed slowing, with the remaining patients unchanged (9). Hollister and Barthel (6) reported that 5 out of 10 patients showed slowing on thioridazine, and Cornu and Hoffet have reported slowing on chlorprothixene (3). The results reported here are in full agreement with these investigations and we would feel that slowing of the EEG is a characteristic finding following the administration of the more potent tranquilizing agents. Reports of paroxysmal patterns and severe dysrhythmias are

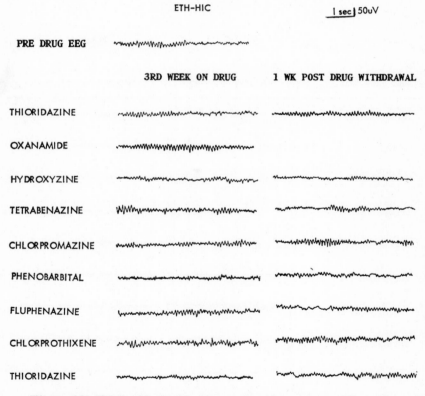

Figure 13. EEG strips of patient who showed essentially no change from her resting pattern during either the time of administration or withdrawal of the eight drugs studied.

also fairly common. Such activity has been seen with chlorpromazine
(**1, 7**), promazine (**8**), chlorprothixene (**3**), and with perphenazine,
prochlorperazine, and triflupromazine (**2**). Our findings are again
in essential agreement with the literature.

The clinical significance of our finding that all of these major tranquilizing agents tend to produce slowing and dysrhythmia may relate
to their effectiveness in the treatment of a group of patients who are
often treated by such other somatic therapies as electroconvulsive
therapy, insulin shock therapy, and lobotomy, all of which produce
similar changes in the EEG. Perhaps for too long, the phenomenon
of EEG slowing has been regarded as a side effect of tranquilizing
agents, while in fact these electroencephalographic changes may relate
in some meaningful way to the mode of action of these drugs.

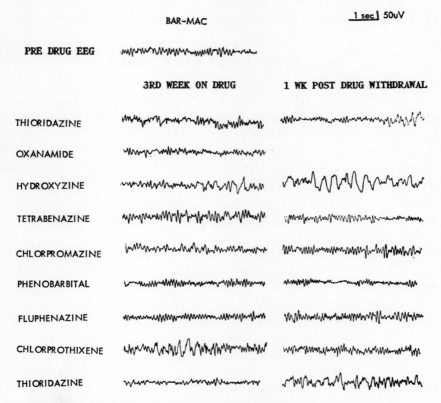

Figure 14. Strips from the EEG records of a patient who
showed a wide variety of responses to the administration of
some drugs and to the withdrawal of others.

We have found that two drugs, tetrabenazine and chlorpromazine, were distinguishable from the other drugs studied in terms of long duration of EEG effect following drug withdrawal. A number of studies have established that the behavioral improvement produced by chlorpromazine is similarly maintained for a long period post drug withdrawal. Good *et al.* (5) cite 10 to 12 weeks as the period in which improved behavior is maintained following withdrawal from chlorpromazine. It is suggestive that this was also approximately the time required for reversal of the EEG changes produced by this drug in our sample.

As suggestive as these findings are, meaningful correlates of EEG patterns and behavior can be obtained only by more elaborate and carefully controlled studies. It is our hope that some of these questions may be answered by the use of electronic quantification of the EEG and more sensitive and objective measures of behavioral change.

SUMMARY AND CONCLUSIONS

Serial EEGs were taken on 21 chronic psychiatric female patients, who received eight tranquilizing drugs successively over a period of 15 months. EEGs were taken prior to medication, during the week of maximum drug dosage, and weekly thereafter while drug effects persisted. Each medication was administered only after the effects of the previous drug were no longer evident in the EEG. Changes in the EEG were noted by comparing the total baseline record with the total experimental record.

Our results indicate that:

1. Changes in the EEG occurred with all agents.

2. Different drugs can be distinguished as having different effects upon the EEG.

3. Some individuals reacted in the same manner to all drugs. There was a relative lack of EEG change in some, but a marked and consistent reaction in others. Other patients were characterized by the diversity of their response.

4. Drug-induced EEG changes in the dose schedules here studied are reversible within at most a ten-week period.

5. Pretreatment basic EEG types influence the type of response seen.

6. The EEG response to thioridazine after a time interval of 15

months, and with intervening treatment with other psychotropic drugs, shows essentially the type of response seen initially.

7. The problems of the relationship of EEG change to behavior is fraught with many complications. The need to control and systematically vary dose, time of administration, and basic EEG type and to use quantitative EEG analysis is stressed.

BIBLIOGRAPHY

1. Barrett, O., Jr. Convulsive seizure after administration of Chlorpromazine, *J. Amer. Med. Ass.* **166**: 1986–1987, 1958.
2. Bennett, J. L., and Kooi, K. A. Five phenothiazine derivatives: Evaluation and toxicity studies. *Arch. gen. Psychiat.* **4**: 413–418, 1961.
3. Cornu, F., and Hoffet, H. Clinical experience with Taractan. *Dis. nerv. Syst.* **22**: 40–44, 1961.
4. Fink, M. A selected bibliography of electroencephalography in human psychopharmacology. *Electroenceph. clin. Neurophysiol.* Supp. **23**: 68 pp., 1964.
5. Good, W. W., Sterling, M., and Holtzman, W. H. Termination of chlorpromazine with schizophrenic patients. *Amer. J. Psychiat.* **115**: 443–448, 1958.
6. Hollister, L. E., and Barthel, C. A. Changes in the electroencephalogram during chronic administration of tranquilizing drugs. *Electroenceph. clin. Neurophysiol.* **11**: 792–795, 1959.
7. Mauceri, J., and Strauss, H. Effects of chlorpromazine on the electroencephalogram with report of a case of chlorpromazine intoxication. *Electroenceph. clin. Neurophysiol.* **8**: 671–675, 1956.
8. Reinert, R. E. EEG changes with promazine. *Amer. J. Psychiat.* **115**: 742–743, 1959.
9. Swain, J. M., and Litteral, E. B. Prolonged effect of chlorpromazine: EEG findings in a senile group. *J. nerv. ment. Dis.* **131**: 550–553, 1960.
10. Ulett, G. A., Heusler, A. F., Word, V. I., and Word, T. J. Mechanical and electronic techniques in the measurement of psychopharmacologic response. In: *First Hahnemann Symposium on Psychosomatic Medicine.* Lea & Febiger, Philadelphia, Chap. 46, pp. 388–390, 1962.

SUBJECT INDEX

AUTHOR INDEX

265